"Dr. Berkelhammer has written a remarkable book for those who live with chronic illness. He has deftly drawn together the self-healing strands of mindfulness, cognitive defusion, acceptance, and value-driven action to help reduce the unnecessary suffering that so often accompanies medical conditions, and to shift focus toward creating a deeply meaningful life."

—Victoria Lemle Beckner, PhD, assistant clinical professor, Department of Psychiatry, University of California—San Francisco; San Francisco Group for Evidence-Based Psychotherapy; lead author of *Conquering Post-Traumatic Stress Disorder*

"Dr. Berkelhammer's research is broad, drawing on insights from psychology, physiology, mainstream Western medicine and medical research, alternative therapies, and the theories, research, and observational findings surrounding methods of mindfulness training and practices. At the same time, this wide-ranging inquiry has a coherent, pointed focus on the implications for those who face chronic and/or life-threatening illnesses. His research draws on extensive literature reviews as well as insights from his own practices, experiences, and observations as a professional who is deeply engaged in this important arena of health practices."

—John Bilorusky, PhD, president of Western Institute for Social Research, chair of the board of the Association of Private Postsecondary Education in California

"Larry Berkelhammer writes with deep understanding, compassion, and courage about living with chronic illness that is difficult to manage or treat. As a psychologist and a patient, Larry grounds his experience in an exploration of the latest research. Using principles from Acceptance and Commitment Therapy that emphasize the importance of valued living and committed action, he invites us all to consider how to best live in the face of disease and uncertainty."

—Maggie Chartier, PsyD, MPH, clinical psychologist

"Dr. Larry Berkelhammer's thoroughly researched and wonderful book comes to us as the result of years of dedicated work. Larry has achieved significant success in linking diverse fields of medical, mental, and physical wellbeing that have the principle of mindfulness as a core element of their effectiveness. This is a profound and encyclopedic volume that enriches the reader's awareness of these varied approaches."
—Thomas G. Browne, PhD, clinical neuroscientist; founder of Neurenics; author of *Psychophysiological Medicine: A Measurable Metamorphosis of Type A Executives*; past president of the Biofeedback Society of California

"From his own personal journey of healing, as well as the research and evidence-based knowledge to support what he's learned along the way, we can thank Dr. Berkelhammer for writing a book that is a road map for people with chronic illness to help them chart their own way to wellbeing. There's great information here to help anyone bring curiosity and awareness to their healing path."
—Jennifer Buchanan, DDS, diplomate, American Board of Orofacial Pain; fellow of the American Academy of Orofacial Pain

"Larry Berkelhammer describes a practical process for people to assess their mental and physical health and presents practices that can empower them to take control of their own healing process so they can have an optimally healthy life."
—Alan S. Cascio, DDS, fellow of the Academy of General Dentistry; member of the American Dental Association and California Dental Association

"I highly recommend Larry Berkelhammer's new book, *In Your Own Hands*. In this carefully researched presentation, Dr. Berkelhammer addresses the components and dynamics of chronic illness and offers specific strategies and techniques to embolden people living with the challenges of chronic conditions. Having worked as a clinical social worker for many

years, I have come to appreciate how important it is for an individual with a chronic medical condition to feel both hopeful and in control of managing their healthcare process. Dr. Berkelhammer's new book makes a valuable contribution to addressing these vital issues, thus honoring the right of an individual with a chronic medical condition to attain and maintain an optimum quality of life."
—Judy Cress, LCSW, retired, previously at Alta Bates Summit Medical Center

"*In Your Own Hands* blends heartfelt sensitivity with science-based, innovative practices. Larry Berkelhammer provides a road map that people dealing with challenging illnesses can follow to improve their ability to face difficulty and ultimately increase their own wellbeing. This book empowers people with simple and effective tools that often are not intuitive and are typically unknown to the general public. This is an extremely important book that could help millions of people facing illnesses."
—Laura Delizonna, PhD, instructor, Stanford University; founder, Choosing Happiness

"Whether you have a chronic illness or want to optimize your health, *In Your Own Hands* describes the mindfulness-based conceptual framework for understanding illness and health. Most importantly, it offers realistic and pragmatic mindfulness behavioral practices that anyone can use. Although it is based upon science, the concepts and practices have also been tested in depth through the author's own coping with chronic disease. The result is a *must* read book for anyone experiencing chronic disease."
—Erik Peper, PhD, professor, San Francisco State University; director, Biofeedback Health; coauthor of *Fighting Cancer* and *Make Health Happen*

"Dr. Larry Berkelhammer is both an experienced professional with expert knowledge of the field of health psychology and a person living with chronic medical illness. He has a deep understanding of the helplessness and hopelessness experienced by people living with chronic illness. In this book, he reveals how the practices of mindfulness, nonattachment, gratitude, authentic self-expression, and values-based living can help chronically ill people gain new hope and live a meaningful life despite their illness. *In Your Own Hands* provides a comprehensive, practical set of mindfulness-based strategies that can change your relationship to your illness and provide a basis for hope and empowerment."

—Melanie A. Greenberg, PhD, practicing clinical and health psychologist; past professor, Alliant International University, San Diego; author; national speaker; consultant to media and organizations

"*In Your Own Hands* is an exceptional book about the healing power of our minds when used in conjunction with self-management of chronic disease. The book's underlying theme is that it is possible to direct our own health destiny by making conscious choices to live in the moment. Intentionally focusing our awareness on the present helps us accept the current state of our health and allows us to recognize our innate ability to improve our future physical and emotional wellbeing.

In Your Own hands discusses the theory and science behind mindfulness methods and then provides specific techniques and practices to transform our lives. There is real power in taking charge of our own health experiences in ways that are mindful of our individual needs, relationships, and choices. *In Your Own Hands* offers hope and support to those who live with chronic illness and to the loved ones who support them in their health journeys."

—Julia Hallisy, DDS, founder, The Empowered Patient Coalition

"In *Your Own Hands* is a valuable guide for anyone living with chronic illness who wishes to take their life into their own hands despite physical limitations. The mindfulness-based practices presented in this book are powerful tools for enhancing wellbeing and reducing unnecessary suffering. For many, this book will be a turning point in beginning to live a more vital, meaningful life."

—Amy Jenks, PsyD, assistant clinical professor, Department of Psychiatry, University of California—San Francisco; director, The Bay Area Evidence-Based Treatment Center

"Psychologist and advanced meditator Larry Berkelhammer shows those of us working with chronic health conditions how mindfulness and commitment to values can reduce suffering and promote wellbeing. This clear, well-organized guidebook offers concrete, evidence-based suggestions to help us find joy in life regardless of physical discomfort and limitations. Informed by his own personal journey, the author demonstrates how approaching medical difficulties with an accepting, empowered heart helps us learn from hardship, build meaningful relationships, and assist others. *In Your Own Hands* reminds us that although health problems are both common and challenging, they don't need to be devastating. Using Berkelhammer's methods, we discover they can actually enhance our appreciation of life."

—Will Meecham, MD, yoga therapy faculty member, Niroga Institute; member, American Society of Ophthalmic Plastic and Reconstructive Surgery; fellow, American College of Surgeons

". . . a treasure of discovery and hope for anyone dealing with a chronic condition."

—Wiveka Ramel, PhD, clinical psychologist, Sevitar and San Francisco Acceptance and Commitment Therapy; teacher, Search Inside Yourself Leadership Institute

"*In Your Own Hands* accomplishes what few other books on the topic of chronic illness do: it proposes a fundamentally optimistic approach toward change that re-establishes a life of meaning, while maintaining a firm stance that one living with chronic illness deserves neither blame nor shame for their struggles. Dr. Berkelhammer's wonderful guidance may be the compassionate, gentle nudge that encourages you to stop waiting for a miracle and reawaken to the possibilities of living fully today."
—Matthew D. Skinta, PhD, ABPP, board-certified clinical health psychologist, private practice, San Francisco

"With sincere appreciation, I recommend this book to anyone who struggles with long-term medical conditions as well as professionals who work in behavioral medicine. Berkelhammer has done a very nice job linking chronic medical conditions and mindfulness-based interventions in a friendly manner that allows the reader to capture the benefits of these interventions. All chapters on practices have a nice balance between learning a new skill conceptually and practicing it right away. I have no doubt that *In Your Own Hands* will make a significant difference for those struggling with a medical condition by helping them discover new ways of living that are consistent with what truly matters to them."
—Patricia E. Zurita Ona, PsyD, founder, East Bay Behavior Therapy Center; coauthor, *Mind And Emotions: A Universal Protocol for Emotional Disorders;* adjunct faculty, The Wright Institute

In Your Own Hands

In Your Own Hands

New Hope for People with Chronic Medical Conditions —Mindfulness-Based Practices for Mastery and Wellbeing

Larry Berkelhammer, PhD

The Empowered Patient Coalition Press

Printed in the United States of America

Design by Meadowlark Publishing Services
Cover photo ©IStock.com/ooyoo
Interior photos ©IStock.com/bgfoto
Author photo by Greg Wilker

ISBN 978-0-9912437-0-9

This book was written in the hope of inspiring, informing, and supporting readers in their efforts to cultivate and live with a sense of self-efficacy, mastery, and wellbeing. The skill-building practices herein should never be used as alternatives to medical treatment or psychotherapy. On the contrary, a primary aim of this book is to help readers partner with their medical professionals.

Published 2014 by
The Empowered Patient Coalition Press
595 Buckingham Way Suite 305
San Francisco, CA 94132

For Irma

Contents

Preface ix
Acknowledgments xv

Part I: Toward Mastery and Wellbeing 1
1   Toward Mastery and Wellbeing 3
2   What Causes Disease? 11
3   Theories of Suffering 15
4   Cognitive Fusion 25
5   Experiential Avoidance 39
6   Living with Chronic Illness 53

Part II: The Fundamental Mastery
and Wellbeing Practice: Mindfulness 63
7   A Brief Introduction to Mindfulness 65
8   The Health Benefits of Mindfulness Practice 77
9   Practice Mindfulness 101

Part III: Valued-Action Practice 117
10 Practice Living by Your Personal Life Values 121
11 What Are You Choosing? 127
12 What Are You Practicing? 139

Part IV: Mindfulness-Based Mastery and Wellbeing Practices . . . 147
13 Practice Gratitude 149
14 Practice Loving Self-Care 157
15 Practice Self-Acceptance 169
16 Practice Authentic Self-Expression 181
17 Practice Cultivating Meaning and Purpose 197
18 Practice Connection and Service to Others 205
19 Practice Building Relationships 219
20 Practice Finding Humor 237
21 Practice in the Eye of the Hurricane 243
22 Practice Something Different 255

Part V: Medical and Home Healthcare Self-Efficacy 269
23   Medical Self-Efficacy and Advocacy:
     An Essential Aspect of Self-Care Mastery 271
24   Mastery and Wellbeing Practices for Family Caregivers. 295

Appendix A: Some Science Behind the Mind's
     Influence on the Body. 315
Appendix B: Conscious Breathing, Heart Rate Variability,
     Respiratory Sinus Arrhythmia, and Health. 343

Notes 351
Bibliography 387
Index. 411
About the Author 429

Preface

I was fifty-three in 2000 when I finally received correct diagnoses for the multiple chronic conditions I had been living with for many years, some of them since childhood. At last, after decades of wrong turns, bewilderment, and feelings of shame, I learned through conclusive testing that none of my varied symptoms were in my head. No doctor had previously ordered any of these very specialized tests, and now I could actually see that specific lab values were way out of normal range.

This was the "good news" concerning these diagnoses. There were names for the illnesses I had, other people had them too, and I was now able to comprehend the physiological processes that underlay my health problems and seek treatments for them.

But right on the heels of these diagnoses came the bad news about my chronic conditions: there were no known cures for any of them.

Not only that, but there were few effective treatments. In fact, I learned that some of the recommended treatments, should I choose them, would cause me further harm. For example, the best treatment available for my three autoimmune diseases (ankylosing spondylitis, subclinical inflammatory bowel disease, and immune thrombocytopenic purpura) would worsen a fourth disease I had, which was a primary combined immunodeficiency disease. I also learned that the treatment I'd been using to alleviate debilitating headaches interfered with calcium absorption and exacerbated my fifth disease, a severe malabsorption syndrome, making my sixth illness, a dangerously severe case of osteoporosis (T-score of -4.6), even worse. The malabsorption could also cause electrolyte imbalances, exacerbating the cardiac dysrhythmias I experienced.

It seemed I had few options left.

Yet every moment of life offers opportunities and decisions. At the moment of my diagnoses, I had a couple of things in my favor.

First, by nature I have always been interested in finding solutions for problems that appear to have none. This is a characteristic of what I now refer to as living with mastery and wellbeing. When the realization sank in that no cures for any of my conditions were likely to appear during my lifetime, I approached my situation mentally as a very complex puzzle that I could potentially solve. I had begun reviewing the medical literature on psychoneuroimmunology and psychophysiology in the early 1990s. Then, late in that decade, I had focused more specifically on evidence-based clinical interventions for working with chronic illness patients. Now I wanted to explore whether mind training could play a role in helping me feel better. I already ate a nutrient-dense diet, got more than an hour of daily exercise, slept six to eight hours each night, and had practiced some form of meditation for almost thirty years; I had all the lifestyle choices I knew about covered. But since I liked science, I searched for evidence related to this topic in refereed journals in order to learn all I could about mind training and health, and also to see if there were any other lifestyle behaviors I hadn't previously considered.

The second thing I had going for me was that nine years before receiving these diagnoses, I'd had a life-altering experience that taught me volumes about the power of the mind to heal disease.

I was watching a karate tournament on television around 8 p.m. one January night in 1991 when I suddenly experienced extreme fatigue, full-body muscle aches, chills—all the classic symptoms of influenza. I felt angry about it because with everything I had going on in my life at that time, I couldn't afford to be laid up in bed for a week. For the next two hours I became very emotionally involved in the tournament, so much so that I felt my whole being become increasingly energized and exhilarated as I watched the contest. I felt as if I was in the tournament fighting that night. In fact, I was fighting! I was leading my immune system into battle, and I knew we would win. I remember defiantly saying aloud, "I am not going to get sick. I refuse! It's not going to happen!" These weren't just empty words or wishful thinking; in my mind, I was convinced that I would fight off the viral invasion.

By 10 p.m. I felt fine.

I had made a complete recovery! And my understanding of the power of the mind to effect profound physiological changes had undergone a transformation. I suddenly knew that many of the bizarre anecdotal stories I had read about inexplicable phenomena such as voodoo death and faith healing were probably true. They made more sense to me now because I'd had this surprising and unsought personal experience of the mind's healing power.

I have tried unsuccessfully to use this same method to overcome illness several times since 1991. I have tried it for spondyloarthropic inflammatory flare-ups, pneumonia, and colds, and I have never been able to repeat the success I had that night. I think it's because of the trying. The night I vanquished influenza, I wasn't trying at all; I knew it was going to happen.

Though I hadn't been able replicate it since, in 2000 the memory of that single experience of spontaneous and complete recovery added to my curiosity and impelled me to learn more about the power of the mind to improve health where no other treatments can be brought to bear.

I decided to review all the evidence-based research on the mind's ability to effect positive physiological changes. I started with Michael Murphy's encyclopedic *Future of the Body*. Then I devoured hundreds of papers in refereed journals and dozens of books in the medical and behavioral sciences, and took two years' worth of science courses at local colleges. After that I trained with several world leaders in psychoneuro-immunology, psychophysiology, and psychooncology. I was a psychotherapist at this time with a practice focused on people who had serious medical conditions. Learning about the mind from all these disparate quarters, I began to put together the evidence that would eventually form the foundation for this book.

As I gathered hard data, the patterns that emerged were both remarkable and undeniable. The conclusions this wide array of researchers had come to—that the mind influences health in intriguing, astonishing, and demonstrable ways—were solidly rooted in the scientific method and had far-reaching implications that seemed tailor made for people such as myself: people living with chronic medical challenges who have the willingness to engage in mind training practices. I knew from what I had observed in clinical training and in my psychotherapy practice that this knowledge would prove useful to others if they were made aware of it. I also knew that my personal experiences dovetailed perfectly with the psychoneuroimmunology research data I was uncovering.

Mind Journeys

My explorations of the mind date back forty years. I learned the techniques of Transcendental Meditation in 1972, Zen in 1978, and samatha vipassana in 1980, but there were many periods when I had trouble sticking with daily practice. In 1994, I became infatuated with biofeedback—especially electroencephalography (EEG) biofeedback—and the published studies proving its efficacy as a form of mind training.

In the mid-nineties as I experimented with biofeedback, I also trained for several years with one of the founders of the American existential-humanistic psychotherapy movement, Dr. James F. T. Bugental. After that I studied hypnosis at the Milton H. Erickson Foundation and the Academy for Guided Imagery. I also completed three years of training at the Simonton Cancer Center. Then, in 2008, I began to study and train in Acceptance and Commitment Therapy (ACT), one of the newer mindfulness-based psychotherapies.

Suddenly, here was a system of psychotherapy—ACT— that had the solid scientific foundation I so highly valued yet was in perfect harmony with my existential training too. This radically altered not only my psychotherapy practice but even my personal mindfulness practice. The philosophy and science of functional contextualism upon which ACT is based gave me a way of offering mindfulness training to clients who would not otherwise be interested. The emphasis on identifying personal values and taking action in harmony with those values resonated with many more of my clients than did the Buddhist approach to mindfulness. I witnessed the difference it made for the chronically ill people I worked with in my practice.

Over the last several years I have continued my studies of the mind and health, reviewing fascinating data on new discoveries in cognitive neuroscience, psychoneuroimmunology, and other scientific disciplines. At the same time, I have dedicated myself to daily, moment-to-moment mindfulness practice, building and strengthening my awareness that virtually all my behavior, including the smallest act, impacts my health and happiness—for good or ill. Like a trio of parallel tracks running through my life, brain science, behavioral science, and applied mindfulness have moved me ever forward toward greater understanding and helped me build skills in mastery and wellbeing: the belief in my own capability to handle life as it comes. And it has been my increasing sense of mastery and wellbeing, developed through engaging in the practices I offer in this book, that has allowed me to live with far greater wellbeing than you might imagine possible for someone with so many chronic medical conditions.

Committing to the mindfulness-based mastery and wellbeing practices put forth in this book can dramatically improve quality of life, and sometimes even health. I have seen the efficacy of these practices in the studies I have reviewed,

in my psychotherapy practice, and in my own life. I firmly believe that continual commitment to these practices in my own
life has made all the difference in living with chronic illness,
allowing me to stabilize certain conditions that are considered
degenerative and even improve others.

Taking my health into my own hands in this way has
enabled me to live a much happier, healthier, and more satisfying life than I ever thought possible at the time when I
received my correct multiple diagnoses. It is with the hope
that you will find the information and practices I have gathered here equally transformative that I offer this book to you.

Acknowledgments

This book is the product of a personal and professional journey spanning many years. Here I would like to acknowledge and appreciate a few of the people along the way who most strongly influenced the evolution of my thinking and the content of this book.

James F. T. Bugental, PhD, was one of the founders of the American existential-humanistic psychotherapy movement. I had the great fortune to train with Dr. Bugental over a period of six years, and I give him substantial credit for my effectiveness in behavioral medicine. Jim, as we knew him, was relentless in his insistence that we all accept responsibility for living according to our values, making conscious, intentional choices from moment to moment. It was during this training period that I committed myself to the primary goal of empowering others to cultivate self-responsibility and self-efficacy. Jim taught us to have enormous respect for the people who came to see us. He lamented our use of the terms *psychotherapist* and *patient* because those terms were disempowering to those who requested our help; he wished we could call ourselves *evocateurs*. It was this philosophy that shaped my work with those who came to me for help. My personal as well as professional life has been greatly enhanced by those six years, and I still benefit daily from his guidance.

My appreciation goes out to research and clinical psychologist Dr. Steven Hayes as the driving force in the creation of Acceptance and Commitment Therapy (ACT): a new science- and evidence-based form of contextual behavioral science. Like Bugental's existential-humanistic philosophy, ACT strives to empower clients to identify their personal life values and then take congruent action in the form of behavioral change. Both approaches emphasize acceptance of our inner events—our thoughts and feelings, regardless of their nature—and both promote living fully in the present moment. ACT has given me vital tools with which I can help make life better for others.

Dr. Lawrence LeShan devoted his entire career to helping cancer patients become proactive in their battles with the disease, providing numerous case studies showing that the act of becoming proactive itself improves health outcomes. Key to his psychotherapy work was helping cancer patients identify what matters most to them and find ways, within the limitations of their disease process, to pursue goals that matter. I had long been a student of Dr. LeShan's work through his writing when I finally got a chance to spend time with him in New York, having private consultations with him and his protégée, Dr. Ruth Bolletino—now a world renowned authority on psychotherapy for cancer patients. I attended a residential retreat with both of them as well.

During most of Dr. LeShan's career, the traditional oncology community failed to appreciate the value of his work, yet today we have ample epidemiological studies as well as psychoneuroimmunology and psychooncology research that validate the clinical work he began with advanced metastatic cancer patients more than sixty years ago. Many other research psychologists have explicated the relationship between states of mind and physiological functioning on an intellectual level, but being around Larry, as he liked to be called, felt qualitatively different—sort of like being on the mother ship, because he so lived what he taught. His warm, soothing presence somehow nourished self-acceptance in all those lucky enough to get to know him.

O. Carl Simonton, MD, was a brilliant maverick who created the Simonton Method to empower cancer patients to become proactive. At weeklong retreats, patients of the Simonton Cancer Center are taught various forms of mind-training skills that they can practice at home to improve their states of mind, which then improve their odds of recovery. The center also provides professional training, and I spent three years training with Dr. Simonton. I most appreciate that he taught me to pursue what I knew to be true, even when mainstream thinking sometimes went in a different direction. He was bold and courageous, and being around him taught me how to take professional and personal risks.

Like LeShan's, Dr. Simonton's work was not understood or appreciated by mainstream oncologists. Throughout his career he was accused of instilling *false hope* in cancer patients. However, since ancient times, empirically based clinicians have known that hope improves physiological functioning and increases the odds of recovery. I have Carl to thank for my ability to instill hope in people today. Those of us who trained with him, and the cancer patients who went through his program, all left his retreats with newfound optimism and a new set of beliefs about what was actually possible.

In a year-long training and in private phone consultations with Jeanne Achterberg, PhD, I learned about the power of the images in our minds to improve physiological functioning, and how to improve health outcomes by working with self-created healing images. I was fortunate to work with her personally, and Dr. Achterberg lives on through her extraordinary book, aptly named *Imagery in Healing.*

Psychologist Dr. Erik Peper is one of the world's authorities on psychophysiological self-regulation and was one of the early biofeedback pioneers. I have trained with him, received countless biofeedback sessions from him, and recorded several inspiring video interviews with him, available free of charge at www.larryberkelhammer.com. As much as anyone I have ever known, Dr. Peper walks his talk, continually using a variety of psychophysiological self-regulation methods on himself. Simply being around him is invigorating because he is so vibrant and curious about virtually any experiments on changing the parameters of physiological functioning using the mind. My commitment to psychophysiological self-regulation as a way of life is something I owe to Dr. Erik Peper.

Though I only had the opportunity to train with psychologist Dr. Donald Moss during one two-day workshop at an annual Association for Applied Psychophysiology and Biofeedback conference, I have had conversations with him at various conferences and have been helped by the sincerity of his teaching, wisdom, and guidance. He seems to exude a love of helping others, and I am lucky enough to have had some of this enthusiasm rub off on me.

More than twenty-five years ago, before I became a licensed psychotherapist, I trained with Ron Kurtz and Pat Ogden in Hakomi Therapy, which made me a better clinician. Yet the most profound and life-altering learning for me came from just being around Ron and Pat and observing their creativity and inventiveness. They inspired me to follow my heart rather than the traditional, standardized path to becoming a psychotherapist.

John Bilorusky, PhD, cofounder and president of the Western Institute for Social Research, taught me the value of doing really good qualitative and action research.

To cofounder and medical director of the Institute for Health and Healing at California Pacific Medical Center, William Stewart, MD, thank you for providing the motivation for me to write this book.

Marshall Rosenberg, PhD, created Nonviolent Communication (NVC). His concept of *needs consciousness* allowed me to later expand on the Acceptance and Commitment Therapy (ACT) concept of *values-based living.*

Robert Gonzales, PhD, provided me with the concept that we are practicing something all the time; he proposed a mindfulness practice of asking ourselves throughout the day: *What am I rehearsing?* This planted the seed for my later teaching of the mindfulness practices of asking ourselves throughout each day: *What am I practicing?* and *What am I choosing?*

Retired anesthesiologist and friend David Benefiel, MD, read the physiology-laden sections of the manuscript and corrected me on some of my biochemistry.

Poet, retired oculoplastic surgeon, and friend Will Meecham, MD, also advised me on my biochemistry.

Thanks to the members of the San Francisco Bay Area chapter of the Association for Contextual Behavioral Science for their collegial support. Special thanks to the members I interviewed for an action research project: Norm Cavior, PhD, Michael Vurek, LCSW, Megan Oser, PhD, Maggie Chartier, PsyD, Kelly Werner, PhD, Wiveka Ramel, PhD, Matthew Skinta, PhD, and Patricia Zurita Ona, PhD.

Finally, I would like to acknowledge my editor. As I worked in partnership with Sheridan McCarthy, the editing of this book became one of the most satisfying, stimulating, and rewarding projects I have ever been involved in.

I had written the original manuscript as a reference book for physicians and psychologists in behavioral medicine. Very early on in the project, Sheridan became convinced that the material in the manuscript could help a lot of people dramatically improve the quality of their lives, and we set about a two-year collaboration to transform the book I had written into a self-help book for the educated general public that would be useful to clinicians and patients alike. That deep belief on her part nourished me during those times when I started to feel overwhelmed by the task. The title of the book was Sheridan's suggestion and I cannot imagine a title that better describes the basic message I want to impart to readers. And though I had heard disquieting stories from other authors about editors who work with a heavy hand, Sheridan retained my personal writing style and vocabulary throughout the book.

When I think of the possibility of writing another book, my primary motivation is to have another opportunity to work in partnership with Sheridan McCarthy.

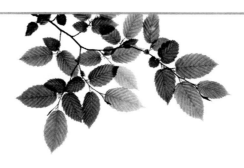

Part I

Toward Mastery
and Wellbeing

Dedication to the mindfulness-based practices in this book will lead to a powerful and life-changing result: mastery — *the felt sense of being the master of your life.* If you commit the time and effort, you will see for yourself that the feelings of helplessness and hopelessness you sometimes experience as a result of your illness will give way to a sense of optimism and great wellbeing — and that this remarkable transformation of your feelings is always in your own hands.

Before you dive into these practices, we need to lay some groundwork, and that is the job of Part I. Here you will learn important context that is a prerequisite to practice. To begin, you will get better acquainted with the concepts of mastery and wellbeing. Then you will explore the nature of illness and the *unnecessary* suffering that often accompanies chronic illness, and you'll be introduced to two of the main causes of unnecessary suffering: cognitive fusion and experiential avoidance. With this framework in mind and a fundamental concept underlying the practices in this book well established — that your mental activity has a powerful influence on the degree of suffering you experience when you are ill — you will finish this section by investigating some commonly experienced aspects of living with chronic physical challenges.

1

Toward
Mastery and
Wellbeing

This is a book for people who live with chronic health challenges. It's especially a book for those who are already getting good medical care and making healthy lifestyle choices and who want to know what more they can do to not only improve their health but live happier, more fulfilling lives. And it's a book for the array of professionals who treat people with chronic health conditions; it offers proven tools based on solid science to inform an effective course of treatment that acknowledges and addresses the realities of living with chronic illness.

According to the Centers for Disease Control and Prevention (CDC), today 133 million Americans, nearly half of all adults, live with some form of chronic illness. Two major categories of chronic illness with which we are all familiar are heart disease and cancer. According to the CDC, 27 million of us are living with heart disease, and the National Cancer Institute estimates about 12 million live with cancer.

There is also a lesser-known category of chronic illness that actually affects more people than heart disease and cancer combined: autoimmune disease. According to the American Autoimmune Related Diseases Association, 50 million Americans, 30 million of them women, live with some form of autoimmune disease. We have known about several of these illnesses for some time—John F. Kennedy lived with Addison's disease, for example, and Dwight D. Eisenhower was diagnosed with Crohn's disease. You have probably seen ads on television touting medications for conditions you may not

Mastery and wellbeing practices have powerful healing properties.

have known were autoimmune illnesses at all, such as psoriasis and restless leg syndrome. The explosion of gluten-free food choices now found in supermarkets is in response to an autoimmune condition called celiac disease, a malabsorption syndrome that is being diagnosed with increasing frequency. So while the term "autoimmune disease" doesn't always come first when people think about the illnesses that afflict us, it is in fact extremely prevalent. There are well over 150 different diseases in this category, affecting more than 50 million people in the US alone, and virtually every organ system in the body can be under attack.

A host of very good treatments have been developed to address almost all forms of heart disease, and although we are still far from finding a cure for most cancers, recent decades have seen significant advances in cancer treatment; as a result, many more people are living longer with the disease than ever before. When it comes to autoimmune diseases, however, the story is very different. With one or two exceptions, there are no cures for any of them, and many of the known treatments have harmful associated risks—some of which can be deadly, including the risk of serious infections and various forms of cancer.

So it is an unfortunate truth that at this time in history, huge numbers of us living with chronic health challenges cannot look to medical science—or, for that matter, to complementary and alternative treatments—for definitive help. While healthcare professionals may be able to assist us in terms of slowing the progression of a chronic disease, mitigating symptoms, or helping us adapt to physical limitations, don't expect cures for your autoimmune disease any time soon.

What, then, can we *do for ourselves* to improve our health

and live full lives despite our physical challenges? I have spent years investigating how to best work psychologically with the subset of patients for whom medicine has no answers, or poor ones. The fruit of my investigation is contained in this book. The answer lies in the healing power of the mind, brought to bear on the challenges of chronic illness by making conscious choices about how we live our lives day to day, moment to moment. The answer, I have found, is to engage in daily, mindfulness-based practices that build mastery and wellbeing.

An Introduction to Mastery and Wellbeing

Mastery can be defined as *the sense that we are in charge of our own experience.* This felt sense of control, in and of itself, has powerful healing properties, and you will find scientific evidence in the book to back this up. In this sense, the degree of mastery and wellbeing we experience is *in our own hands.*

It is a universal human need to feel that we are in control of our own environment. This need is greatly underappreciated, but meeting it is essential for our health and wellbeing. Adolescents need a sense of control in order to learn to step up and take charge of their lives. Prison inmates need it to become rehabilitated. Even in the dying stage of life, the sense that we can still make choices about how we experience our waning days is essential to dying well.

Mastery is especially important for chronically ill people because our physical challenges often appear to rob us of options. Our mobility may become limited; we may tire too easily to engage in favorite activities for as long as we would like; we may have to spend much of our time at medical appointments when we'd really rather be working, being with family or friends, or spending quiet time in solitude. This is why it is essential to accept responsibility for the cultivation of mastery and self-efficacy. Our wellbeing is greatly enhanced once we are able to live with those attributes. Identifying our personal life values and acting in accordance with them can help keep us from succumbing to feelings of hopelessness and helpless-

People who live with mastery and well-being would describe their lifestyle as something they *intentionally created, and that it's in their hands.*

ness, both of which are emotional states that have been shown to lead to declining health and unnecessary suffering.

There is a powerful alternative to descending into such states. By engaging daily in the mindfulness-based mastery practices contained in this book, we can instead experience ever increasing states of wellbeing. We can reconnect with the joys of life and live more fully.

So just what is life like for people who have attained a high degree of mastery and, as a result, a strong sense of well-being? Following are some of the characteristics such people share:

- They hold the belief that they can effectively handle the challenges presented to them each day.
- When things don't go as planned or as they had hoped, they usually recover quickly.
- Their personal and work relationships are satisfying and they can handle difficult interactions and relationships.
- When they occasionally feel overwhelmed by responsibilities and challenges in their lives, they effectively find a remedy.
- Whenever they are dissatisfied with any aspect of their home or work life, they are able to work out an effective way to get beyond the dissatisfaction.
- They are good at managing their home and work schedules and they get great satisfaction from keeping up with daily demands.
- They are effective in finding the types of work, home activities, and relationships that are most satisfying to them.

- People who live with mastery and wellbeing would describe their lifestyle as something they *intentionally created, and that it's in their hands.*

As is the case with developing any skill, the more frequently and successfully we engage in practicing mastery—repeatedly giving ourselves the experience, "I can do this"—the greater mastery we achieve. When we embark on this path, our first task is to locate our mastery skills: to learn the practices and take our first tentative steps with them. Then, as the terrain becomes more familiar, we build those skills, and we are able to strengthen and support ourselves mentally, emotionally, and physically. We develop greater resilience and vitality, and we can feel their surprising effects as our lives become more enjoyable and satisfying. We are better able to manage the choices inherent in the everyday challenges we all face, such as how we will receive bad news or deal with conflict. Mastery skills can be put to use to support us in all facets of daily life, and they are available to anyone who is willing to commit to practicing them.

At some point in our journey toward mastery and wellbeing, we who live with chronic illness arrive at a remarkable discovery: *we are capable of managing our health ourselves.* This is tremendously liberating news for anyone who has suffered with health challenges for any length of time, and even if there were no other pay-off for making the commitment to practice, this alone would make all our efforts worthwhile. This does not mean we can cure ourselves, but it does mean we can maintain a sense of control of our choices.

The Heart of Mastery and Wellbeing: Mindfulness Practice

The single most important practice you can engage in to create mastery and wellbeing in your life, and one that is fundamental to all others, is *mindfulness.* Three chapters are devoted exclusively to this practice, and you will find it referred to frequently elsewhere throughout the book. Mindfulness practice

entails becoming aware of all of the thoughts, images, emotions, and sensations we experience, moment by moment. It
also means becoming aware of all our behavior from moment
to moment. Developing such awareness gives us the power
to consciously choose how we will respond to what life sends
our way, and this is where the felt sense of control that creates
a sense of mastery can be found.

How This Book Is Organized

The book is divided into five main parts. Common to all of
them is information from contemporary studies demonstrating the mind's power to influence health. Scientific evidence
forms the foundation for understanding how the practices in
this book influence physiology and lead to improved health
and happiness. This evidence has been culled from the fields
of psychoneuroimmunology, psychooncology, psychophysiology, positive psychology, contextual behavioral science,
and cognitive neuroscience.

The remaining chapters in this Part look at the nature of
disease and the causes of suffering, with emphasis on the relationship between emotional distress and physiological stress.
We'll examine the psychological processes that actually create
unnecessary suffering for chronically ill people, with special
emphasis on two of these thought patterns: *cognitive fusion*—
entanglement with our thoughts and beliefs—and *experiential
avoidance,* the impulse to reject, deny, or avoid what is happening with us, physically, mentally, emotionally, and be-
haviorally. Part I concludes with a discussion of living with
chronic health challenges, with unnecessary suffering placed
in this context.

Part II, The Fundamental Mastery and Wellbeing Practice:
Mindfulness, explores this topic in three chapters. The first
describes what mindfulness is, as described by the foremost
experts in the field; the second outlines the considerable beneficial impacts of mindfulness practice on health; and the third
explores how mindfulness is practiced.

Next, with Part III, we move into a core application of

mindfulness in three chapters that together form a central aspect of the method I teach: Valued-Action Practice. The key to mastery and wellbeing is to make choices and engage in practices that are in accord with your personal life values, and these chapters describe the three steps involved in doing so: identifying your values—what is most important and meaningful to you; learning to make choices moment by moment that support these values; and paying careful attention to how you are actually behaving relative to your values. We are all practicing something, all the time, and this chapter invites you to become conscious of everything you practice day by day.

In Part IV, I introduce you to a series of extremely beneficial mindfulness-based practices; this Part is a kind of road map to greater mastery and wellbeing. These practices include self-acceptance, loving self-care, authentic self-expression, altruism, and gratitude, among others.

Part V includes two chapters: one for family caregivers and one that introduces the topic of medical self-efficacy—how to achieve mastery in working with your healthcare professionals.

The book concludes with two appendices. The first goes into greater depth concerning the mind's influence on physiology; the second relates to conscious breathing and its effects on health.

ை

Many years of research of the scientific literature, my own experience of creating mastery and wellbeing for myself, and my observations of how these practices have worked for others have shaped *In Your Own Hands: New Hope for People with Chronic Medical Conditions*. I have written it with special consideration for people like me who require an evidence-based rationale for engaging in any practice intended to improve health and wellbeing.

If you are already engaged in some of the mastery practices introduced and described here, I trust that you will find

reinforcement and inspiration through the research findings and case studies demonstrating their sound scientific
underpinnings. If you have not yet considered practices such
as mindfulness, or loving self-care, or altruism to support
your health, I hope you will find ample reason to consider
further investigation. Wherever you may find yourself along
the spectrum of familiarity with the methods introduced in
this book—from complete novice to lifelong mindfulness
practitioner—I invite you to explore this compelling universe.
Greater wellbeing is truly in your hands.

2 What Causes Disease?

Almost everyone I have ever known who was diagnosed with a cancer or any serious chronic medical condition wondered: "Why me?" Most people think they may have done something to cause the disease. To make matters worse, well-meaning friends often ask questions that imply that the disease could have been caused by a particular diet, activity, exposure—or worst of all, by negative thinking. Although mystery is a popular form of fiction, in our real lives we are very uncomfortable with mystery. We tend to think that if we could just solve the mystery of why we developed the disease, we should be able to find the cure. It rarely works out that way. Unfortunately, etiology (cause) is commonly idiopathic (unknown), and so the mystery remains.

In the hope of dispelling some myths about why we get sick, let's start by getting clear on the actual causes of disease. The root cause of disease is *physiological stress*. It can be triggered by physical trauma; infection with viruses, bacteria, fungi, or parasites; some prescription drugs; exposure to environmental or endogenously produced toxins; or temperature extremes. Other potential physiological stress factors include genetic predisposition to disease, epigenetic events, unhealthy behavior, and an endless number of idiopathic pathophysiological processes. Often, disease is the result of an unfortunate confluence of more than one of these physiological stressors.

One thing all medical conditions have in common is that the healing process is influenced by our state of mind. State of mind is a constant variable that helps explain why exposure

When emotional distress becomes chronic, it creates chronic physiological stress that can trigger disease, exacerbate existing conditions, and interfere with healing.

to any particular physiological stressor does not necessarily always confer disease. In fact, reducing emotional distress can mollify the effects of most forms of physiological stress.

Although emotional distress is just one type of physiological stressor and just one of the variables that influence whether we succumb to disease, it is a primary focus of this book because it is the kind of stressor we have the power to mitigate through mastery practices. However, it is not the whole story. Throughout this book, I will also explain how the mind's effect on health goes far beyond the issue of emotional distress.

The Physiological Effects of
Persistent Emotional Distress

It is normal to experience emotional distress brought on by the events and circumstances of everyday life. When this happens sporadically, it is not a problem—the body is resilient enough to fully recover from most transient stressors, emotional or otherwise. When emotional distress becomes chronic, though, it creates chronic physiological stress that can trigger disease, exacerbate existing conditions, and interfere with healing.

Chronic emotional distress can take the form of depression and despair, anxiety, social isolation, or hostility. Ohio State Medical School researcher Janice Kiecolt-Glaser has described how the chronic physiological stress that accompanies these states increases what is called *allostatic load*—cumulative strain on the body—and this in turn increases vulnerability to disease.[1]

Emotion in Context

Our genetics, epigenetics, and other factors can determine the specifics of our future illnesses and the age at which we will be struck down. Those who have exceptional genetics; who get good nutrition, ample sleep, and regular exercise; and who minimize their exposure to environmental toxins will have greater health and longevity than those with a less optimal profile, but no one is immune from the deleterious effects of persistent emotional upheaval.

When I was practicing psychotherapy with people living with chronic or life-threatening diseases, I observed that a large percentage of them had survived childhoods involving an unusually high degree of emotional distress in their families of origin. I began to wonder if it was possible that over a period of many years, their emotional distress had actually created pathogenic (disease-causing) levels of physiological stress, which could have contributed to their autoimmune diseases, cancer, and other debilitating medical conditions. This led me to review the published literature from refereed journals and books by experts in the field, and you will find many of my findings in this book.

Of course, there are healthy adults who grew up in very dysfunctional families who do not succumb to early or midlife chronic illness. What do they tend to have in common? They eat, sleep, and exercise just the right amount, have good genes and supportive friends, and minimize their exposure to environmental toxins. But this disease-free result is exceptional. Among the clients with whom I worked, some had done everything right in terms of self-care, but long years of emotional distress were too much for them and they eventually developed some type of debilitating medical condition. Like those individuals, since the early 1970s when I was in my mid-twenties, I have done everything right in terms of nutrition, exercise, and sleep. Despite this, as I described in the preface, I live with several so-called "co-morbid" chronic conditions. What I neglected until recently, however, despite having a meditation practice that also dates back to the early 1970s, was to engage in the variety of mindfulness-based wellbeing practices I advocate in this book. Outwardly, I had been very successful, but I was out of touch with my inner subjective experience.

Emotional Distress and the Untrained Mind

Emotional distress is often self-inflicted by the untrained mind, the result of *being out of harmony with our inner, subjective experience of the moment.* This happens when we do not allow ourselves to fully experience our thoughts, sensations, or emotions, or to recognize them for what they are: insubstantial mental constructs. It is important to understand that disharmony does not result from unpleasant thoughts or feelings; rather, it occurs when we believe they are things of substance that we must obey, when we fuse with them and allow our thoughts and feelings to dictate our behavior.

This state of disharmony can be substantially eased through mindfulness training, the core practice of mastery.

ʘ

Now that we have briefly considered emotional stressors as one of the underlying causes of disease, let's move on to explore more deeply the ways in which the mind works at cross-purposes to emotional wellbeing, beginning with the next chapter, Theories of Suffering. When we understand the thought processes that trigger emotional stressors and learn to recognize them in ourselves, we become able to consciously intervene in the mental/emotional cycle that creates physiological stress. And we can begin to turn the tide toward greater wellbeing.

3 Theories of Suffering

Many of us living with chronic health challenges often find ourselves thinking that all our suffering stems from pain, fatigue, or physical limitations. But this is not the whole picture. As we saw in the preceding chapter, much of our suffering is inflicted by the untrained mind. Without training, the mind lets us get battered about and bullied by thoughts and feelings. A trained mind, in sharp contrast, observes thoughts and feelings without getting hooked by them, simply observing them as if watching clouds float across the sky. This is tremendously liberating, and it is a proven path out of unnecessary suffering.

Dedication and consistency are required to train the mind, and a committed, lifelong mind-training practice is essential. But the effort invested pays for itself many times over. It enables us, moment by moment throughout the day, to free ourselves from the emotional distress we have needlessly endured, and as you now know, reduced emotional distress equals reduced physiological stress.

The first step to changing our mental patterns is to gain an understanding that these patterns are primarily responsible for our unnecessary suffering. To aid in this understanding, let me cite a few experts in the field of psychology.

Research psychologists Lizabeth Roemer and Susan Orsillo teach that unnecessary suffering results from three related mechanisms:

1. An unhealthy relationship to our inner subjective experi-
    ences, consisting of one or more of the following:
    a. Cognitive fusion—an overidentification with our
        thoughts, emotions, images, and sensations
    b. Judgment—criticism of self and others
    c. Lack of awareness of thoughts, emotions, images,
        and sensations

2. Experiential avoidance: evading unpleasant thoughts,
    emotions, images, and sensations. Our efforts to escape
    these can take cognitive, emotional, and behavioral
    forms.

3. Behavioral constriction or restriction. This occurs when,
    in our quest to avoid or escape distressing thoughts,
    emotions, images, and sensations, we choose not to
    engage in actions we value; we fail to pursue what mat-
    ters most to us, such as a creative endeavor or intimacy
    with others. By constricting or restricting our behavior in
    such a way, we perpetuate the very suffering we want to
    avoid.[1]

We can address all of these causes of unnecessary suffering through mindfulness practice. Let's examine two of them
a little more closely: cognitive fusion and experiential avoidance. They are important enough to an understanding of how
to achieve mastery that I have also devoted a full chapter to
each, chapters 4 and 5.

Cognitive Fusion
The mental state of cognitive fusion is one in which we con-
fuse our thoughts and beliefs with reality; we become so identified with our thoughts that we lose the ability to see them
for what they are—inventions of the mind. Our thoughts
are fleeting, insubstantial things, products of a brain whose
business it is to continually manufacture them. If we cannot
"unhook" or "disengage" from them, they become a kind of

cognitive quicksand that drags us toward suffering. Applying this idea to our experience of illness and health, if I begin to experience intermittent blurring of my vision, I may begin to fear a brain tumor. Having the thought is not the same as having a tumor, but if I am cognitively fused to the idea, it can feel dangerously real, even though the truth is that the only thing I can say with certainty is that I'm experiencing intermittent blurred vision. Here you can easily see how cognitive fusion with thoughts that evoke fear causes terrible emotional distress. The prudent course would be to acknowledge that I'm having a thought that is not based in fact and to see my ophthalmologist as soon as possible to determine the real nature of the problem.

Experiential Avoidance

Experiential avoidance is two-pronged. First, it involves the unhealthy behavior of avoiding any thoughts, feelings, emotions, or sensations we find unpleasant. It also means avoiding taking actions that are life serving in an attempt to avoid such unpleasant emotions as fear, anger, embarrassment, or shame.

Experiential avoidance rarely has the desired effect. As you will see when we examine it more closely in chapter 5, avoiding an experience generally has the effect of giving it greater power. And it denies us valuable opportunities to learn and grow from meeting our discomfort head-on.

Other Causes of Unnecessary Suffering

In addition to cognitive fusion, experiential avoidance, and the other factors Roemer and Orsillo have identified, some acceptance- and mindfulness-based researchers such as Jason Luoma have identified additional causes of unnecessary suffering.[2]

The Dominance of the Conceptualized Past and Future

Part of the human condition involves creating *concepts.* We do this in the hope that they will provide us with understanding and even a sense of predictability. Concepts are essential to our survival and to the ability to live a full life. Unfortunately, the human condition also includes cognitive fusion with our concepts. Without mindfulness practice, we are unable to step back from these concepts and see their fundamental unreality. In such a fused state, we fall victim to regret about the past and worry about the future.

Attachment to the Conceptualized Self

Narcissistic personality disorder is an extreme example of what we all experience throughout life. It involves fusion with the belief that we are a certain way — a certain kind of person. Like the conceptualized past and future, the conceptualized self (also known as the ego) is not intrinsically bad; in fact, it is essential for life. The problem arises when our self-concepts are challenged and we are unable to immediately step back from them and see that they are actually nothing more than secretions of the brain, or as comic George Carlin termed them in the title of his book, *Brain Droppings.*[3]

Inaction and Its Companion, Impulsiveness

Many of us hold ourselves back from doing things that would enhance our lives because we're afraid of embarrassment, shame, or failure. On the other hand, some people, especially those with bipolar disorder or borderline personality disorder, act impulsively in order to avoid the same very uncomfortable feelings. We all do this to some extent, and for most of us, mindfulness practice is one of the best antidotes, because it allows us to embrace our fears and take action that is in harmony with our personal values even while experiencing uncomfortable emotions. It also helps us to live with intentionality and a commitment to the cultivation of mastery.

Lack of Clarity about Personal Life Values

It is impossible to live a rich and rewarding life until we begin to live in full contact with what matters to us most. But in most cultures through-out the world, a large segment of the popula-tion becomes so fused with societal values that they are unaware of their own personal values. In-stead, they unquestion-ingly value what their culture deems worthy.

Much of our suffer-ing is inflicted by the untrained mind. With an untrained mind, we experience more FEAR.

Like many people, in my family of origin I was expected to adopt the family's religious and cultural values and my own were not accepted. In modern Western culture, this problem is ubiquitous in schools, in the corporate world, in government, in all religions, and to varying degrees in every area of work and play.

Sometimes it's easiest to recognize these societal values in the details of unwritten rules we followed in the past—prac-tices from which we've since distanced ourselves. For exam-ple, I remember a time when you couldn't play tennis without wearing white and men couldn't play golf without wearing those silly-looking plaid pants. Though these values—in this case definitions of propriety—may not be terribly important in the scheme of things, they are indications of the extent to which societal values can guide the choices we make and the way we live.

Another Construct to Consider: FEAR

The acronym FEAR provides another picture of the elements of unnecessary suffering, and as you can see in the list that follows, it includes our familiar concepts of cognitive fusion and experiential avoidance. In developing mastery, it can be helpful to keep this FEAR construct in mind.[4]

- *F is for Fusion* (cognitive fusion): As I described earlier, this means holding our thoughts and beliefs to be real things as opposed to creations of the mind. This causes a kind of blindness that limits our ability to live with acceptance, authenticity, and choice.

- *E is for Evaluation:* While the ability to evaluate our surroundings and circumstances is essential to our survival, it has an unhealthy side. We create enormous suffering for ourselves and others when we use this skill to judge people by their race, nationality, customs, beliefs, and even their hair or eye color. We negatively evaluate ourselves as well for an array of perceived transgressions, even for having certain thoughts.
- *A is for Avoidance* (experiential avoidance): Most of us have learned the unhealthy behavior of trying to avoid what makes us uncomfortable, including our unpleasant thoughts and emotions. This tendency even extends to avoidance of healthy behaviors.
- *R is for Reason-giving:* Thinking up reasons, explanations, and justifications for our behavior removes us from our present-moment experience and leads to experiential avoidance, inauthenticity, and considerable suffering.

Core Beliefs

Core beliefs are the deeply entrenched beliefs about ourselves and the world that we carry through life. Very unhealthy core beliefs often originate from our dysfunctional families of origin. This is where we might have learned to believe *I'm not lovable* or *I'm not good enough.* We also carry core beliefs that are the result of the propaganda with which we are bombarded throughout life, propagated in families, school systems, religious institutions, and the media.

As an extension of our core beliefs, and despite all evidence to the contrary, we can easily become deluded into identifying ourselves and others as being a certain way—as more of a static idea than a human being. For example, in the United States we continually hear people described as being "a good person," "a good Christian," or a good anything that we value. On the surface, there might seem to be no harm in this, but there is inherent danger in identifying with labels.

It's just as easy to label people as bad as it is to label them with more positive attributions, and the unfortunate logical conclusion of such labeling is often violence against those determined "bad." There is considerable suffering in this for both the judger and the judged.

Suffering and the Spectrum of Moods

From a psychoneuroimmunology perspective, happy moods are life serving and unhappy moods are unhealthy. But, perhaps counterintuitive at first, happy moods are actually unhealthy as well, and the reason lies in the importance of mindfulness in emotional wellbeing and the nature of mood itself: moods and mindfulness cannot coexist. When we are mindful, our thoughts, images, sensations, and emotions change from moment to moment; we don't reside in a single state. So from a mindfulness perspective, happy moods are destructive because they entail a lack of psychological flexibility. Yes, it is possible to be in a *happy* mood, but a *healthy* mood is an oxymoron.

More About Psychological Inflexibility

I had an insight into my own psychological inflexibility at a workshop I attended at Spirit Rock Meditation Center in rural West Marin County, California. The room was quiet and all attention was focused on Dr. Paul Ekman's presentation (upon whose work the *Lie to Me* TV series was based). Suddenly, someone's cell phone rang. Because we were in a place that tries to maintain quiet, my immediate response was one of annoyance and judgment about the owner of that phone. I suffered because of my limiting belief that *people should be more aware and considerate.* Ekman, however, had other ideas. He paused in his lecture and exclaimed, "Isn't it *wonderful* that there's such great reception out here in West Marin!" This incident is memorable for me because it so exemplifies the extent to which the rigidity of our beliefs and judgments creates our own suffering. I squirmed in discomfort even though the presenter wasn't fazed at all.

Ekman had spent considerable time with the Dalai Lama, and during his lecture I was quite shocked when he told us that His Holiness makes an exception to the Buddhist practice of preserving all life when it comes to mosquitoes—carriers of disease. This was another lesson in psychological flexibility, this time on the part of a venerated leader of world peace. I reflected upon how the followers of such a person can create enormous suffering by developing literal interpretations of the metaphors he or she uses; meanwhile the leader lives with flexibility and clarity and experiences far less suffering.

At the same lecture, Ekman made the point I made here earlier: that there are no constructive moods; all moods are destructive because they are fixed states. He described spending time with well-known monk Matthieu Ricard, the man referred to in Buddhist circles as "the happiest man on the planet." Ricard is known to be able to spend most of his waking hours just watching his thoughts and emotions come and go like birds in flight.

Reining In the Mind to Reduce Suffering

As the case studies I present throughout the book demonstrate, every thought or image, every product of the imagination we spin out as we move through the day, has physiological correlates and effects upon our state of health. When we are fused with these machinations of the mind, we are helpless to avoid being affected by them—psychologically, emotionally, and physiologically—and we allow them to rule our behavior. This is why mindfulness is so important. Through mindfulness practice, we are able to disengage and dis-identify from all these products of the mind, which is good for our health and allows us to make better decisions in our lives.

Much of our emotional distress is the result of our thoughts residing in the future or the past. For many of us, the majority of our thoughts have to do with worries about future events or replaying of past events, especially those about which we have regret. The fusion with those mental constructs leads to emotional distress. And as we have learned, emotional distress leads to physiological stress, and chronic physiological stress eventuates in disease.

Mindfulness practice offers a powerful intervention in this vicious cycle. When we train ourselves *to be aware of and fully present with what is,* we do not have to live with the anxieties of past and future or their deleterious effects on our health. We can instead cultivate an ever increasing sense of wellbeing.

When We Seek Help

Interestingly, Roemer and Orsillo's research shows that the most common complaints people bring into their psychotherapy sessions have as their root cause cognitive fusion, lack of acceptance of self and others, experiential avoidance, or failure to take valued action.[5] In light of our discussion of unnecessary suffering, this is not surprising, as we have seen that these are all common causes of it. They are at the root of the pain that drives people to seek help.

∞

In the next chapter, we will follow this overview of the causes of unnecessary suffering with a deeper exploration of one of the prime culprits: cognitive fusion.

4 Cognitive Fusion

Thoughts are electrochemical events, taking place within nerve cells, and these chemical changes inevitably invoke parallel chemical and hormonal changes throughout the body.
—Alastair Cunningham, PhD

B y now you are becoming acquainted with the concept of *cognitive fusion,* the unnecessary suffering it creates, and how chronic suffering is deleterious to our health. In this chapter we will look more closely at what it is, how it works, and the role of mindfulness-based wellbeing practices in overcoming it. It is important to understand cognitive fusion, because learning how to recognize and respond to it is a prerequisite to achieving mastery of your experience—and this may be the single most important contributor to wellbeing.

Cognitive fusion is the state of mind in which we are so fused with our thoughts that they appear to be synonymous with fact: the literal truth.[1] In this state, we have such strong identification with and/or attachment to our thoughts and beliefs that we are unable to see what is *in fact* the literal truth—that our thoughts are transitory and without substance. We can become so entangled with our thoughts, images, sensations, and emotions that we fall into a type of *trance,* or *altered state of consciousness* (ASC). This is the result of not being in full contact with the present moment, and, unfortunately, most of us are in this state of disconnection most of the time.

This is a problem, because when we are out of touch with our moment-to-moment, inner subjective experience, we have no choice but to react to the machinations of the mind.

Mindlessness, Mindfulness, and Cognitive Fusion

Mind*less*ness—which exists whenever we are not actively practicing mindfulness—is a mind state wherein we tend to rely upon rigid categories and distinctions we acquired in the past. New events and situations are classified according to old, timeworn labels. Our attitudes and behaviors develop out of these rigid constructs of the mind, and we wind up acting according to what amounts to a formalized set of rules of our own creation.[2]

For example, our conversations and interpersonal interactions commonly fall into very predictable patterns, both with particular people and in general. This provides a sense of safety and predictability; after all, when we are in full contact with the present moment, nothing is predictable. But staying locked in these predictable patterns limits our range of choices in how we interact.

This mind*less* state is in contrast to mind*ful*ness, wherein our attitudes and behaviors develop out of our moment-to-moment subjective experience. When we are mindful, we are able to create new approaches to events and situations and are no longer bound by the past. This allows us to explore our world with fresh and varied perspectives.[3] It is essential in breaking free of cognitive fusion.

The danger with cognitive fusion—which, again, is a state most of us dwell in most of the time—is that our thoughts exercise enormous power over us. In fact, they control us completely because we labor under the mistaken belief that they must be obeyed; this is the opposite of mastery and true well-being.

How, then, do we "cognitively defuse" or disengage? The first step is to recognize our fused, unconscious state. There are telltale signs.

Forms of Cognitive Fusion

Cognitive fusion takes place in several common categories of thinking. Learning these categories is a first step to recognizing their influence in your life.

The Conceptualized Self

The conceptualized self, touched on in the last chapter, is a term used to describe the self-identity or self-concept that we have identified with throughout life, usually since childhood. For example, my view of myself as being too introverted and not social enough has a ring of truth, yet I am much more than those characteristics. My self-concept cannot possibly give a true picture of the depth of my thoughts, emotions, and behavior. Like a photograph that can't possibly convey the experience of a live scene, the conceptualized self is a fixed, rigid concept that only tells part of the story. Whether it is positive or negative, fusion with this conceptualized self serves to limit the ways in which we can experience the world and ties us to a static sense of self.

Here's one example of how this type of cognitive fusion leads to suffering. If we are fused with a conceptualized self— a fixed idea of "who we are"—and someone intentionally says something insulting about "us" in our presence, our experience is that the one making a nasty comment is challenging the very person we are, and that hurts. But if we are able to take a step back and decouple from our notions of who we are, we can simply let the slur fly by. Because we have no attachment to a rigid idea of who we are, the comment has nowhere to "stick."

Now, we all have ideas about who we are, and the point here is not to *get rid* of the conceptualized self. The problem arises when we are so thoroughly fused with our self-concept that the slightest insult causes great suffering. The conceptualized self can be addressed, as can all our thoughts and beliefs, *by learning to hold such concepts lightly* so we can easily let them go.

Core Beliefs
As I also mentioned in the last chapter, beginning early in our lives many of us developed very unhealthy core beliefs about ourselves, such as that we weren't good enough or that we were unlovable or flawed in some significant way. These beliefs about ourselves cause immense suffering if we are in a state of fusion with them and they can be so thoroughly entrenched in the psyche that trying to alter them is an exercise in futility. This is why the antidote is not to waste our energy trying to dispute them, but rather, through mindfulness practice, to learn how to view them as insubstantial mental constructs.

Rumination
Another kind of cognitive fusion is rumination: repeatedly and perhaps even compulsively turning over an idea in the mind. The Latin root is "chewing," and you might think about a cow with its cud or a dog worrying a bone—we are capable of "chewing over" our mental constructs seemingly without end. A related idea is resentment, a word that holds the literal meaning "to feel again and again."

We all find ourselves ruminating about various challenges in life from time to time—and you may have noticed for yourself that this often leads nowhere. Far from getting us to effective solutions, our ruminations build upon themselves as they circle around in a closed loop. In fact, ruminations can catalyze progressively more intense emotions. As psychologist Rebecca Crane points out, once our internal style of thinking and experiencing has developed into a particular pattern, the pattern becomes entrenched and reinforced in direct proportion to the number of times we repeat that line of thinking.[4] This serves to perpetuate our rigid patterns.

According to psychologist Zindel Segal, rumination has been found to be the primary mechanism responsible for relapse in major depressive disorder as well as in dysthymia (chronic, low-grade depression).[5]

When we are not practicing mindfulness, we are not able

to observe our moment-to-moment inner experiences and we rely instead upon intellect and language to interpret and attempt to influence the world around us—hence our endless inner chatter. This places our perceptions squarely amid our static thoughts and beliefs, and in that situation, we base our behavior on judgments stemming from what we are taught is *right*. This is a recipe for perpetuating cognitive fusion and suffering, both for ourselves and for those with whom we interact.

Fusion with Attributions

In understanding the deleterious effects of cognitive fusion, it is important to explore how the *attributions* we assign to all stimuli directly influence our physiology and health. We assign attributions when we connect a quality, character, or cause to a particular event—often with little awareness that we are doing this. Attributions assigned to both the actions of others and to internal stimuli can create rage, fear, anxiety, depression, frustration, sadness, shame, and even a sense of hopelessness within us.

For example, if I attribute an adverse medical outcome to a doctor's or nurse's carelessness, I am likely to experience rage, whereas if I attribute it to something beyond anyone's control, I am more likely to accept it. If I attribute a doctor's abrupt manner before a procedure to his or her disregard for me, I'm likely to feel fear. If instead I attribute it to his or her complete focus on making sure everyone on the team and all the necessary instruments and equipment are in place, I may feel gratitude.

Much of the suffering we experience with chronic medical conditions is less a result of the seriousness of a medical diagnosis or the degree of physical pain or disability we experience and more a product of the attributions we assign to diagnoses and symptoms as well as to our identification and cognitive fusion with those attributions.[6] In my own experience, I notice that when I get a certain type of back discomfort, immediately I am flooded with images of possible renal hypoperfusion (decreased blood flow through the kidneys). As soon as I disengage from those images, I feel better.

Attachments to Outcomes
Attachment to outcomes is another form of cognitive fusion, and this is tricky terrain. When we are ill, we need to strike a balance between non-attachment to specific health outcomes and actively doing everything possible to improve our health. We need to create a good environment for healing without becoming attached to a particular result, such as complete cessation of a chronic condition. Interestingly, research psychologist Ellen Langer has found that the idea of *battling and fighting* illness—the determination to conquer it completely—can have a paradoxical effect, resulting in a state of mind wherein we give the illness even greater power over us.[7]

Examples of the Extreme Danger of Cognitive Fusion
A researcher by the name of Herbert Specter did an experiment about twenty years ago when he was the head of molecular biology research at the National Institutes of Health. He injected mice with a chemical called Polyisee, which stimulates the immune system, while at the same time exposing them to the smell of camphor. After a while, when the mice smelled camphor, their immune systems were activated.

Specter gave some other mice psychlophosphamite, which is a chemical that destroys the immune system; once again, he paired the drug with the smell of camphor. When those mice smelled camphor without the chemical present, they became functionally immunodeficient, quickly developing pneumonia and dying when exposed to pneumococci bacteria. Exposure to carcinogens also led to swift and certain death.

In the first group, meanwhile, exposure to pneumococci and carcinogens had no effect. What was the crucial difference between survival and death in these mice? It was the *interpretation of the memory of the smell* of camphor. Lacking the human ability to recognize that they were fused with the pairing of a

stimulus (camphor) and the drug—and also lacking the ability to disengage from it even if they could somehow become
aware of their plight—the mice were helpless victims of the
unconscious associations made in their brains.

Another example of the extreme danger of cognitive fusion impacts humans. One of the most disturbing comments
that hospitalists and nurses hear is when someone who has
been brought into the emergency department says, "I'm not
going to make it through the night." Whenever they hear such
an announcement, the medical staff gets worried because,
statistically, these patients are usually dead by morning. It's
not that patients can predict the future. It's that the belief that
they are going to die, and their inability to disengage from
this belief, is more powerful than most of the treatments they
receive. This is especially true in hospitalized patients because being in the hospital can be so frightening that patients
automatically go into an altered state of consciousness, and
ASCs dramatically interfere with executive function, resulting in extreme cognitive fusion. Unfortunately, the various
drugs given to hospitalized patients compound this problem
of trance.

Similarly, when patients are told that they have three to
six months to live, most comply and die within that time period. When someone has just been given a cancer diagnosis
by a physician, the patient almost invariably enters an ASC
and goes into cognitive fusion. When hospitalized patients are
given a poor prognosis while in this state of cognitive fusion,
their health will be negatively impacted. The only antidote at
that point is to get the assistance of someone who can help
them disengage from that state.

Cognitive Fusion Run Rampant

In the 1970s, I read about an incident involving nearly two
hundred people who were watching a high school football
game at a stadium and suddenly had to be rushed to area hospitals by ambulance. It seems that a handful of people had
developed nausea and vomiting, and believed they must have

Red flags signalling cognitive fusion include words like *should, shouldn't, right, wrong, good, bad,* and similar evaluative language.

been poisoned by the food at one of the concession stands. After a little investigation, it was determined that all those who had fallen ill had consumed soft drinks from a dispensing machine located under the stands. School officials feared that the syrup in the machine had somehow become contaminated, so they made an announcement over the loudspeaker system warning the crowd to avoid that machine.

The moment the announcement was made, a couple of hundred people in the stands suddenly began suffering nausea and vomiting, and many fainted. Ambulances from five area hospitals were called and remained busy for some time transporting the unusually high number of ill people. As each hospital struggled to manage treatment of a huge influx of emergency room patients, the physicians were stymied, not just by the number of people affected but also by the unusually rapid onset and severity of the illness. A few hours later, while the sick fans were being treated, the soft drink syrup was tested.

There was nothing wrong with it.

As word spread through the hospitals that the soda had never been contaminated after all, two hundred people suddenly made complete recoveries. Everybody got up and went home.

This is a dramatic example of both the power and the danger of cognitive fusion. The hospitalized football fans had experienced a series of thoughts: *several people got sick; they all drank sodas from a contaminated dispensing machine; I drank soda from that same machine—I've been poisoned!* Their physical symptoms were undeniable. But it was fusion with the thought—*I've been poisoned!*—that had catalyzed the physiological processes involved. If these people had instead developed the mindfulness skills to be able to recognize this series of thoughts as thoughts and nothing more, they would not have gotten sick.

Recognizing Cognitive Fusion in Language— and Using Language to Disengage

Cognitive fusion commonly involves entanglement with *categorical and judgmental* thought.[8] Red flags are words like *should, shouldn't, right, wrong, good, bad,* and similar evaluative language. They indicate that we are fused with our mental constructs and out of touch with actual moment-to-moment reality.

Other reliable indicators that we are fused with our thoughts are words like *I, me,* or *mine.* When *I am* is followed by the word *anxious* or *depressed,* it is a sign that we are suffering in a fused state—and more often than not, it creates a self-fulfilling prophecy. The hypnotic and physiological effects of saying *or even thinking* "I am depressed" are well known in cognitive neuroscience and in psychoneuroimmunology.[9] *I am depressed* = depression.

When I say, *I'm depressed,* my mind hears the words as a hypnotic suggestion: *Be depressed.* This in turn affects every cell in my body and I actually reinforce the depression.[10] The same has been shown to be true of physical pain; expecting and identifying with pain reinforces the existing neural pathways for pain and creates new ones, thereby increasing the likelihood of experiencing increased pain.[11]

Now let's look at shifting the language. It may seem a subtle distinction at first, but *I'm depressed* is very different from *I'm interpreting my sad, uncomfortable feelings to mean I'm depressed,* or *I'm having the thought that I'm depressed.* These latter statements reflect awareness of one's state *and* do not contribute to remaining trapped in it. The same dynamics come into play with anxiety. The fused position of *I'm overwhelmed and will not get my work done in time* is very different from the disengaged position of *I'm aware that I'm having the thought that*

I'm overwhelmed and will not get my work done in time. The second way allows us to step back and have room to breathe a sigh of relief. Also, this second way causes less physiological stress as a result of less emotional distress. This is how mindfulness, which allows us to take a disengaged position, has the ability to improve physiological functioning and possibly even health outcomes.

An Approach to Cognitive Fusion with Beliefs

During my three years of training at the Simonton Cancer Center, there were many retreat participants who claimed they were willing to do whatever it took to get well, but such a commitment was not always evident in their behavior. Often, their prognoses were optimistic and they expressed several reasons why they wanted to continue living, yet they seemed apathetic.

Then there were those whose prognoses were dismal, who had been told by their oncologists to go home and get their affairs in order. Many of these participants continued to live with enthusiasm, vitality, and purpose. In fact, some in this cohort went into long-term remission.

Two distinguishing characteristics described this second group. One was that they had fighting spirit and a strong will to live. The other was a sense of mastery: the belief that what they did could make a difference.

The way we worked with the apathetic participants was to explore their beliefs about their situation. Often, the reason they lacked fighting spirit was that they were cognitively fused with the very unhealthy belief that there was nothing they could do to influence the course of their illness. We worked with them to help them disengage from this belief, thereby teaching them a fundamental skill in developing mastery.

CR

In this chapter we have seen further evidence that it is never the content of our thoughts, but rather our relationship to, or fusion with, our thoughts that creates suffering.[12] Changing our relationship to our thoughts requires an ongoing mind training practice in the form of acceptance and mindfulness, which we will explore in depth in future chapters.[13]

An Opportunity to Examine Cognitive Fusion

The following questions are designed to help you start thinking about how cognitive fusion typically contributes to your own suffering. Remember, this is something we all experience, and it is vital that we each get acquainted with how it plays out in our daily lives. The way you answer these questions will depend on your ability to recognize when you are fused with your beliefs and your ability to disengage from them. Note that one way to recognize that you are cognitively fused with an idea or feeling is to notice when you find yourself making unhealthy choices.

1. Are you self-aware when you feel tense, angry, or frustrated or are experiencing some other unpleasant emotion?
   a. If so, how do you know?
   b. Do you know because of how you're behaving, or do you know by being able to correlate specific sensations with certain emotions?
2. If you say or do something that you later regret, see if you can recall a moment that had occurred just before you did that. Was there an instant when you had some awareness that you had a choice?
   a. Do you have a sense of how you would like to respond the next time you're presented with a similar situation?
   b. How hopeful are you that you can do something different next time?

3. When you feel sad or depressed, can you think of any precipitating thoughts that may have gone through your mind and contributed to the feeling?

4. When you have self-deprecating thoughts, can you sometimes see that they are just thoughts, not fact? Or does your negative self-talk seem like immutable truths?

5. When you feel an unusual pain or other unpleasant sensation, do you often imagine that it could mean a tumor or worse?

   a. When you imagine this, are you sometimes able to laugh about it, recognizing the thought as just something your brain likes to manufacture.

   b. Are you able to calm and reassure yourself when you imagine such a thing, or do you obsess over those thoughts?

   c. Are you able to differentiate between the *thought* that this is what the pain *might* mean and the need for medical care?

6. When you don't feel like doing your daily exercise routine:

   a. Do you skip the exercise?

   b. Do you do it just to get it done?

   c. Are you able to see the desire to skip it as just an insubstantial mental construct? Can you then proceed with the exercise with enthusiasm and with the feeling of wellbeing that results from making conscious, healthy choices?

7. When you find yourself acting on unhealthy impulses:

   a. Are you able to think of a possible early warning signal that could have helped you avoid acting on the impulse?

   b. Are you able to recognize that you aren't behaving in a way that best supports your health?

   c. Are you able to see the connection between the behavior and the thoughts that led to it?

    d. Are you able to change to a healthier behavior?

    e. Are you able to calm and reassure yourself when this happens?

5 Experiential Avoidance

If you are not willing to have it, you will.
—Steven Hayes, PhD

The term *experiential avoidance* originated in contextual behavioral science research.[1] It refers to a common psychological pattern to which we are all naturally susceptible: the attempt to avoid unpleasant thoughts, images, feelings, sensations, and emotions.[2]

Experiential avoidance prevents us from being accepting of and present to our natural inner impulses, and this is problematic in a number of respects. In detaching us from feeling, experiential avoidance interferes with the very function of emotions, which is to inform us of our inner subjective experience. And because our inner experience is what informs our conscious choices, experiential avoidance has the effect of limiting our options. It prevents us from acting on opportunities to pursue the personal values that give our lives meaning and it undermines the pursuit of mastering our experience.[3]

Habitual experiential avoidance can be terribly debilitating. In fact, studies have shown that it is a common trait found in people who have difficulty making normal, everyday decisions. Research psychologist Michael Twohig and his team found that decision making becomes challenging for such people precisely because they are out of touch with their inner cues and direct experience.[4] Imagine forgetting to go to bed because you can't tell that you're tired, or forgetting to eat because you don't know you're hungry.

Experiential avoidance is
orthogonal to acceptance
of feelings.

In addition to limiting our choices and even making the act of choosing more difficult, experiential avoidance carries another danger: it repeatedly reinforces the message that *we are not strong enough to withstand our more painful feelings.* This kind of self-denial is the underlying cause of much of the current epidemic of depression in the industrialized world.

Feelings of sadness, anger, frustration, anxiety, and grief—the emotions we are most likely to try to avoid—are normal and healthy; in fact, we cannot function very well when we are out of touch with them. Our inner world informs us of our needs and wants, and it is through our inner experience that we interact with our environment.[5] If we tamp that experience down, we cannot live fully, nor can we grow. The tragedy of experiential avoidance is that when we deny our inner life we deny our aliveness—our very existence.

Keys to Overcoming Experiential Avoidance

Becoming aware of our avoidant behavior is an essential first step in practicing healthier behavior, and mindfulness practice is an excellent way to increase awareness of this tendency. Psychotherapy with an Acceptance and Commitment Therapy (ACT) therapist can also be extremely beneficial because therapists in this field are trained to help people improve mindfulness, identify and pursue personal life values, and reduce experiential avoidance.

Whether we achieve awareness of our avoidant behavior through mindfulness practice on our own or with the additional help of an ACT therapist, once we have brought this destructive behavior into the light of day, mindfulness-based mastery and wellbeing improve.

A Self-Attenuating Habit

Experiential avoidance involves psychological rigidity, and it is this rigidity that often prevents us from behaving in ways that are in harmony with our personal life values, such as pursuing activities that offer a sense of meaning and purpose.[6] I can give you an example of how this works from my own history with experiential avoidance.

I tend to feel uncomfortable when I'm in a group setting with people I don't know. To avoid that experience, I might decide not to accept an invitation to a party, or not to sign up for a workshop on a topic that interests me. I may make this choice despite knowing that these events offer opportunities to enjoy being in community with others, and that they will give me a sense of belonging—and these are both life values that I hold dear. I have made such choices despite knowing full well that my discomfort will be accompanied by an opportunity to grow, which is another personal life value of mine. Attending the event would be an act of loving self-care, and dealing with any emotional discomfort while I'm there would give me the opportunity to strengthen mindfulness-based mastery and wellbeing. All of these benefits are lost to me if I engage in the self-attenuating behavior of avoidance.

Exploring Avoidant Behaviors

We avoid uncomfortable inner experience in myriad ways. What follows are just a few.

Addictions

Addictions of all types lead to a very constricted and restricted lifestyle that is necessarily centered around avoiding thoughts, mental images, sensations, or emotions. This is why people who have lived with addictions often appear to be psychologically and emotionally underdeveloped, regardless of their age. They have instinctively distracted themselves from the precious growth opportunities that uncomfortable feelings present. Compounding this, the shame associated with addiction contributes to self-hatred and low self-esteem, in effect multiplying the impulse to avoid their inner subjective experience.

Tics and Twitches

Except in neurological diseases, tics and twitches are often unconscious attempts to evade our experience, and interestingly, obsessive-compulsive behaviors of many kinds, including seemingly insignificant nervous tics, have a similar effect on self-esteem as do addictions.[7] They develop into nervous habits because they are effective in providing a distraction from unwanted thoughts or feelings, but they work at great cost. As with all forms of experiential avoidance, they interfere with our ability to fully experience our aliveness and they are at cross-purposes to building mindfulness-based mastery and wellbeing.[8]

Resisting Memories

Our imagination allows us to reexperience past events. In fact, vivid memories are commonly associated with the same physiological changes we experienced during the original event, which is why vivid pleasant memories are so welcome. Likewise, vivid disturbing memories can sometimes make us feel just as bad as we did when we went through the original experience, and we quite naturally go to great lengths to avoid them. Unfortunately, here we run into the great paradox that accompanies all forms of experiential avoidance: trying to suppress unpleasant memories *strengthens them and increases their damaging effects.* The antidote to reexperiencing the unpleasant memory is not to attempt to shut it out; the antidote is to invite it in and explore it—not by analyzing it, but rather by allowing ourselves to learn that the feelings associated with the memory are *survivable.*

As I said earlier, it is natural to want to avoid painful experiences. It is also natural to believe that we *cannot survive* certain intense feelings. But the reality is that we can endure even the most dreaded thoughts, images, sensations, and emotions, and we become stronger when we summon the courage to al-

> When we courageously commit to staying
> with uncomfortable thoughts and feelings,
> we build mindfulness-based mastery and
> wellbeing.

low ourselves to be in full contact with them.

When memories of traumatic events, such as witnessing or being the target of violence, intrude into our minds on a regular basis, the resulting psychophysiological responses can ruin our health. Unfortunately, a large segment of the population suffers from posttraumatic stress disorder (PTSD). The original event can be a war experience, a gang-related experience, rape, ritual abuse, any type of child abuse, or a traumatic car accident. The antidote to PTSD always includes learning to be present with the traumatic memory rather than avoid it and recognizing that the content of our imaginations is not the same as present-moment reality. This takes time and is best accomplished by working with someone who has extensive professional experience with PTSD.

"Healthy" Avoidance Techniques

Many practices that are generally considered healthy, such as yoga, tai chi, or other physical disciplines, *when practiced in order to avoid unpleasant thoughts, images, emotions, or sensations,* limit our ability to live a full and rich life. While we may gain some health benefits by engaging in such practices, if what moves us to practice is the desire to escape the fullness of our experience, those practices can also have harmful effects. And there is another down side: when we engage in favorite activities as a way to avoid experiencing distressing thoughts and feelings, our experience is usually not as joyful or satisfying as it would be otherwise.[9]

Discomfort: An Invitation to Mastery

We have seen that the more energy we expend on avoiding our unwanted inner subjective experiences, the further we get from developing mastery. By contrast, when we courageously commit to staying with uncomfortable thoughts and feelings, we build mindfulness-based mastery and wellbeing. Let me give you another example.

A few years ago I was asked to do a demonstration of my therapeutic work in front of an audience of peers. Like many people facing the prospect of performing before a group—and in this case a group of professionals—when I got to the venue, I was terrified. My first impulse was to seek ways to avoid the anxiety that was surging through me. Rather than embrace it, I tried to counteract it with cognitive restructuring and mental imagery. The result? I became *more* anxious!

Finally, exhausted from the effort, I abandoned that strategy. I gave up trying to control my anxious sensations and instead allowed myself to fully experience them. I decided to accept my anxiety as a part of the full range of emotion I'm capable of feeling, and when I opened myself to the experience in this way, I not only felt calmer, I actually felt incredibly energized. By accepting my anxiety I became more accepting of myself and my humanity. This kind of acceptance, embracing an uncomfortable emotion as part of the full range of human experience, is a key component of mindfulness-based mastery and wellbeing.

By the way, my dilemma—attempting to avoid anxiety and inadvertently escalating it instead—is not unique. And here again, we find the paradox of experiential avoidance. The more importance we place on avoiding anxiety, the more we develop *anxiety about our anxiety*. This is believed to be the mechanism behind panic attacks.[10]

Further Investigations of Paradox

Let me expand a little further on the paradox of experiential avoidance with a few more examples. In each case, the experience we are seeking to avoid becomes magnified because this is where we have placed our attention.

When we attempt to analyze uncomfortable thoughts and feelings, we raise an inherent problem: using language to try to think our way through problems that were created by language in the first place. Here I'm referring to the beliefs and self-concepts described in previous chapters that are at the root of much suffering. As with anxiety, the degree to which we defend against or grapple with our suffering by analyzing it is in direct proportion to the amount of suffering we experience.[11]

Most of us have expended great amounts of energy in trying to solve our problems by attempting to think things through, changing our thoughts, or suppressing them.[12] Yet studies conducted by research psychologist Daniel Wegner have shown that analyzing, suppressing, disputing, and substituting thoughts all result in magnifying the very thoughts that so disturb us.[13]

Just as I described with my own experience of anxiety, attempts to suppress our unpleasant emotions have the same amplifying results as attempts to suppress our thoughts.[14] What's more, there can be *interplay between thought and emotion* that further exacerbates the problem: Working with researcher Richard Wenzlaff, Wegner found that attempting to suppress a thought in the presence of an emotion eventually *causes the emotion to evoke the thought*.[15] We become further trapped in a magnifying loop.

There are of course physical corollaries as well. Most of us have had the experience of trying to not dwell on an uncomfortable physical sensation only to notice that trying to not feel it is like trying not to think of an elephant. The more we try to avoid feeling a bellyache, a headache, or an itch, the worse it gets. This is because we're focusing all our attention on the discomfort.[16]

Experiential Avoidance and Intimacy

The avoidance of life experiences is the most serious
of all the psychological processes.
—Steven Hayes[17]

One of the real tragedies of experiential avoidance is that it makes intimacy in relationships impossible.[18] Our true emotions allow us to communicate with others and maintain healthy relationships with them. Whether we avoid and conceal our emotions consciously or unconsciously, we deny ourselves the possibility of validation, understanding, and empathy—necessary ingredients for health and even survival.

This happens even among professionals who "should know better." Therapists are not immune to the impulse to distance themselves from their inner world. For example, I've met weekly in a group for psychotherapists for more than sixteen years. Even after all this time, some of us still occasionally feel frustrated with the lack of empathy we get when we describe a personal struggle. But this is invariably the result of our own failure to reveal our true feelings. When we are able to express our authentic feelings, those around us are more likely to feel and freely express their empathy for us.

When Experiential Avoidance Is Healthy

Although attempting to avoid our inner, subjective experiences is usually problematic, there are some rare situations in which it's healthy. During acute traumatic experiences, distraction can be a beneficial choice. For example, in the past, I've experienced tremendous emotional distress in enclosed spaces such as an MRI scanner. Therefore, sometimes I intentionally go into a trance and imagine I'm watching a performance of Kodo drummers or some other percussion group; in this way, I'm able to transform the booming MRI sounds into something I find nonthreatening.

I have also used my imagination rather than mindfulness just before going into the operating room for surgery because the pre-op period before administration of general anesthesia is a very emotionally distressful time.

Any behavior that results in increased mastery and well-being is healthy. This is why the conscious decision to dissociate from reality and use the imagination in order to have a more palatable experience during invasive medical diagnostic or treatment procedures can be a healthy choice.

So, *dissociation* and *distraction* (both forms of experiential avoidance) are, on some rare occasions, effective techniques and can sometimes even contribute to mastery and wellbeing, and you will read more about this in chapter 21, Practice in the Eye of the Hurricane. But in everyday situations, they have not been found to be nearly as effective as the development of mindfulness and acceptance skills and the willingness and ability to be present with all of our inner subjective experiences. And in most cases, the paradoxical effect of experiential avoidance is in full force, regardless of whether the unwanted experience we wish to escape is a thought, belief, image, emotion, mood, or physiological sensation.[19]

In sum, when choosing mindfulness versus experiential avoidance techniques such as dissociation or distraction, it is important to consider the severity of the situation: dissociation and distraction can be most effective in minimizing acute physical pain or terror, but they are not effective in dealing with chronic physical or emotional pain.[20]

Effects on Health: The Physiology of Experiential Avoidance

Now let's take a look at the effects of experiential avoidance on health so we can see why it's so important for those of us with chronic medical conditions to become aware of this tendency and strive to reduce it in our lives. Our health is already compromised; we cannot afford to worsen it needlessly.

Suppression of thoughts and feelings is associated with sympathetic arousal (fight or flight), including hypertension, increased heart rate and respiration, vasoconstriction, and all the other usual effects of stress.[21] We can contrast this with the opposite of experiential avoidance: acceptance. Acceptance of our experience is associated with physiological homeostasis. When the autonomic activity involved in suppressing thoughts and emotions is allowed to quiet down, balance is restored to the immune system, which does not function well during strong autonomic activity. Functioning of the neuroendocrine system, gastrointestinal tract, and cardiovascular system improves when stress levels diminish, as does overall physiological functioning.

Research by psychologist James Pennebaker confirms these effects: his studies reveal that when we stop suppressing memories of our past traumas and instead write about them in a journal, we can experience profound improvement in physiological functioning.[22]

The suppression of unpleasant thoughts, emotions, images, and sensations results in a constriction contributing to dis-ease, which eventuates to disease. This constriction not only causes the chronic sympathetic arousal I just mentioned; it also affects brain function and the workings of every cell in the body.[23] And so we see the paradox of suppression playing out on a physiological as well as emotional level. A fascinating study conducted by research psychologists James Gross and Robert Levenson in the 1990s dramatically illustrated this fact: When study subjects were instructed to conceal their emotional expression while simply watching an emotional film, they experienced a paradoxical increase in sympathetic drive.[24]

In other studies where subjects were instructed to control their physiological sensations, they, too, reported increased emotional distress and evidenced increased sympathetic drive. When subjects were instructed to accept the sensations, on the other hand, they reported reduced emotional distress and evidenced quieting of sympathetic drive.[25]

It's interesting to consider the polygraph test in this light. There are many people who can fool a polygraph. One very famous Watergate conspirator was able to do that and perform many other feats that seem impossible to most people. But no one can fool the polygraph *by trying to control physi-*

ological sensations because, as we have seen all along in this discussion, this has the effect of increasing the stress response the subject is trying to suppress: the equipment will register the stress and the subject will flunk the test. (Excluding psychopaths, those who can fool the polygraph are highly skilled in psychophysiological self-regulation. They have practiced extensively while hooked up to biofeedback instrumentation or have used a polygraph itself as their biofeedback training device.)

It has also been shown that the physiological effects of experiential avoidance worsen with repetition. Repeated efforts to control our thoughts, images, feelings, emotions, and bodily sensations *increase our negative judgments of these internal events when they recur,* and this leads to even more concerted efforts to control them. A 2004 study revealed that this cycle of progressively increasing reactivity leads to chronic sympathetic arousal, and this can have devastating impacts on health.[26]

In general, pain and physiological functioning worsen in proportion to the degree of resistance to what we experience.[27] We heal faster when we are more open and accepting of our situation.[28] This is why pain medications can sometimes actually speed healing and recovery; they allow us to relax into our experience.

Further insight into the physiological effects of experiential avoidance can be found in the helping professions. Helping other people is a behavior that has consistently been associated with improved health outcomes. However, many people in the helping professions help others as a way to avoid their own distress, and researchers have discovered that this can negate the positive effects that helpers usually enjoy.

An Opportunity to Examine Experiential Avoidance

As I close this chapter, I'd like to leave you with a writing exercise from *Get Out of Your Mind and Into Your Life* by Dr. Steven C. Hayes. This exercise can help build awareness of the impact and cost of experiential avoidance in your life. Keep in mind that we are all blind to some of the ways we engage in experiential avoidance; for that reason, it is valuable to work with a psychotherapist—especially an ACT therapist.

The memories and images I most avoid include:

_____.

Avoiding these memories and images costs me in
    the following ways:

_____.

The bodily sensations I most avoid include:

_____.

Avoiding these bodily sensations costs me in
    the following ways:

_____.

The emotions I most avoid include:

_____.

Avoiding these emotions costs me in the following ways:

_____.

The thoughts I most avoid include:

_____.

Avoiding these thoughts costs me in the following ways:

_____.

The behavioral predispositions or urges to respond that I
    most avoid include:

_____.

Avoiding these behavioral predispositions or urges to
    respond costs me in the following ways:

_____.

଼

Now let's retrace our steps thus far in Part I. In chapter 1 I introduced the theme of the book: your power to take mindfulness-based mastery and wellbeing into your own hands by engaging in the scientifically sound practices I offer here. We took a brief look at the causes of disease in chapter 2. Then, in the subsequent chapters, we explored the primary causes of unnecessary suffering—essential concepts to grasp so you can begin to free up much-needed energy for healing. This is all important information to take with you as you enter the final chapter in Part I, Living with Chronic Illness.

6 Living with Chronic Illness

When people are told they have a chronic, incurable disease or condition, especially if the diagnosis is potentially life-threatening or extremely debilitating, they understandably react with shock, terror, disbelief, anger, and grief. For some people, the diagnosis also serves as a wake-up call and they begin to live life more fully than ever before. A number of people in groups I've facilitated have told me that their diagnosis of AIDS or cancer actually served to improve the quality of their lives. Sure, they wanted nothing more than to recover from the disease, but they also expressed strongly that their diagnosis helped them take a fresh look at their priorities and explore whether they were truly living by their most important life values.

Most of these people had no formal mindfulness practice. The diagnosis itself served to open their eyes to the truth of the ubiquity of change and impermanence that eventually becomes evident with such a practice. I saw many of them begin to pursue their personal life values with greater intentionality.

Those of us living with serious chronic conditions are often more motivated than healthier people to practice developing the mind training skills that will help us live more fully. It becomes more important to recognize states of cognitive fusion and experiential avoidance, because being ill often involves fear and dread. We can all too easily succumb to these feelings if we don't actively and consciously train our minds to recognize the thoughts flitting through them as insubstantial, mental constructs—secretions of the brain. The practices contained in this book serve as potent counterweights to cognitive fusion and experiential avoidance and, in this way, significantly reduce the unnecessary suffering that often accompanies chronic medical conditions.

I do want to emphasize that these practices address *unnecessary* suffering. Based on my personal experiences with mindfulness and chronic illness, along with my experiences working with hundreds of cancer patients and people living with all types of chronic health challenges, I believe that to a certain extent, *suffering is in fact an inherent part of pain.* So while cognitive fusion indeed adds considerable suffering, some suffering is an unavoidable component of pain, fatigue, malaise, and other disabling conditions. Mindfulness will not help you relieve all suffering, but I have witnessed its power to lift much of the burden of suffering from many, many people who are chronically ill.

I will describe a few experiences that are unique to chronically ill people. Let's examine them in the light of all we have learned so far.

The Temptation to Put One's Life on Hold
While healthy people are out and about in the world, working full-time jobs, spending time with family, or simply having fun, many people with chronic medical conditions are not well enough to live this way. It is a challenge to live with the vicissitudes inherent in a life where we often do not feel well, and a life that revolves around always struggling to feel better. We face a reality that often entails some combination of unremitting fatigue, malaise, pain, and disability. We often can work no more than a few hours a day (if at all), and it is difficult to maintain relationships with spouses, family, and friends or to parent our children. Not only can these limitations lead to ruined careers and family life, they present challenges in terms of involvement in the kinds of activities that give life meaning.

Anyone who has been down with a bad cold has had the experience of needing to put life on hold for a few days. It

Putting our lives on hold when we have a bad cold or fever helps us rest and get well; doing so with a chronic condition makes us feel worse.

can be inconvenient, and stressful; while we may need to stop and rest, the many demands on our time rarely cease. But at least we know that we'll be back on our feet soon. For those of us who are chronically ill, though, there is no end in sight. If we wait for things to improve before engaging with life, as tempting as that idea can be ("Once I feel better, then . . ."), we could wait forever.

We simply cannot afford to put our lives on hold because at this time in history, modern medicine has very few cures for us. We need to face the truth that, for many of us, our physical condition is not likely to improve. And let's be realistic: even in healthy people, the normal process of aging means that chronic health challenges eventually touch almost everyone.

I have been living with two forms of arthritis since my early thirties and with other medical conditions since childhood, and I've found that putting my life on hold every time I don't feel well only makes me feel depressed. Over the decades, a few colleagues have recommended to me on occasion that I try antidepressants. I am pleased to say that I have never taken any antidepressants, and that I have found a much more effective path to greater happiness. The idea of "anti"—trying to get rid of something undesirable—is never as effective as going toward one's goals and personal values, unless perhaps we're talking about antibiotic, antifungal, or antiviral medications.

A healthier alternative is to start living in the moment, right now, and that means engaging in the pursuit of mindfulness-based mastery and wellbeing practices. Mindfulness training and practice, and all of the other practices I offer here, add to the skill set that allows us to live healthier, more fulfilling, and happier lives despite living with health challenges that in most cases are not going to go away.

Those of us who are chronically ill would act differently if painful thoughts, sensations, and emotions were no longer an obstacle. It is worthwhile to consider these questions, and how you would address them: What projects or activities would you be engaged in if you were not so consumed by discomfort? What might you attempt if negative, pessimistic thoughts and beliefs were not an issue? The answers to these questions can help you understand what you value and that you have choices other than putting your life on hold.

Chronic Illness and Unnecessary Suffering

In chapter 3, I presented theories of suffering, describing several mental patterns in which the untrained mind can easily become trapped. Here I will tighten the lens and examine unnecessary suffering specifically as it pertains to people living with chronic health challenges.

The Greatest Source of Suffering: Identification with the Illness

> Much of the suffering in this population is related not to the symptoms, but rather to identification with the symptoms, and to identification of oneself as an ill person.[1]

As I mentioned earlier, pain, disability, and fatigue do cause suffering, but our suffering is magnified when we fail to recognize the thoughts related to symptoms as transient and insubstantial. When we are fused with those thoughts, mistaking them as factual, we create *preventable* suffering. Fortunately, we can learn to disengage from those thoughts.

It's common to hear people talk about *my* cancer, *my* Crohn's disease, *my* Lyme disease, *my* pain, *my* fatigue, or *my* disability. It's also common to hear people say *I'm depressed.* Yet as we have seen, assuming *ownership* of an illness or a state of mind takes a terrible toll emotionally, and from a psychoneuroimmunology perspective it is very damaging to your health because the emotional distress creates physiological stress. Identifying with your illness is one of the quickest ways to exacerbate it, and this is why mindfulness training, which enables us to see this identification as a mere thought, is such an essential skill for those of us living with day-to-day health challenges.

Attachment to Getting Well

While it's true that with a dedicated mindfulness-based, mastery and wellbeing practice we may be able to improve our health—and we can certainly experience greater wellbeing and a better quality of life—being attached to a return to full health only causes further emotional distress and physiological stress as our cognitive fusion with this ideal collides with reality. It's better to take the approach that we fully intend to live the best life we can, moment by moment.

Cognitive Fusion with New Symptoms

Another source of distress relates to panic over new symptoms. Even experienced mindfulness teachers can find it difficult to recognize that the frightening attributions they assign to new symptoms are usually not based on facts. It can take years of mindfulness practice to appreciate the reality that all of our thoughts and beliefs are without substance—including those concerning symptoms of illness. This is a very difficult concept to grasp until one has engaged in mindfulness practice for a certain period of time.

Although it's not a substitute for mindfulness practice, a new science-based form of psychotherapy I have mentioned before, known as ACT, or Acceptance and Commitment Therapy, is a powerful way to learn to disengage from troubling thoughts about the meaning of a new source of pain or discomfort. In addition, ACT's focus on personal life values builds mastery and wellbeing.

Depression and Anxiety

Living with chronic health challenges and the accompany-ing experience of loss often lead to increased depression and anxiety, and further suffering. If you think about the impacts chronic illness has on people's lives in the following list, it becomes obvious why this happens.

- Increased loneliness
- Loss of income
- Loss of relationships
- Loss of the ability to be a provider
- Loss of career
- Loss of the ability to engage in favorite activities
- Loss of the ability to engage in activities that provide a sense of meaning and purpose
- Chronic physical pain or discomfort
- Chronic fatigue
- Chronic malaise
- Chronic disability of any type

Feelings of shame and many other factors also contribute to anxiety, depression, and immense misery. Bear in mind that depression is epidemic in the *healthy* population.[2] It is even more rampant in the growing population of people who live with chronic diseases and conditions, including several forms of cancer.[3] And aside from preventing people from living a full life, depression results in poorer attention to self-care.[4]

Almost everyone who has ever experienced a serious ill-ness, especially if it involved a dire diagnosis, a long hospital stay, or a long period of feeling awful, has experienced hope-lessness, physical and emotional exhaustion, resignation, and depression.[5] All of these are the result of no longer being able to engage in the activities that give our lives meaning, pur-pose, and joy. This is why it is so essential to identify what we value and, through taking on mindfulness-based mastery and wellbeing practices, seek alternative ways to find fulfillment and create a rewarding life.

Isolation and the Need for Support

People living with chronic health challenges rarely receive the emotional and psychological support they need.[6] They need to feel *seen* and *appreciated,* and both are hard to achieve when you are no longer well enough to engage in the kinds of activities for which people are normally appreciated. And without ongoing support, a sense of mastery and wellbeing is difficult to develop and maintain.

The Need for Understanding

Friends and family, and healthcare providers too, often feel frustrated because they want to help, yet all too often, *nothing* seems to help. Behind their frustration is the fact that they usually have not learned how to listen to the ill person without treating him or her with either pity or sympathy; neither is what the person needs. I believe that no one except a fellow traveler on the path is truly capable of understanding what life is like for the chronically ill. There is a sense of isolation that is damaging to health and state of mind, so seeking support of the kind you genuinely need is essential. For this reason, one of the mindfulness-based mastery and wellbeing practices that will be discussed is referred to as "relationship building."

Support Groups, Victimhood, and Mindfulness-based Empathy

You must seek such support with great care. I have both attended and facilitated numerous support groups for people with chronic as well as life-threatening medical conditions over the years, and I have come to the conclusion that identification with your diagnosis or symptoms is the greatest source of unnecessary suffering. I also reached another, initially surprising, conclusion: I came to understand that many support groups actually exacerbate this problem, inadvertently supporting *the suffering itself* rather than practices that can reduce suffering.

In many illness-based support groups, members talk about their suffering while the rest of the group offers either advice or empathy. Most often, compassion, empathy, and understanding are far more valuable than advice. Most of us find it very validating to share our troubles and receive empathy and understanding. The need to be seen, heard, and understood is what drives us to talk about our struggles, but it has a dark side: *without incorporating mindfulness-based mastery and wellbeing practices, support groups can devolve into an orgy of victimhood.* Much of what goes on in many of these groups is a festival of complaints: about pain, fatigue, malaise, disability, and limitation of life activities, a kind of self-pity party.

The activity of sharing our complaints with the group serves to bolster our identification with and attachment to the very things about which we feel compelled to complain. And it increases our identification with and attachment to being a member of a group of sick and helpless *patients*. ("Patient" is an important term to use intentionally. I use it to refer to someone who passively receives a medical or complementary treatment. When used to describe people in psychotherapy or any form of skill-building group, the word "patient" is inappropriate and disempowering because it implies passive receipt of a treatment that actually requires conscious effort and participation.)

Support groups are healthy when the facilitator guides participants in how to empathize with each other's *feelings* rather than with *the facts of their situations.* Another feature of a healthy support group is that it incorporates skill building into every session. The lives of the group members improve when there is a focus on building mindfulness-based mastery and wellbeing, leading to a sense that we can make a difference in our lives and in the lives around us through our actions.

"I'm Terminal" Is a Dangerous Use of Language
It's common to hear someone with very advanced cancer say, "I'm terminal." In the last stages of the disease, this acceptance of death is healthy and allows for a more peaceful dying process; the dying phase is a time to accept and make peace

with dying. But identifying and attaching to a diagnosis or prognosis when there is still a chance of recovery can cause unnecessary additional suffering; it is not conducive to health and wellbeing. In my training at the Simonton Cancer Center, I occasionally met program participants who referred to themselves as being "terminal" at a stage when it was still reasonable to hope for recovery. Perhaps you can see that this is a slippery slope because although it is important to maintain hope, it is also important to not become attached to getting well. Mindfulness-based mastery and wellbeing practices offer a way to negotiate this complex terrain.

Attempting to Live a Normal Life

Some people living with debilitating chronic medical conditions are committed to going about their lives as if they were healthy, and this works fine for some people. Others of us can do this for a certain percentage of the time but are then struck down with fatigue, malaise, or some other disabling condition that makes living the life of a normal, healthy person impossible.

Although people with chronic illness would certainly like to live as everyone else does, the reality is that sometimes we can and sometimes we can't. Still, a large percentage of us are able to have productive careers, a rich family and social life— and a lot of fun. We may simply have to do these things a little differently from the way healthy people do them, taking into account our limitations.

Interactions with the Healthy: Vulnerability and the Illusion of Control

It is very frightening to think that no matter what we do to take care of ourselves, we are still vulnerable to serious medical problems. One time when I was trying on a new pair of shoes I got talking to a young woman who looked like a world-class athlete. I asked her what sport she competed in and that discussion led to my sharing about having been involved in ski racing in my teens and twenties, and the fact that I hadn't skied since age thirty. She asked why I had quit skiing at such a young age, and I decided to tell her about the very debilitating connective tissue problems that had led to my giving it up, among other things. Whenever I get into a conversation like this with athletes, at some point they invariably want to know what *caused* all my health problems. I can tell by the way they ask that their concern relates to their belief that such things will never happen to them because they eat the perfect diet, exercise properly, get enough sleep, and manage their stress. The conversation always takes a negative turn when I explain that I was already doing everything right prior to developing serious health problems; they begin to look worried and the conversation ends abruptly.

Even if we do everything right, we cannot control our health, but we can learn how to disengage from the types of thoughts that otherwise lead to fear of illness and death. As my first Buddhist meditation teacher once said, "You can't stop the waves, but you can learn to surf."

CR

Our examination of living with chronic medical challenges concludes Part I. By this point in the book, you have gained a good understanding of the causes of unnecessary suffering and the common patterns of suffering that chronically ill people experience. But unnecessary suffering is by definition preventable, and now it's time to start learning how to alleviate it. In Part II I will introduce you to the mastery and wellbeing practice of mindfulness: what it is, how it benefits health in myriad ways, and what the practice entails.

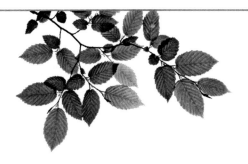

Part II

The Fundamental Mastery and Wellbeing Practice: Mindfulness

Mindfulness is the core skill you need to develop in order to engage in all the other practices introduced to you throughout In Your Own Hands. This Part contains three chapters devoted to mindfulness. The first will familiarize you with what it is, the second with why it's important to your health, and the third with how it is practiced. While this is not a "how to" — and in fact I recommend you register for a mindfulness training — it will give you a good grounding that you can then take further on your own.

7 A Brief Introduction to Mindfulness

In Part II we begin to delve into mindfulness-based mastery and wellbeing practices. To get us started, in this chapter I offer perspectives on the nature of the foundational practice—mindfulness—drawing on the words of some of its chief investigators. I will also briefly touch upon some associated terms you may run across as you explore the topic further. My aim is to help you become familiar with the principles of mindfulness before you consider how to apply it in your daily life.

What Is Mindfulness?

To answer this fundamental question, it is probably best to start with some of the ways Dr. Jon Kabat-Zinn describes mindfulness. More than anyone else in the world, he has been successful in integrating mindfulness into mainstream Western medicine.[1]

Kabat-Zinn uses the term to refer to both a *state* of mindful attention and a practice, which he describes as a *way of life* that involves a deep commitment to the study of direct experience. He defines mindfulness as "the awareness that arises through paying attention on purpose in the present moment, nonjudgmentally." This definition encompasses the cultivation of mindfulness through numerous practices, including both formal sitting meditation practices as well as informal attentional practices. In his view, mindfulness is both a method and an outcome. In other words, practicing mindfulness

The essence of mindfulness is denatured or lost if it is viewed as a concept rather than as a practice and way of life.

will make you more mindful, which means that you will more fully experience life.

Kabat-Zinn makes it clear that *the essence of mindfulness is denatured or lost if it is viewed as a concept rather than as a practice and way of life.*[2] As he puts it, the practice aspect "emphasizes that it is a living, evolving understanding, not a fixed dogma relegated to a museum honoring a culturally constrained past." Here he refers to this "dogma" as a limited, conceptual Buddhist study of mindfulness that offers none of the benefits that are available through direct practice.

Researchers Dr. Shauna Shapiro and Dr. Linda Carlson give us the following description of mindfulness:

> Mindful awareness is fundamentally a way of being. It is a way of inhabiting one's body, one's mind, one's moment-by-moment experience. It is a natural human capacity. It is a deep awareness, a knowing and experiencing of life as it arises and passes away in each moment. Mindful awareness is a way of relating to all experience, positive, negative, and neutral in an open, receptive way. This awareness involves freedom from grasping and wanting anything to be different. It simply knows and accepts what is here, now. Mindfulness is about seeing clearly without one's conditioned patterns of perceiving clouding awareness, and without trying to frame things in a particular way. It is important to learn to see this way because how a person perceives and frames the moment generates one's reality. ...Thus, mindfulness involves simply knowing what is arising as it is arising without adding anything to it, without trying to get more of what

one wants (pleasure, security), or pushing away what one doesn't want (e.g., fear, anger, shame).[3]

Shapiro and Carlson's definition provides a window into the life of someone who has had a serious commitment to mindfulness practice for many years. That degree of bliss does not come without very hard work.

Another definition, by psychologist and mindfulness researcher Dr. Scott Bishop, is particularly inclusive: "Mindfulness is the self-regulation of attention so that it is maintained on immediate experience, thereby allowing for increased recognition of mental events in the present moment; this includes adopting a particular orientation toward one's experience that is characterized by *curiosity, openness, and acceptance* [emphasis mine]."[4] Most experienced meditators have discovered that these qualities are the direct result of formal, mindfulness meditation practice. Bishop adds that it is wise to intentionally cultivate them.

Research psychologists Dr. Alan Marlatt and Dr. Jean Kristeller define mindfulness as "… bringing one's complete attention to the present experience on a moment-to-moment basis."[5] They go on to say that the practice includes observing your experiences with an attitude of acceptance and lovingkindness. Lovingkindness goes beyond acceptance; it refers to actually embracing your thoughts, emotions, and sensations while not analyzing them.

The following description by psychologist Dr. Jeffrey Greeson and psychiatrist Dr. Jeffrey Brantley is especially complete because it includes an actual method of practice in the last line:

Mindfulness is a word that refers to a basic human capacity for non-conceptual, non-judging, and present-moment-centered awareness. This awareness arises from intentionally paying attention, from noticing on purpose what is occurring inside and outside of us, with an attitude of friendliness and acceptance toward what is happening while it is happening. Mindfulness has been cultivated by human beings using *inner technologies* of meditation in various spiritual contexts for literally thousands of years.

... [Mindfulness is] an intentional willingness to fully and completely engage with one's direct experience of living, on a moment-to-moment basis, with whatever pleasant, unpleasant, or neutral events that arise. The central goal of living mindfully is to open to the fullness and richness of each moment, and not to add, subtract, or modify any part of one's psychological or physical experience. At its core, mindfulness is intended to help one live a life of deep meaning, value, direction, and purpose even when emotional or physical pain is present. *By awakening to the possibilities available in the present moment, one often becomes empowered to choose a wise response in the face of an upsetting internal experience or external event, as opposed to having an upsetting experience or event dictate how one responds* [emphasis mine].[6]

Research psychologist Dr. Sona Dimidjian and Dialectical Behavior Therapy founder Dr. Marsha Linehan break mindfulness into these components:
- Observing, noticing, bringing awareness
- Describing, labeling, noting
- Participating

They describe the characteristics of the practice using these terms:
- Nonjudgmental, accepting, allowing
- In the present moment, with beginner's mind
- Effective[7]

In this construct, *observing* refers to seeing clearly without evaluation. *Noticing* simply refers to having one's eyes and ears open. *Bringing awareness* means directing and focus-

Mindfulness disengages automatic sub-conscious programs so the conscious mind can generate behavior that is coherent with our intentions.

ing your attention on your sensory input. When they talk of *describing, labeling,* and *noting,* they mean naming what you perceive in order to more easily and clearly experience it. *Participating* means that this is not simply a passive process where all you are doing is observing. Finally, they list *effective:* taking action to effect a change.

Nyanaponika Thera, a Western-born Buddhist monk, makes clear that the term *mindfulness* encompasses the practice itself as well as the end result of it: "Mindfulness then, is the unfailing master key for *knowing* the mind, and is thus the starting point: the perfect tool for *shaping* the mind, and is thus the focal point; and the lofty manifestation of the achieved *freedom* of the mind; and is thus the culminating point."

Then we have this description of Buddhist mindfulness practices by cell biologist Dr. Bruce Lipton and Steve Bhaerman, more commonly known as Swami Beyondananda, which may be particularly appealing to the Western mind:

> One of the most ancient practices to regain conscious control over one's life is Buddhist mindfulness. Fundamentally, mindfulness is a training exercise to rein in the conscious mind's wandering into the past and future in order to focus on the present moment and make aware choices in the now. Essentially, mindfulness disengages automatic subconscious programs so the conscious mind, the seat of our personal wishes and aspirations, can generate behavior that is coherent with our intentions.[8]

Let's break this statement down and examine its elements more closely. That mindfulness is a *training exercise* is critical: it is not a philosophy. The conscious mind's *wandering into the past and future* is natural and automatic, yet it undermines your quality of life. It is *present-moment* inner awareness that allows you to live with intentionality, disengaging the *automatic subconscious programs* that lead to unhealthy behavior. Your *personal life values* are the precious values that give your life meaning, and mindfulness gives you the opportunity to *behave* in accordance with them.

Research psychologist and cofounder of Acceptance and Commitment Therapy Dr. Steven Hayes frames mindfulness in three categories, which I have summarized in the following list:

- *Observing* the experience of the present moment by simply noticing current emotional reactions, bodily sensations, thoughts, or other experiences.
- *Describing* the experience of the present moment by describing the facts of the situation or experience without using constructs, labels, judgments, or inferences. A possible area of confusion here is Hayes's exclusion of "labels." This is a matter of semantics. When Kabat-Zinn and others include a labeling step, they are referring to labeling in order to gain clarity, but *without any evaluation or judgment* of what is being labeled. There are many mindfulness practices that do not include formal labeling, yet all mindfulness practices improve our ability to objectively observe and accept all internal and external stimuli—with or without naming them.
- *Participating* in the present experience by allowing yourself to be fully engaged in the activity of the moment, without self-consciousness. This is what research psychologist Dr. Mihali Csikszentmihalyi refers to as flow.[9] Committed mindfulness practitioners have the ability to live in this state no matter what activity they engage in, in proportion to the quality and quantity of their practice.

Now that you have an overview of what constitutes mindfulness practice and a few different perspectives and models to consider, let's briefly clarify a few terms that are closely associated with mindfulness.

Related Terms

In the context of mindfulness, the terms *insight, wisdom,* and *self-knowing* refer solely to what you experience from *moment to moment*. Hence, from a mindfulness perspective, insights about the self are very different from *intellectual* insight. An example of intellectual self-knowledge would be the knowledge that the reason you have a low opinion of your ability to achieve great things is that when you were growing up, your parents treated you as if you were incompetent. In contrast, self-knowing would be the awareness in the present moment that you are still telling yourself the same horrific, unhealthy story about your incompetence that your parents told you. To a mindfulness practitioner, insight and wisdom are neither theoretical nor intellectual; they are experiential. Self-knowledge is valuable and useful, but it doesn't usually lead to the vibrant life that can be gained through the practice of moment-to-moment self-knowing. This is why the new mindfulness-based psychotherapies such as Acceptance and Commitment Therapy (ACT), Mindfulness-Based Cognitive Therapy (MBCT), and Dialectical Behavior Therapy (DBT) are dramatically influencing the older forms of psychotherapy.

Another important term to understand is *present experience,* which appears in various definitions of mindfulness. Present experience includes your thoughts, images, sensations, and emotions as well as the events going on around you.

Beginner's mind means to see things clearly and without any evaluation. A baby sees things with beginner's mind because it does not yet have the ability to evaluate and judge what it is experiencing. While we adults need the ability to evaluate our surroundings in order to survive and thrive, we often carry that skill too far; judging others, ourselves, and events leads to immense suffering. Such judgments do not disappear with mindfulness practice, but we learn to dis-entangle from them. We learn to view our judgments with curiosity and nonattachment, recognizing them as transient mental events of no intrinsic consequence. We can even begin to see the humor in our unnecessary criticisms of people and situations.

Finally, note that I do not often associate the term "medita-tion" with mindfulness. This is because the term can be terri-bly confusing. It is used synonymously with religious prayer, mantra type meditations such as TM or Relaxation Response, various forms of mental imagery, concentration practices such as staring at a candle flame, counting the breaths, lovingkind-ness meditation, and many more practices, all of which are often simply referred to as meditation. All the different types of meditations produce different results, and "mindfulness practice" is the accurate term for the kind of mind training we are concerned with in this book.

The Value of Mindfulness

The benefits of a mindfulness practice are many, including considerable benefits for health; I will go into some detail about those in the next chapter. For now, let's look at the ben-efits more generally.

Psychology and mindfulness researcher Dr. Fabrizio Di-donna offers his perspective on one of the chief benefits:

> The possibility to disidentify ourselves from our own thoughts can free us up from one of the strongest and most deeply rooted attachments—the attachment to thinking for the sake of thinking, that is, being depen-dent on the incessant mental conversation that goes on in our minds.... When we realize that our thoughts are non-concrete and have no substance, that their true nature does not necessarily have anything to do with reality, we have overcome the obstacle of attach-ment and the possibility that it will degenerate into the negative effects of rumination.[10]

Through mindfulness practice, we learn to focus so intently on present-moment experience that obsessing on the past and worrying about the future gradually diminish. This is because the mind cannot simultaneously be fully present and dwell in the past or future.

Mindfulness practice especially develops the ability to be a neutral observer, including neutrally observing ourselves engaged in observing. Mindfulness of our thoughts, feelings, and behavior provides us with a wide range of choices that we cannot access when we lack such awareness.

The goal of mindfulness practice is a way of life in which all the senses are heightened, yet there is no attachment to any sensory input. The practice involves the conscious, detached observing of sensations, feelings, thoughts, mental images, and even our reactions to those things in real time. By reducing unnecessary processing of what we see, hear, smell, taste, and feel, we experience an increase in clear, intense, direct perception of raw, unprocessed sensory information from all sources. Ordinarily, sensory input is subjected to filtering, selecting, and abstracting. With mindfulness practice, the sensory input registers simply as pure stimuli, completely absent of attributions.

By observing fleeting thoughts and corresponding physiological sensations without reacting in our typical mindless, learned, rigid ways, we begin to recognize that all experiences—including rumination, anxiety, and even pain—are transient and impersonal.

Mindfulness and Explanatory Style

Your *explanatory style* refers to how you explain unwanted events or unwanted results. This is important for even minor events like dropping your fork on the floor while you're eating. Those who shrug it off and simply get another fork are less stressed than those who berate themselves for being clumsy or instinctively decide this means they're having a bad day. A mindfulness practice allows you to notice the ways you typically respond to things that do not go as you would like them to go, and the resulting awareness of your reactions allows you to develop choice and a sense of control over your life that is not possible otherwise.

Mindfulness and Mastery

Mindfulness practices help free you from knee-jerk reactions to your thoughts and feelings and external events. You develop the ability to respond by choosing rather than reacting automatically. This helps you stop reinforcing what you do *not* want and start reinforcing what you *do* want. If your intention is clear, all you need to do is bring attention to your inner experiences and sensory input, and positive change will happen.

By increasing your ability to control your attention and focus objectively on various levels of cognition, emotion, sensation, and behavior, you can discover new aspects of anything that may be troubling you.[11] More importantly, this practice leads to a greater sense of self-control, self-efficacy, and well-being.[12] This is living with mastery.

For example, imagine yourself caught up in a vicious argument. Without the ability to sustain attention on your values and your inner subjective experience, you will tend to react defensively, escalating the divide between yourself and the other person. But through mindfulness practice, you can gradually develop the skills to be able to observe all your intense feelings without becoming completely fused with them.

Mindfulness and Personality

Since the 1970s there has been an ongoing discussion of whether mindfulness practice can help people improve their personality traits. Consider this excerpt from a Kabat-Zinn report:

> These characteristics [such as, for example, the Type A time-pressured personality or the procrastinator-type personality] have traditionally been seen as associated with deep and stable personality structures and are not usually thought to be amenable to change,

particularly in a short time period. The changes we are seeing in these personality variables in the people who go through the stress clinic [MBSR] suggest that training in mindfulness meditation can have a profound positive influence on one's view of oneself and of the world, including an ability to be more trusting of oneself and others.[13]

Although he does not specify the process by which personality characteristics change, I would explain it this way. When we are able to recognize that our thoughts are not reality, we no longer get as triggered as we used to by stressors or other people's actions. This enlightened view results in a much more pleasant personality. Although it can be adopted quite easily on an intellectual level, to be able to avoid biting the hook when our buttons are pushed requires a serious commitment to mindfulness practice.

For example, when I was in my teens and twenties, I was known as a hothead because I was quick to go into a rage. I would say things to people that I consistently regretted later, and I lived with intense frustration and shame because I didn't know how to change my behavior. Gradually, I developed the skills to be able to observe my thoughts and feelings without acting them out. I developed a dramatically more pleasant personality—not by trying to do so, but by practicing stepping back from my thoughts and feelings, honoring them but not acting on them. There was no longer any need to act on them as I developed the ability to see that they were not me—they were simply what I was experiencing.

ೞ

And so we have seen what mindfulness practice is, and that there are many benefits to be gained from it from psychological and emotional standpoints. These benefits also include profound and in some cases even life-saving physiological effects, which we will explore in the chapter that follows.

8 The Health Benefits of Mindfulness Practice

This is an exciting time for those of us who appreciate the power of mindfulness practice to improve our health and who also value evidence-based data. A growing number of neuroscience researchers are now providing us with solid findings that support the efficacy of mindfulness practices that have been around for thousands of years. And while people generally follow a mindfulness practice primarily with the aim of living a fuller, happier life in general—not with the specific aim of better health—these scientists have found that greater health and wellbeing are often wonderful side effects. In this chapter you will learn the results of numerous studies on the connection between mindfulness practice and health and delve into some of the underlying physiology, with particular emphasis on the workings of the brain.

Hundreds of studies have shown that mindfulness practice normalizes heart rate, heart rhythms, blood pressure, and oxygen consumption. It changes countless physiological parameters, such as normalization of blood lactic acid levels. Studies have shown that it lowers salivary bacteria levels; reduces pain; and improves vision and hearing and reaction times involving responsive motor skills.

One of the greatest health benefits of mindfulness practice is that it helps you become aware of your unhealthy habits and problematic behaviors; thought processes that have been operating below the level of your awareness become increasingly observable as you practice mindfulness.[1] When you are paying attention to your thoughts, feelings, and sensations throughout the day, you cannot help but observe these things about yourself. This awareness opens up choices that were not previously available to you, and you can choose to do those things that help you feel better. We will delve deeply into this topic in chapters 10 through 12 on Valued-Action Practice. For now, just consider that instead of being a victim of environmental stressors or stressful situations, you can choose to respond in healthy ways to the challenges of life. And you will become more stress-hardy and resilient when you do.

Mindfulness involves learning to connect patterns of thinking with mood and state of mind. This is important because our state of mind significantly influences our state of health. A rapidly growing number of studies over the last ten years have shown that through mindfulness practice, psychological and emotional flexibility improve.[2]

Mindfulness offers the opportunity to become aware of your explanatory style, which we examined briefly in the preceding chapter. And again, here you have a choice: you can continue your "self-talk" in a similar vein and, if it tends toward the negative, continue to tolerate its effects, or you can intervene and recognize your inner chatter as rambling thoughts that may not support your health. Studies have shown an association between long-term negative explanatory style—the tendency to harshly judge yourself or others when faced with a difficult or unpleasant situation—and poorer health.[3] The more aware you become of this habit through mindful observance, the greater your ability to positively influence your health by holding such thoughts more lightly.

In fact, as brain researcher Dr. James McGaugh writes, as you gain emotional distance from your thinking—a healthy "side effect" of mindfulness practice—you become better equipped to devise the most reasonable strategies for resolving all kinds of conflicts, both intrapsychic and interpersonal.[4] This is an important aspect of mastering your life experience because when you are emotionally distressed, your mind lacks both the clarity and the acceptance it has when you are calm and centered.

Mindfulness-Based Stress Reduction (MBSR) Classes and Better Health: General Findings

Research psychologist Paul Grossman performed a meta-analysis of Mindfulness-Based Stress Reduction (MBSR) studies. After analyzing data from twenty of them, he concluded that MBSR is effective in treating symptoms associated with a broad range of chronic medical problems, and that it also has beneficial effects on psychological and physical wellbeing.[5]

Similarly, in a large, randomized, controlled trial, research psychologist Michael Speca and his colleagues found that MBSR resulted in significant decreases in total mood disturbance, emotional distress, and anger. And it supported greater vigor (see the brief section on energy to follow). They also found that, compared with controls, MBSR participants had reduced cardiopulmonary symptoms of arousal, central neurological symptoms, gastrointestinal symptoms, and anxiety. And they enjoyed an increase in psychological flexibility, an important quality to cultivate to more easily negotiate the life challenges associated with chronic physical limitations.[6]

Psychology researcher Dr. Linda Carlson has done extensive research on MBSR and found that patients participating in a single eight-week MBSR program experienced improved immune functioning. Carlson and her colleagues also discovered that both during the program and at the six-month follow-up point, these patients exhibited fewer cardiopulmonary symptoms of arousal (meaning better overall, systemic oxygenation and perfusion), reduced central neurological symptoms (which could translate into improvements in the functions of every organ system), fewer gastrointestinal symptoms, improvement in habitual stress-related behavioral patterns, less anxiety and fear, and improved overall emotional flexibility.[7]

Another finding was that approximately 40 percent of the participants showed a decrease in afternoon and evening cortisol levels. These lower levels of stress hormones translated into a generally improved quality of life, including sleep patterns. In a one-year follow-up, cortisol levels were found to

MBSR and other mindful-
ness practices are as effective as drugs in treating
hypertension.

continue to decrease, im-
mune function continued
to improve, and systolic
blood pressure continued
to decrease and normal-
ize.

Problems with the
hormone melatonin are
associated with distur-
bances in sleep/wake cycles, increased cancer, and decreased
immune function. Massion et al found that those who engaged in a formal mindfulness practice had the highest rates
of normal melatonin regulation.[8]

A study by research psychologist Laura Van Wielingen
found that MBSR participants were able to sustain drops in
systolic blood pressure of 15.5 mmHg; *this finding shows that
MBSR is as effective as antihypertensive drugs in treating hypertension.*[9]

A Core Benefit: Freeing Up Vital Energy

As I mentioned earlier in the book, energy is essential to health
and mindfulness practice frees up enormous stores of it.[10]
This is because we no longer need to expend so much energy
processing events that actually do not require our attention.[11]
Psychotherapy offers a good example. In traditional psychotherapy, considerable time and expense are spent analyzing
troubling thoughts. The new science- and evidence-based
psychotherapies like Acceptance and Commitment Therapy
teach clients how to use mindfulness practices to simply *disentangle* from their troubling thoughts instead of burning up
energy in chasing them back to their origins and analyzing
them.

Outside of the therapeutic context, as we simply go about
our day-to-day lives, we find that when we do our activities
mindfully, without getting caught up in our thoughts and
beliefs about them, even the more unpleasant tasks cease to
drain our energy. In allowing us to release unhelpful ideas

and images throughout the day, mindfulness practice unlocks vast reserves of energy that we are then free to dedicate to supporting our health.

Good Sleuthing: Detecting Prodromes

Another key health advantage of mindfulness practice is that it allows us to detect *prodromes:* early, subtle signs and symptoms of illness. This gives us the opportunity to care for ourselves in ways that can lessen the severity of illness—to rest instead of going out, for example. It also gives us a chance to see a doctor early, when treatment can often be most effective. Many types of illness, especially cancers, are more treatable when diagnosed sooner, and in the very early stages can even be cured. Also, self-treatment of many conditions becomes possible. For example, I have developed the ability to convert cardiac dysrhythmias such as atrial fibrillation by changing my breathing as soon as I experience the first, very subtle preatrial or preventricular contraction. The longer any cardiac dysrhythmia continues, the more difficult it is for me to self-convert it to normal sinus rhythm.

Given the frequency with which colds and more serious diseases follow episodes of emotional distress, it is useful to view *the signs of emotional distress themselves* as prodromes of illness. Of course, we must first learn how to develop the awareness that we are in fact feeling distressed, and this, too, is where a mindfulness practice proves useful. This is an important element of loving self-care practice, the topic of chapter 14.

The theta brain wave state (4 to 7hz) allows for a quietness of mind that includes our most creative moments, and it has been found to be common to some Buddhist mindfulness practices such as vipassana.[12] Alpha/theta (neurofeedback) training as well as vipassana lead to the integration of different aspects of our lives. This in turn results in an enhanced body consciousness that *allows us to tune in to physiological processes that would otherwise not reach our awareness.* This consciousness, coupled with creative aspects of the mind that are common to the hypnagogic state found in theta, can contribute to homeostasis and physical healing.

Using Internal Feedback Loops

Sensory feedback is the process of tuning in to all sensory input and then using that information to make conscious choices. The ability to pay attention to sensory feedback provides us with awareness of physiological events, and this affords us the power to effect healthy changes in them. This direct awareness is referred to as an *internal feedback loop*.

Physical and emotional pain, as well as all signs and symptoms of any medical condition, can be used as a natural, sensory feedback system. These sources of sensory feedback can serve as an early warning system, alerting us to the need to change something. Simple examples include putting on warm clothes as a result of feeling cold, eating after feeling sensations of hunger, responding to feelings of sleepiness by going to sleep, going to the bathroom as a result of feeling bladder or bowel pressure, and intentionally relaxing as a result of recognizing symptoms of stress. Mindfulness practice *with special attention to sensing* can make dramatic differences in our quality of self-care as we learn to act on the prodromes that precede overt symptoms.

Sensing Prodromes and Correcting Physiological Imbalances

University of Arizona psychophysiology researcher Gary Schwartz teaches that all signs, symptoms, bodily sensations, and emotions can be used as biological forms of biofeedback. He writes that when we attend to these red flags, connect them to consciousness, and express them appropriately, we can correct physiological imbalances.[13] For example, headaches could mean that our breathing is suboptimal. Anger could be a sign that we are projecting our thoughts and feelings onto others. The disharmony that results from ignoring such red flags contributes to illness. Also, when we do not attend to these warning signs, we become sympathetically aroused, and the resulting cortisol and norepinephrine create a very unhealthy situation for the cardiovascular system in particular and for physiological functioning in general.

∞

It can be useful to keep a journal of symptoms in order to develop the ability to detect prodromes of the symptoms; correlate cognitive processes, behaviors, and moods with your symptoms; and *notice* prodromes that would otherwise go unnoticed.

Deeper into the Physiology: Mindfulness and the Brain

Dramatic information has emerged about the impact of mindfulness practice on brain function. Creswell et al concluded from fMRI studies that this activity is associated with increased and widespread prefrontal cortical activity and reduced activity in the amygdala, bilaterally.[14] The act of naming or labeling our thoughts, emotions, and sensations—which is at the core of mindfulness practice— contributes to the upregulation of the prefrontal cortex (which translates into increased ability for rational thought) along with a downregulation of the amygdala (which translates into greater mastery over the emotions.)

The anterior cingulate cortex (ACC) is another neuro-anatomical structure to undergo improvements through mindfulness practice. Neuroimaging studies have consistently shown increased ACC activation. According to Treadway and Lazar, this may mean enhanced integration of attention, motivation, and motor control.[15] Numerous other researchers have found a direct correlation between mindfulness practice and improved brain functioning.[16]

Researcher Dr. Richard Davidson, head of the functional brain imaging lab at the University of Wisconsin, used electroencephalography (EEG) to demonstrate that subjects who completed an eight-week MBSR class had experienced a slight right-to-left hemispheric shift in activity in their resting EEG.[17] Since depression and anxiety are associated with greater right hemispheric electrical activity in the resting state, this could explain the phenomenal success of the new acceptance- and mindfulness-based psychotherapies in treating mood disorders. This may also be one of the explanations for the extraordinary ability of very experienced mindfulness practitioners to experience negative events with far less autonomic reactivity than less-experienced mindfulness practitioners.

Farb et al also found dramatic differences in concentration abilities over just an eight-week period. Areas of the brain that correlate with present-moment experience were activated in the graduates of an eight-week MBSR class. When mindfulness-naïve controls received the same instruction, those areas were also activated but not as much as the areas associated with memory of past events.[18] Shapiro and Carlson have analyzed many such studies and have offered convincing evidence that mindfulness practice allows us to disengage and disentangle from the products of the mind.[19]

Although Buddhist monks have generally achieved greater mastery of mindfulness practices than the rest of us, the health benefits can accrue even in beginners. A study divided a group of executives from a large biotech firm into two smaller groups. The controls went about their lives as usual. The experimental group was trained in MBSR. After eight weeks, the controls had no increased activity in the left prefrontal cortex (PFC)—the area of the brain associated with positive affect, optimism, curiosity, gratitude, and other attributes that correlate with health and happiness. Those who had set aside a brief time each day to practice evidenced increased PFC activity.[20]

When the Dalai Lama first invited Richard Davidson and his colleagues to Dharamsala, the researchers fitted monks with 256 EEG sensors. They were stunned by the results. Just fifteen seconds into a meditation session, all the monks registered sustained bursts of high gamma activity. This was shocking because it had previously been believed that mindfulness practices slow brain waves from beta to alpha. These readings were in the 25 to 70 hertz range. At first the monks were in high-amplitude beta, then high-amplitude alpha (8 to12hz), and then briefly back to beta, and then to gamma. *Such high-frequency brain waves are generally associated with deep levels of learning and great flashes of insight.* The object of attention in the monks' meditation in this case was compassion for all beings.[21] This type of meditation, known as *metta,* is common to Theravada Buddhism and is different from mindfulness practice, where the object of attention is the pure observation of thoughts, emotions, and sensations. Yet these results indicate the profound impacts of dedicated, long-term mind training of various types on the workings of the brain.

Davidson discovered that at high-amplitude gamma, large areas of the brain begin to synchronize: the monks' brains were operating at peak intensity. The rapidity with which the monks were able to enter such a state of rapt attention could only mean that their neural processing had been permanently altered by years of intensive Buddhist meditation practices. It is believed that their high brain function, even in the resting state, was the result of advanced and highly focused forms of Buddhist practices they had been engaging in for many hours a day for twenty years or longer; the highest amplitude gamma was recorded with the most experienced monks. During periods of deep meditation, the monks' brain waves resonate in a frequency range that occurs in non-meditators *only during periods of ecstasy.* This seemed to be true for mindfulness as well as metta forms. Studies using fMRI revealed that the monks' left PFC was more developed. *This is significant because it can help explain what seems to be the greater depth of joy in life that had been observed in the monks.* Interestingly, it had also previously been believed that mindfulness practice slows the heart rate, yet monks experienced increased heart rate during their intense meditation sessions.[22]

One conclusion was that the monks had developed and reinforced neural networks that are the result of consciously tuning in to happiness most of the time. But Davidson also discovered that brain-wave patterns are altered early on. For example, at the University of Wisconsin, students who had been practicing mindfulness for as little as two months were put in fMRI scanners and their brains revealed findings consistent with new elevations in mood. The type of mindfulness training they practiced involved exceptionally intense concentration.

Using fMRI and PET, Creswell et al found that mindfulness practitioners had greater PFC activation and less amygdala activation during an experiment in which they were asked, while in the scanner, to name the affect, or mood, of people in photos they were shown. The researchers showed that the PFC in mindfulness practitioners regulated emotional reactivity in the limbic system. Many of us who have practiced mindfulness for a length of time have observed that senior teachers seem to have a degree of happiness and equanimity that pervade their lives.[23] This and research by Davidson and others are now providing us with a scientific explanation for the happiness and equanimity we have observed in our teachers.[24]

Brain scan studies of the minds of long-term mindfulness practitioners reveal that mindfulness practices actually result in neuroanatomical and neurophysiological improvements as well. For example, Lazar demonstrated that the brain regions related to attention and sensory processing are more highly developed in long-term mindfulness practitioners than in non-practitioners and that older practitioners had greater cortical thickness and more gray matter than age-matched non-practitioners.[25] In a similar finding, Pagnoni and Cekic found greater attention performance and gray matter volume in older practitioners than in age-matched non-practitioners.[26]

Richard Davidson studied the brains of Tibetan Buddhist monks while they were engaged in mindfulness practices in the fMRI scanner. They were asked to create various states of mind at will while Davidson's team mapped the resulting psychophysiological changes. Some of the monks were able to produce several distinct brain states on command. For example, some were able to activate a region of the brain that is known to light up with the experiencing of positive emotions.[27]

According to the research of Creswell et al, mindfulness practices result in increased activation of the medial PFC along with simultaneous decreased activation of the amygdala. These researchers hypothesize that mindfulness practices correlate with enhanced prefrontal regulation of limbic responses.[28]

Hölzel found increased gray matter density in the insula, hippocampus, and left temporal gyrus in neuroimaging of mindfulness practitioners.[29] Using high-resolution MRI, Lazar studied cortical thickness in twenty experienced mindfulness practitioners and fifteen non-practitioners. The mindfulness practitioners had increased cortical thickness in the anterior insula, sensory cortex, and prefrontal cortex.[30]

Mindfulness meditation subjects have consistently shown high-amplitude, low-frequency alpha brain waves. The significance of this is that low-frequency alpha (7 to 9 hertz) is associated with states of very calm, clear, creative thinking. Many studies have also shown that the two hemispheres of the brain become synchronized in mindfulness practitioners.

Neuroplasticity: Sculpting the Brain
Davidson conducted studies with Kabat-Zinn in 2003 and with Dr. Antoine Lutz in 2008, both of which demonstrated that mindfulness practices capitalize on neuroplasticity, leading to anatomical and physiological improvements in the brains of long-time mindfulness practitioners.[31]

New research in the neurosciences now makes it clear that what we think and feel directly sculpts the brain and shapes the mind. For that reason, it is healthy to cultivate practices and activities that result in feeling good in order to program our brains to have more of those experiences. This can be a slippery slope, though; if we focus too much attention on lighting up the reward circuits in the brain, increasing dopamine synthesis, we risk becoming attached to those mind states and can even start engaging in addictive behaviors.

Mindfulness Practices and Aging: Reductions in Cognitive Decline

Lazar et al have shown that a serious mindfulness practice protects against the cortical thinning that normally occurs in old age. Her 2005 study of people who practice the vipassana form of mindfulness demonstrated that one small region of the PFC showed none of the age-related cortical thinning that would have been expected.[32] A later study replicated with practitioners of Zen (a Japanese form with slightly different practices) produced the same results.[33]

Nursing Home Studies

Dr. Ellen Langer of Yale and her colleague Dr. Judith Rodin of Harvard have been researching the effects of mindfulness practices on aging for the last thirty years. In one study they assessed a meditation intervention in promoting longevity. Seventy-three residents of eight nursing homes were assigned randomly to one of four groups: a no-treatment control group, a relaxation-only control group, a transcendental meditation (TM) group, and a mindfulness group. All participants except those in the no-treatment group practiced as instructed for twenty minutes twice a day.[34]

After three months, those in the mindfulness group significantly outperformed all the other participants on cognitive flexibility as well as health measures such as blood pressure and fasting glucose. Eighteen months after the study started, nurses providing patient care who were blind to the participants' experimental condition were asked to rate the mental health of the patients. Participants in the TM and mindfulness groups received significantly higher ratings than those in the two control groups. Interestingly, improvement in psychological flexibility correlated with improved physical health. This is not surprising since psychological flexibility—how well we are able to "roll with the punches" of daily life—cor-

Mindfulness practices capitalize on neuroplasticity, leading to anatomical and
physiological improvements in the brains
of long-time mindfulness practitioners.

relates with lower levels of emotional distress and therefore
lower levels of sympathetic arousal, and this translates into
improved physiological functioning.

Based on this study and some of their other research,
Langer concluded that *mindfulness may be not only central to
cognitive functioning but central to physiological functioning as
well.* She believes that mindfulness practice can free us from
unhealthy scripted beliefs and behaviors we have about aging. She came to the realization that while we are practicing
mindfulness, there is no separation between the psychological and the physiological, and she concludes that the most
extreme consequence of mind*less*ness could be a belief in natural limitations on human potential; these are actually self-
imposed restrictions that never reach conscious awareness.[35]
Elimination of these self-imposed restrictions is an especially
important goal for psychotherapists working with cancer patients or with people who have any debilitating chronic medical condition.

The most significant finding came three years after the
study began: *the survival rate of participants in the TM and mindfulness groups significantly exceeded those in the two control groups
as well as the average survival rate of the eight institutions studied.*
The percentage of those who were still alive after three years
is as follows: 100 percent of the TM group, 87.5 percent of the
mindfulness group, 77.3 percent of the non-treatment control
group, and 65 percent of the relaxation-only control group.
This is compared to 62 percent for the overall population of
the eight nursing homes.

Langer and Rodin offered no hypothesis as to why the
control group had fewer deaths than the relaxation group, or

A serious mindfulness practice protects against the cortical thinning that normally occurs in old age.

why the TM group did better than the mindfulness group. As for why the relaxation group did worse than the control group, it is possible that the relaxation group may not have actually succeeded in relaxing, instead drifting into a preoccupation with worrying about their circumstances. This variable could have been addressed using biofeedback, which would have provided objective, quantitative data in real time on the levels of relaxation achieved.

What was more surprising to me was that the TM group did better than the mindfulness group, because mindfulness practices are generally more highly regarded than TM among the majority of serious mind training researchers. The reason mindfulness is generally held in higher regard than TM is that TM primarily builds concentration, whereas mindfulness practice builds both concentration and insight. Conceivably, post-intervention interviews with the test subjects could have revealed more information to explain some of the unexpected results, but here is my hypothesis: TM is a simpler technique that is considerably easier and faster to learn, and this would render it more effective in the short term. It's also possible that TM's simplicity is more efficacious for a nursing home population.

In fact, Langer and Rodin concluded, "It is important to note that the mindfulness group would have done even better if they had used the usual (greater) amount of time that is taught for mindfulness meditation."

Besides psychological flexibility, blood pressure, and cortisol levels, the researchers collected data on measurements of impatience and perceived control. Participants in the mindfulness group scored significantly higher than those of the other groups on the revised Locus of Control Scale—which measures such things as cognitive processing, autonomy, and resistance to social influence—but did not differ significantly from the controls in the impatience measure. Rather than accepting a given situation, the mindfulness group appeared interested in mastering it.[36] Mastery has been found in numerous studies to be inversely correlated with chronic medical conditions in middle age.

The Benefits of Mindfulness Practice for the Immune System

> *The immune system is a mirror to life, responding to its joy and anguish, its exuberance and boredom, its laughter and tears, its excitement and depression, its problems and prospects. Scarcely anything that enters the mind doesn't find its way to into the workings of the body. Indeed, the connection between what we think and how we feel is perhaps the most dramatic documentation of the fact that mind and body are not separate entities but part of a fully integrated system.*[37]

Psychoneuroimmunology (PNI) researchers explore the relationship of cognition and emotion to nervous, endocrine, and immune system functioning. This field was born in the early 1980s when new technology allowed researchers to discover that there are nerve receptors on immune cells. It is important to have a very basic understanding of this connection in order to appreciate the impact that the mind can have on physiological functioning. Although various methods of mind training have been evolving for thousands of years, the sciences of psychoneuroimmunology and psychophysiology now support what has been known empirically by healers of various cultures throughout history.[38]

Considerable research now reveals that immune function improves with mindfulness practice.[39] Mindfulness practice has been associated with positive neurological changes and immune and endocrine enhancement.[40] These positive neurological changes have also been associated with some neurofeedback (EEG biofeedback) protocols. This should not be surprising because neurofeedback protocols have been developed to allow us, through operant conditioning, to create states of mind that look very much like those we can create through mindfulness practice.

Dr. Richard Davidson and his group administered an influenza vaccine to an MBSR group and to a control group. At the end of the eight-week course, the MBSR subjects had mounted a significantly more robust immune response to the vaccine than the controls. The durability of the response was evidenced by higher antibody titers at two later dates (meaning the body made greater numbers of antibodies in response to the vaccine). The mindfulness students evidenced greater leukocyte activity and reduced cortisol, inflammatory cytokines, tumor necrosis factor (TNF-alpha), and interferon gamma. They had all increased their interleukin-10 (IL-10). In a nutshell, participation in the MBSR course dramatically improved the immune systems of the participants by improving activation of immune cells, reducing stress hormone secretion, and making communication between immune cells more efficient.[41] The cytokine reductions can reduce autoimmune disease.

Davidson's team found that this stronger immune response in the experimental group was found to correlate with increases in activity in the left PFC, the significance of which is that the increased activity in that area of the brain correlates with increased wellbeing.[42] In a longer, sixteen-week study, TM instead of MBSR was taught to subjects with heart disease and metabolic syndrome. As they learned to practice TM, their blood pressure, insulin resistance, and various cardiac measures normalized.[43]

Another researcher, Solberg and his team, measured the effects of mindfulness practice on the immune system after physical stress, working with six runners who practiced mindfulness and six runners without a mindfulness practice. Observing that the increase in CD8 lymphocytes after oxygen consumption (VO2max) was significantly less in the experimental group than in the control group, the researchers concluded that mindfulness practice may modify the suppressive influence of strenuous physical stress on the immune system. Excessive stress is immunosuppressive regardless of whether it results from very strenuous exercise or from invasive surgery. The Solberg study looked at CD8+ T lymphocytes (which secrete perforin and proteolytic enzymes in order to attack viruses and anything else identified as foreign). This type of study provides evidence for the efficacy of mindfulness practice to mollify the otherwise harmful effects of physiological stress from physical stressors.[44]

In a study of medical patients with moderate to severe psoriasis (an autoimmune disorder), Kabat-Zinn observed that those who listened to mindfulness practice audiotapes during individual phototherapy (UVB) and photochemotherapy (PUVA) sessions showed significantly quicker clearing of their skin (Mdn = 65 days) than those who received light therapy alone (Mdn = 97 days).[45]

The Benefits of Mindfulness Practice for Chronic Pain and Fatigue

When we become aware of our thoughts and emotions simply as thoughts and emotions, and feature the sensations themselves center-stage in the field of awareness, and learn to rest in awareness of the bare sensations, our entire relationship to them can change on its own. We may actually come to see and know deeply that we are not our pain—we are much bigger than it is—and that there are many different ways we can choose to be in relationship to intense sensations and even limitations that can help us to live and live well with things as they are in the only moment we ever get in which to live, which is this one.
—Jon Kabat-Zinn

By practicing mindfulness, it is possible to live a full and satisfying life despite chronic pain, fatigue, disability, and all manner of other chronic health challenges. As we have seen, the practice of mindfulness acts to catalyze dramatic improvements in the functioning of the brain and the entire nervous system, as well as the immune and endocrine systems.[46] It is important to understand that mindfulness practice does not involve *striving* to improve health. In fact, any attachment or striving to get well can negate the benefits otherwise derived from this practice.

In numerous efficacy studies of mindfulness practice as treatment for chronic pain, participants reported reductions in pain, anxiety, and depression along with increases in emotional, social, and physical functioning. They also reported less disability and greater ability to participate in activities that were important to them. Self-esteem, which tends to diminish as a result of living with chronic illness or chronic pain, improved. Participants also reported needing less analgesic medication. Across the board, they experienced reductions in medical as well as emotional challenges.[47] Morone et al found that older participants were better able to focus on tasks and pace their activities, gained greater insight into their emotional processing, were able to come to peace with their limitations, became more engaged in activities, and enjoyed improved overall physical functioning.[48]

One of the many diseases for which medicine has not found an effective treatment is the painful condition of fibromyalgia. When Grossman et al and Sephton et al taught mindfulness practices to fibro patients, they evidenced reduced pain and fatigue along with improvements in coping, mood, and quality of life. In a three-year follow-up, the improvements had proven to be durable.[49]

One of the most helpful aspects of mindfulness practice for chronic pain patients is that it leads to an acceptance of pain and disability along with an ability to disengage and detach from the pain. What is remarkable is that the pain does not even need to diminish for suffering to ease and quality of life to improve. This is because, as we explored earlier in the book, a lot of suffering is from the negative attributions we assign to the pain and not from the actual sensations of pain.

Acceptance of pain is directly correlated with improved emotional, social, and physical functioning. It also correlates with improved work status and reduced medication use.[50] Jon Kabat-Zinn, in the foreword to a book by Gardner-Nix discusses what he has found by practicing mindfulness fairly regularly over time: "paying attention in a particular way to the very sensations, emotions, and thoughts that together constitute the experience of pain—in the present moment and as nonjudgmentally as possible (which may be very judgmental a good deal of the time)—actually has within it the seeds of freedom from suffering."[51]

Reduction in Symptoms
Managed care organizations in the US and in national healthcare systems elsewhere are learning that mindfulness training helps contain costs by decreasing the number of medical visits.[52] McCracken and Vowles found a direct correlation between symptomatology and level of mindfulness practice. Their patients who practiced mindfulness the most evidenced the greatest reductions in pain, depression, pain-related anxiety, and physical disability. In their study, 171 chronic pain patients received a combination of individual treatment with Acceptance and Commitment Therapy (ACT) along with a mindfulness-based group treatment. This was an unusually intense treatment; the patients met for six and a half hours a day, five days a week, for almost a month. These patients had fewer medical visits and were able to return to work much faster than expected.[53]

The Effects of Mindfulness Practice on Cancer
Cancer has many causes. In most people, it is the result of a complex interaction between many factors. It can be the result of having contracted certain viruses thirty or forty years before the onset of the disease. It is commonly the result of exposure to environmental toxins; just living in the modern world exposes most of us to a constant bombardment of

toxins in our air, water, and food. However, the identical level of toxic exposure in any group of people will have clinical significance in only some of the people because of different genetics and many other variables. One of these variables is the level of emotional distress with which we all live. And this is where mindfulness practice can come in.

The Carlson Studies

Carlson et al found increased antitumor activity against breast cancer among mindfulness practitioners. MBSR classes were offered to breast cancer and prostate cancer patients who were three months or more post-treatment.[54] The researchers discovered that the MBSR graduates who continued to practice mindfulness had increased T-cell production of IL-4, a decrease in interferon gamma, and a decrease in NK-cell production of IL-10—all changes that are consistent with improved immune function. Their one-year follow-up revealed a lasting response in improved immune function as evidenced by a continued diminution in pro-inflammatory cytokines.[55]

Cancer survivors commonly have increased cortisol levels; in this study, cortisol dropped to normal levels. Also, the toxicity of chemotherapy negatively impacts cardiovascular health, but during the course of the eight-week MBSR class, blood pressure also decreased—a sign of improved cardiovascular health.

In one study, MBSR classes were offered as an intervention to attempt to reduce mood disturbance and other symptoms of emotional distress in ninety cancer patients (with a mean age of fifty-one years) using a random wait-list controlled procedure. This differs from a no-treatment group in that the wait-list subjects get the identical procedure but they get it after their test results are compared with those of the treatment group. The wait-list method is used when the treatment (MBSR) is considered so efficacious that it would be unethical to deny treatment to the controls. Those in the treatment group reported significantly lower scores on total mood disturbance and subscales of depression, anxiety, anger, and confusion, as well as more energy than controls. The treatment group also had fewer stress symptoms, fewer cardiopulmonary and gastrointestinal symptoms, less emotional irritability and cognitive disorganization, and fewer habitual patterns of stress. The overall reduction in mood disturbance was 65 percent, with a 31 percent reduction in stress symptoms. Subsequent follow-up measures showed that these changes had been maintained six months later.[56]

The Meares Studies

In the 1970s, Ainsley Meares, MD, an Australian psychiatrist, provided documented case studies of seventy-three of his cancer patients. Five of those patients went into full remission just by practicing a very simple breathing-focused mindfulness practice he taught them.

These patients were not expected to recover even with standard of care, and they had all refused any medical interventions. Another five, also not expected to recover and who had also not received any medical interventions, went into partial remission.[57]

One of Meares's full-remission patients, Ian Gawler, was diagnosed with very advanced osteogenic sacrcoma with lung and brain metastases. Because of his training in veterinary medicine, he knew exactly what was happening to him. He showed marked regression of metastases through intensive mindfulness practice. Most importantly, Gawler let the effects of the intense and prolonged practice enter into his experience of life. When he was seeing Meares, he was practicing a mindfulness formal sitting meditation for five hours every day. Dr. Meares said that Gawler's extraordinary low level of anxiety was obvious, and he believes this inner tranquility gave an enormous boost to his immune system so that it could get rid of the cancer.

Meares reported that Gawler had an extraordinary will to live and had sought help from all the alternatives to orthodox medicine that were available to him. These included acupuncture, Philippine faith healers, laying on of hands, and yoga in an Indian ashram. After his first diagnosis he had begun to receive treatment with radiation and chemotherapy, but he quit and refused to finish these treatments against medical advice. Instead, he adopted the diet and enema treatments popularized by Max Gerson in the 1940s, which have since been proven to lack any efficacy. Gawler also had extraordinary help and support from his girlfriend, which would have had a positive effect on his outcome.

Meares had travelled very extensively in order to study with shamans, Zen masters, and all manner of mystics. Given the number of mystics Meares consulted, it is especially telling that he makes the following remark about Gawler: *"He developed a degree of calm about him which I have rarely observed in anyone, even in oriental mystics with whom I have had some considerable experience."*[58]

Gawler has written and mentioned in interviews that he believes it wasn't the formal sitting mindfulness meditation practice per se that catalyzed his remarkable and complete recovery from the precipice of death. Rather, he is clear that one must adopt mindfulness practice *as a way of life*, not just for the formal mindfulness sitting meditation periods each day. There is no evidence that mindfulness practice cures cancer. However, it can dramatically improve quality of life and state of mind, and this is certainly conducive to improvements in health in general. Gawler now runs a large cancer center in Australia.[59]

Obviously, there is no way to prove that Gawler or any of Meares's other patients would not have gotten well without practicing mindfulness. Still, statistically, it is unlikely that more than a couple of those patients would have survived without medical interventions. Gawler believes that his ability to develop inner peace and tranquility through formal sitting, coupled with other mindfulness practices such as practicing being fully present with all his daily activities, cured him, cured other Meares patients, and continues to cure many of his own patients.[60]

Several additional fascinating case studies emerged from

Meares's investigations, and as I find them of great interest, I have included them in appendix A at the back of the book.

ℭℛ

We have seen ample evidence of the efficacy of mindfulness practice in improving health and wellbeing, impacting a wide array of illnesses and conditions. In the next chapter, we will round out Part II and our discussion of mindfulness with a look at how it is practiced.

9 Practice Mindfulness

Meditation provides a way to quit living in the potent mental movies of disaster, regret, anger, and fear that not only rob your peace of mind, but can sometimes trick the body into believing that they are really happening.
—Joan Borysenko

The practice of mindfulness is available to everyone. And as we saw in the first chapter of Part II, it isn't complicated. Still, it is not easy; it requires an uncommon level of commitment. To become skilled at it, you must apply strong intention, clarity of purpose, and enormous self-discipline every day. As Jon Kabat-Zinn and others maintain, this cannot be an intellectual exercise in which you explore the *concept* or *philosophy* of mindfulness. No amount of academic study can substitute for the practice itself.

But for people who have chronic medical difficulties, making an extraordinary commitment to mindfulness practice carries the promise of extraordinary rewards. No matter what kinds of health challenges you're living with, this practice can improve your health and wellbeing by helping you become better able to navigate the vicissitudes resulting from chronic medical conditions. It works by allowing you to disengage from unhealthy thinking patterns. This has the effect of decreasing your emotional distress, which decreases the kind of physiological stress that can exacerbate or even create disease. The result is improved physiological functioning.

Many people mistakenly think the goal of mindfulness

meditation is to relax, and it is true that relaxation can be a result as emotional distress decreases. But while some other forms of meditation aim for relaxation as the primary goal, the goal of all mindfulness practices is to learn to live in full contact with the present moment.

The Value of Neutral Observation or Mind-Watching

Mind-watching is the most important thing we can do.
—Dalai Lama

Mindfulness practice entails neutrally observing thoughts as they come and go. In this way you gain insights into your unhealthy thinking patterns and behaviors. This helps you understand your motivations and worldview as well. It is not about developing a running commentary on your thoughts and feelings; instead, it is a way to lovingly observe and be fully present with your thoughts, emotional states, and sensations and the entire gestalt of your life experiences.

It is all too easy to get tangled up in a series of reactions to your thoughts: arguing with them, trying to be positive, trying to distract yourself, and getting anxious and frustrated about your inability to stop them. Mind-watching is fundamental to learning to experience your thoughts differently—in a new, objective context—and give yourself the opportunity to act in new ways relative to them.

Over time, you learn to perceive the arising and passing away of all phenomena, including the thoughts the brain generates. You become aware of all sensations without becoming attached to pleasant ones or trying to push away painful ones. Equanimity and nonattachment become common experiences.[1]

Being aware of the nature of the wanderings of the mind without judging or attempting to change them leads to acceptance of not only your most unpleasant thoughts, but of situations and other people as well. This creates a sense of

Many people mistakenly think the goal
of mindfulness is to relax, but the goal of
mindfulness practices is to learn to live in
full contact with the present moment.

connection with others, which is one of the most important
contributors to health, wellbeing, and mastery. Chapters 18
and 19 explore the value of connection in detail.

Getting Started

Although it's possible to maintain a mindfulness practice on
your own once you have attained a certain stage of practice,
in the early years you will need a teacher. Despite the simplicity of the practice, it is almost impossible to stay on the path
without ongoing guidance and support. This is because your
neural pathways for entanglement with your thinking processes have been reinforced since childhood; it takes a teacher
to intercede in this entanglement by repeatedly offering alternatives to it.

The best way to get started is to attend an introductory
workshop at a Buddhist meditation center or take an eight-
week Mindfulness-Based Stress Reduction (MBSR) class.
MBSR classes are a wonderful entry point to the practice and
are offered in almost every major city in the developed world.
After you receive this initial instruction, residential retreats
are usually the best way to deepen your practice. You can begin with a weekend retreat and then move on to longer ones.

Some people are able to create their own solitary retreats
instead of taking part in an organized one. I know one physician who spends his vacation time camping in the desert
and practicing mindfulness, far from any sign of civilization,
and it works for him. The advantages of organized retreats,
however, include the guidance of an experienced teacher and
the support of going through the process in community with
others.

Both options, group and solitary retreats, give you an extended, uninterrupted time away from all the distractions of
daily life. Solitary retreats should be free of contact with your
day-to-day world, including email, social media, phone, and
all other media. This allows you to come face-to-face with the
workings of your mind, including all your thoughts, sensations, and emotions, in ways that are not possible through a
brief daily sitting meditation practice.

The single most important mindfulness practice, however, also happens to be the most difficult one. This is the
informal practice of mind-watching as you go through your
day—every day. Your formal sitting meditation practice and
retreats make it possible to persevere with this daily informal mind watching because when you sit formally, you do
it in a quiet environment you have designated for that purpose. This makes it easier to create and reinforce the neural
pathways associated with the ability to observe cognitive and
emotional processes. I will have more to say on the distinction between formal and informal practice a little later, but
first I'd like to introduce you to a main category of mindfulness practice: *vipassana, or insight meditation.*

Vipassana
There are several varieties of vipassana, and different kinds
of practices within each type. Some are appropriate for beginners and others are achievable only after years of intensive
work. The practice I follow is called *samatha vipassana.* Each
word refers to a component of the whole practice. *Samatha*
refers to the concentration component in which you *focus intently on something,* often the sensations of breathing. When
you notice that your mind has wandered from this object of
focus—and that is inevitable because sensory distractions
abound and the mind continually generates thoughts—you
return your attention to the object. You do not judge the fact
that your attention wandered away; you simply notice that
this has happened and gently bring it back.

The other component—the *vipassana* aspect—is the development of insight. Here you not only return to the object of focus but also carefully notice *where your mind went* when it wandered off and what thought, emotion, or sensation you experienced while wandering.

So insight meditation usually involves riding the waves of the breath, being fully present to the full duration of each in-breath and out-breath without doing anything to control the rate or depth of either. You also notice the still point between each breath. Then you notice when your attention wavers from this point of focus, observe where it went, and bring it back to the breath.

Labeling

I mentioned that you notice your mind's distraction *without judgment.* In practicing mindfulness, you notice all sounds and other sensory input that have caught your attention. But as with your thoughts, you merely *note* everything you become aware of, without analyzing the source or nature of the stimuli, and without becoming attached to them. An intricacy of the practice is what you do when judgment arises — as it will despite your intention. When you realize you are judging, you simply label it so: *judging.* You don't assign a judgment to the fact that you're judging. This builds acceptance and mastery of your experience.

We touched on this topic of labeling in the last chapter. It is important that there be no struggle to identify and label thoughts. Many mindfulness practitioners never label them, and it is not necessary to do so; labeling is simply a tool that many people have found helpful, as I have. How do you know whether labeling is appropriate for you in your practice? For some people, the process of labeling their thoughts can put them in an analytical frame of mind, and this is not what is desired. For others, labeling thoughts in real time, if it can be done from the perspective of an objective observer, serves to provide great insight into the workings of the mind. This noticing of the mind's activity is known as *bare attention.*

Here is an example. If I become aware that I'm

thinking about a future event, by identifying and labeling these thoughts as *planning,* I'm able to see that planning is something the mind naturally does. I can then accept this and not become cognitively fused with and lost in the *contents* of the planning. It is enough to observe my mind engaged in planning; now I can go back to observing my breath.

If you use labels, you can use any you like. The ones I use in my own practice include *planning, rehearsing, reviewing, ruminating, judging, negativizing,* and *gobbledygook.* When I notice my mind has wandered from my breath, I describe my thoughts with one of those labels.

Gobbledygook, by the way, is the label I came up with for those times when I cannot easily identify my thoughts. Sometimes, for example, when I'm doing my formal daily sitting meditation, my mind goes into a dreamlike state where my thoughts are no longer logical. I don't want to try to make sense of them; instead, I simply label them as gobbledygook and then immediately return to following the sensations of respiration. In this way I develop the skill of taking my thoughts less seriously.

Disengaging
The practice of insight is in many ways a practice of disengaging or disentangling from your thoughts and beliefs; mindfulness allows you to see their intrinsic insubstantiality. Even the most internalized core beliefs, no matter how awful they may be, cease to be problematic after a certain amount of mindfulness practice. This is because moment-to-moment mindfulness dissolves conceptual judgments and beliefs, including the ones you have about your diagnosis, your prognosis, and a host of other mental constructs associated with living with chronic illness or being a cancer survivor.

Formal and Informal Practice
Let's return to the topic of formal versus informal mindfulness practice. Samatha vipassana is just one of many *formal* sitting meditation practices that are generally done at an ap-

pointed time each day. All such formal practices can serve as the essential foundation for moment-to-moment mindfulness practice *throughout the day,* known as *informal practice.* It casts a much wider net because it consists of nonjudgmentally observing all of your naturally arising thoughts, sensations, and emotions as you go through the day instead of becoming entangled or fused with them, and then returning to the activity at hand. Instead of getting caught up in concepts and constructs—the usual province of the mind—you focus on the direct, felt, sensory experience of the moment, no matter what may be occurring. And rather than relentlessly trying to interpret your experience, you set an intention to accept and be curious about it without analyzing or judging it. You engage in loving, nonjudgmental acknowledgment of all your waking moments.[2]

Each time you acknowledge thoughts as transient events in the field of awareness, you reinforce your ability to be mindful in the future. Your practice builds and deepens. And there are infinite opportunities to reinforce your practice because every activity, without exception, offers the choice to be present to the moment.[3]

A Word About Self-Consciousness

Many people think that observing your thoughts throughout the day must lead to self-consciousness, or a preoccupation with yourself. But the truth is that self-consciousness is caused by thinking *about* the self rather than actually experiencing it. Mindfulness involves stepping back from self-absorption and viewing your thoughts and feelings without getting caught up in them. You are not thinking about yourself; you are calmly and objectively observing your experience of self with kindness and curiosity—an entirely different quality from self-absorption.

Self-consciousness diminishes when you stop claiming ownership of thoughts, sensations, and emotions. Mindfulness practice allows you to distinguish between thoughts and the thinker of the thoughts. Put another way, when you think about yourself as the thinker of the thoughts and judge yourself for having such thoughts, you increase self-consciousness. When you observe thoughts as simply products of the mind, and do not struggle to try to get rid of them, troubling thoughts cease to be troubling.

Is a Formal Daily Sitting Practice Necessary for Everyone?
Although a formal daily sitting meditation practice is considered the foundation of mindfulness practice and living a mindful life, not everyone who has practiced mindfulness has had such a practice. One of the most revered mindfulness teachers of the twentieth century, Jiddu Krishnamurti, never practiced or taught this method; in fact, he was very critical of sitting meditation. He wrote, "The meditative attitude must be directed toward the whole of one's living, not invested in precious, encapsulated practices."[4] But he was quite unusual. It would be almost impossible for most of us to maintain a serious mindfulness practice without setting aside time each day for formal sitting. Though I have occasionally met people who claim to be able to practice mindfulness without a formal practice, when I dig a little deeper it usually becomes apparent that they are really intellectualizing about mindfulness and mistaking this for practice.

Using Symptoms in Informal Mindfulness Practice

Because informal mindfulness practice involves noting all your thoughts and sensations, the symptoms of illness provide wonderful opportunities to practice noting the connection between thought and sensation. Symptoms often occur or worsen as a result of what's taking place in the mind. If you feel a bellyache, headache, or backache when you engage in certain thinking patterns, you can be assured that those patterns are not healthy for you.

Opportunity in Discomfort

Uncomfortable bodily sensations, like uncomfortable thoughts and feelings, are not only difficult to avoid, but attempting to do so results in a form of self-rejection. All forms of discomfort—physical, mental, and emotional—are opportunities to practice acceptance. Mindful awareness of bodily sensations is very important because it is through them that you identify emotions.[5] Becoming aware of contractions in the shoulders, neck, chest, abdomen, or face can provide you with valuable insight into your emotional states. In fact, it is through the contraction of specific facial muscles that you know whether you're feeling happy or sad. A rise in skin temperature of the face, neck, chest, or other places tells you of other feelings.[6]

When you observe yourself sighing, groaning, tensing up, or feeling the first stirrings of pain, you can choose how to respond to those sensations in the moment when they occur. For example, you can ask, *Am I trying to avoid a thought or feeling?* Avoidance of unpleasant thoughts and feelings often results in sympathetic (fight or flight) arousal, which, long-term, contributes to chronic physiological stress and disease. With practice, you can learn to note that you have just had a certain unpleasant thought or feeling, that you instinctively resisted it, and that you then experienced the sensations of sympathetic arousal.

Another way to respond is with a statement that begins *I am having the thought that . . .* For example, as soon as I become aware that I'm feeling tense, or that I'm experiencing a symptom that I associated in the past with a certain line of thinking, I take note of my thinking process. If I'm thinking something unhealthy—such as *I'm just going to keep getting more decrepit and die a horrible death!*—I can preface this thought with: *I am having the thought that . . .* The new statement is *I am having the thought that I'm just going to keep getting more decrepit and die a horrible death.* When practiced every day, this informal mindfulness technique of acknowledging even the most upsetting thoughts for what they are—merely thoughts—can be an effective antidote to cognitive fusion.

It is particularly important to become an observer of your nonstop self-talk and to be especially mindful of any negative or self-deprecating automatic thoughts. This will increase your awareness of the extent to which you have them, and will help you discover that much of your negative self-talk repeats the same themes. One common theme for cancer survivors is *That pain in my side* (or wherever it is felt) *could be my tumor coming back.* A common theme for many of us living with autoimmune disease is *Why is my immune system attacking me?* Or for those of us living with various chronic, progressive, debilitating conditions, a common theme is *I'll never be normal,* or *I'm just going to keep getting worse.* The more you reinforce these themes, the stronger they get. Through intention and mindfulness, you can reverse the trend and diminish their power, and in so doing, cultivate mastery.

Here are a few more useful prefaces you can try when you notice physical discomfort:

I am having the feeling of

_____.

I am having the emotion of

_____.

I am having the mood of

_____.

I am feeling the bodily sensation of

_____.

(Describe the nature and location of the sensation.)
I am noticing the tendency to

_____.

(Describe any behavioral urge or predisposition.)

What's the Story?

Uncomfortable emotions also offer opportunities to practice. We all have our own unique triggers: certain situations or people that push our buttons and upset us. When you find yourself about to have an encounter with a person or circum-

stance that you can pre-
dict will leave you feeling
angry, sad, embarrassed,
or ashamed, or experienc-
ing some other unpleas-
ant emotion, you have an
opportunity to practice
mindfulness. As you be-
gin to enter the conver-
sation, be on the lookout

> Becoming an observer of the non-stop chatter in your mind allows you to step back and disentangle from it.

for your thoughts and feelings and stay present with them as they come up.

In becoming aware of an unpleasant emotion, it can be helpful to ask the following question: *What story am I telling myself?* Asking this question serves to increase your aware-ness of why you feel a certain way in any given moment. It helps you establish a direct cause-and-effect relationship be-tween thoughts and feelings. The advantage of referring to your thoughts as a story is that it helps you recognize that your thoughts truly are fiction—you make them up. Here are some examples of how you can make use of this technique:

- When you're feeling depressed, the question can help you discover a story you're telling yourself that involves self-judgment.
- When you're feeling frustrated about performing a task, the question can help you discover a story related to a belief that the task should be easier.
- When you're feeling angry, the question can help you discover a story that involves a belief that someone or something *should* be different from the way she, he, or it is.

Exploring Mortality

Now I would like to touch on another form of mindfulness practice that is commonly done and is one I recommend. This is the practice of exploring your own mortality. It involves observing thoughts, emotions, and sensations as you ponder your own inevitable death. This particular practice strengthens your intention to practice living in full contact with the present.

To do this practice, spend time observing your thoughts and feelings as you call up images of yourself dying or already dead. I did this each morning for a year and found that it helped me bring greater presence to my daily activities. When I imagined myself at the end of life, I felt very deep regret that I had not lived more mindfully, and with that realization came gratitude that I actually have the opportunity to live a more mindful life *right now*. This strengthened my resolve to live fully in my present-moment experience.

At the Simonton Cancer Center, we helped patients appreciate that they could live more mindfully regardless of how little time they had left. The following set of three questions is adapted from my training with Dr. Lawrence LeShan and Dr. Carl Simonton. You can answer them even if you have never formally practiced mindfulness and they will help strengthen your intention and commitment.

When I find myself at the end of my life, what will I most regret?
What will I wish I had done differently?
What will I regret never having attempted?

Psychiatrist David Spiegel is known for his research showing that women with metastatic breast cancer who participate in weekly groups live much longer than those who don't; he now believes he can explain their greater longevity: honestly facing one's own mortality and making rational choices about how to live one's life has an invigorating effect and catalyzes the immune system to function optimally.[7]

The simplest and most powerful way to create more joy and deep fulfillment in your life is to recognize that the choices you make today can have profound repercussions, now and later. Exploring your mortality helps you examine whether or not you're spending your remaining time living the way you most want to live, right now in this moment.

Suggestions for Practicing Mindfulness

Here are some instructions for practice based on the work of research psychologist Steven Hayes that will give a clear idea of one of the ways in which mindfulness is used to de-fuse from your thoughts and your private experiences.[8]

> When your mind wanders and you find yourself getting angry or sad or imagining something you want to say to someone and slipping into fantasy, just notice that you have wandered off and bring yourself back. Notice how you get sucked into the content of your thoughts and start to fuse with them; notice your analytical, judgmental mind. Simply notice and bring yourself back again, gently and without judgment. Whenever you have judgments about how well or how poorly you are doing, just notice these too. All there is for you to do is simply follow and observe whatever you notice without any analyzing or judging. When you discover that you have been analyzing or judging, neutrally observe that as well.

Further Suggestions for Formal Practice
- Take some time every day to sit quietly and follow the sensations of breathing. Try to notice your thoughts without analyzing them. Whenever you become aware that your mind has wandered off, have some appreciation for your ability to notice that, and return your attention to the sensations of breathing.
- If you are too tired or sleepy to practice while seated, walk very slowly for fifteen minutes, putting all your concentration on the sensations of walking.
- At other times, lie down, and without moving at all, take a tour of your body. Tune in to sensations in each toe, each leg, your low back, middle back, upper back, your

head resting on the floor. Concentrate fully on each area in turn.

- Tune in to any pain, fatigue, malaise, or other chronic symptoms you experience. Allow yourself to remain in full contact with those sensations without trying to make them go away and without trying to *not* feel them. See how the sensations change as you fully allow yourself to experience them. Notice the thoughts related to the sensations that come and go. Allow yourself to fully experience these thoughts.

- Practice mindfulness by training yourself to maintain your brain waves in the six-to-eight-hertz range with the help of EEG biofeedback (neurofeedback) training sessions. This has not been well researched, yet I have personally found this experience to promote an exceptionally deep level of mindfulness abilities. Although it would not be realistic or even a good idea to go through the day in that state of mind, I believe it can be very healthy to spend a few minutes each day practicing mindfulness in that particular brain-wave state.

Further Suggestions for Informal Practice
- As you go through the day, maintain a strong intention to concentrate on the task at hand, whether it's doing the dishes or doing surgery.
- Throughout the day, notice your emotional state and describe to yourself the physical sensations that allow you to know what you are feeling.
- Whenever you notice a strong emotion, notice too what thoughts seem to be associated with this feeling.
- Each time you realize that your mind has wandered from the task at hand, feel appreciation for your ability to realize that your mind had wandered, and return attention to the task.
- Throughout all your waking moments, remind yourself of your intention to be as fully awake as possible in all your endeavors, from the simplest to the most complex.

- As you go through the day, notice how you identify with any symptoms or with a diagnosis you may have received.

An Unstructured Body Scan Meditation to Work with Pain

When there is pain or discomfort anywhere in the body, just observe it. Also observe other sensations throughout your body; do the same with itches, twitches, tickles, and gastrointestinal shifting sensations. Observe any tight muscles—especially of the forehead, eyes, and jaw. Do not resist any sensations; allow your attention to stay with whatever sensations are calling you. Observe them without attachment, analyzing, or judging.

When you feel pain, accept it. If you find yourself resisting it, notice how that tends to increase the pain. Even just naming it as pain can do that as well. When you accept pain as simply a bodily sensation, it is more likely to diminish.

When your mind wanders away from the body, gently return it to bodily sensations, including any pain or discomfort you may be feeling, again without any analyzing or judging. You can learn a lot about pain by dealing with it through mindfulness.

This body scan is an excellent daily practice that leads to a very sensitive and acute ability to discern physiological sensations that need attention from those that do not. This valuable skill also serves to develop your ability to detect prodromes, early signs of illness. Every illness and condition is much easier to cure if detected in the prodromal stage.

In addition to helping you detect problems in the prodromal stage, you can also use the body scan to reduce symptomatology when it serves no useful function. The reason for this is that as you become more skilled at tuning in on a very sensitive level to bodily sensations, you gradually acquire the ability to discern symptoms from normal healthy sensations. For example, pressure, pain, or heat could be a red flag that requires medical attention or it could be a perfectly nor-

mal physiological sensation that doesn't indicate anything of
concern. With time, you will become increasingly able to tell
the difference. Once you can, you no longer need to get entangled with the fear and unhealthy thoughts that arise when
the mind is allowed to ruminate and catastrophize. Because
this will reduce your emotional distress, it will eliminate some
of the physiological stress that can lead to new symptoms.

CR

In this chapter I have given you an overview of mindfulness
practice, delved into some important facets of it, and described
the promise it holds for people living with chronic illness. In
the next three chapters I will introduce you to a unique, three-
step mindfulness-based method I developed to create greater
mastery and wellbeing: Valued-Action Practice. While this
practice stands on its own, and I have found it tremendously
helpful in coping with my own illnesses and living a healthy,
happy life, it can certainly be enhanced by a daily, formal
mindfulness-based meditation practice.

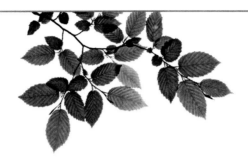

Part III

Valued-Action Practice

As I pointed out early in the book, emotional distress and its accompanying physiological stress are less the result of external events than of the attributions you assign to those events—your thoughts and beliefs about them—and your cognitive fusion with those attributions. The antidote to this suffering is mindfulness practice, which provides you with the skills to be able to disengage from your unhealthy thoughts and beliefs.

There is another approach to emotional distress that I have found highly effective, both in my personal life and in my professional practice. It, too, involves mindfulness, but in a different way, and it is a core practice I recommend to achieve mastery and greater wellbeing in your life. I call it Valued-Action Practice, and it is the subject of the three chapters that comprise Part 3.

This method addresses the fact that the vast majority of the time, most of us go through the day more focused on what we *don't* want than what we *do* want. When anything at all doesn't go as we would have liked, we end up thinking about what went wrong, magnifying its importance. When we don't feel well, we focus on not feeling well. When any condition exists that we don't like, we focus on that condition. In this way, we create even more emotional and physiological stress than our condition or illness itself generates. We also reinforce the neural circuits for negativity, thereby increasing the odds of experiencing more of what we don't want. This reinforcing of what we do not value has another deleterious effect: it distances us from our personal life values. And being out of touch with our values leads to the types of thoughts, feelings, and behaviors that can be very destructive to our health.

The reason we engage in this counterproductive, paradoxical practice is that, since ancient times, we have mistakenly believed we need to focus on what we don't want in order to figure out how to keep bad things from happening. We've vividly imagined the tiger's approach in order to help us prepare to ward off an attack. Still, although most people throughout the millennia have focused on what they didn't want, there has always been a tiny percentage of individuals who were able to keep their attention on those things they held most dear—their personal life values. Other factors being equal, they have always tended to live with better health and greater wellbeing.

There is nothing to stop you from learning and employing the brilliant strategy these healthier people have used and weaving it into the fabric of your life. You, too, can develop the skill of focusing on your most deeply held values in every waking moment.

10 Practice Living by Your Personal Life Values

L et's begin our exploration of Valued-Action Practice by examining what values actually are and how they differ from goals.

A goal is something you desire to achieve. This can involve acquiring a material thing—a new car, for example—or it can involve achieving a certain quality of life, such as being free enough of pain or disability to be able to resume golf, tennis, dancing, or hiking. But it is always a thing or an end result; you will know when you have met your goal.

A life value cannot be achieved; it can only be lived. It is a way of being or a human quality you value. These ways of being and qualities are golden; when you identify them and then consciously engage in the mindfulness practice of living in harmony with them, you tap into a wellspring of health and happiness—this is what is meant by mastery. The mere act of focusing on what you value can shift your entire experience of life.

Though they are different in nature, values and goals can intersect. You can base what you desire to achieve on your most closely held values, thereby ensuring that those values are always at work in your life, expressed through action.

Although focusing on values sounds simple, it contains a big challenge: how do you determine which life value to focus on at any given time? One approach might be to make a list of what you value, review it during the day, and try to make sure your most deeply held personal life values are covered in how you live that day. This would be a methodical approach,

> To identify your personal life values, observe the thoughts and feelings you have after each action you take.

but perhaps not a very realistic one.

The alternative I have learned, used, and taught, which works very effectively, is to first identify your personal life values and then learn how to determine which one is most pertinent *in any given moment*. You can actually do both steps simultaneously by engaging in the mindfulness practice of observing your emotional reactions to people and events. You can also see your values reflected in the activities you choose. Following are some examples.

- If you feel irritated when a doctor or nurse tells you you'll never recover, this signals that you value hope. On the other hand, if you feel irritated when a doctor or nurse tells you that you'll be fine after you've just been diagnosed with a stage IV cancer, this reveals that you value authenticity.
- If you feel warm and satisfied after providing needed support, hope, or active listening for other people dealing with a disease or condition you have managed to live well with, this shows that you value serving others.
- If you suffer as a result of self-criticism, it means you value acceptance.
- If you feel better after offering your heartfelt thanks to someone, you value gratitude.
- If you admire people who are very much in control of their lives despite living with a degenerative condition, you probably value the sense of being in control of your own life.
- If you practice mindfulness meditation or some other form of mindfulness, one of your values is presence, or living in full contact with the present moment.

- If you look for opportunities to share information and emotional support with others who know from personal experience what it's like to live with chronic health challenges, social support is one of your values.
- If you are someone who likes to look for the humor in a situation, you value laughter and a lighthearted approach to life.

I offer these particular examples of values because they line up with the behaviors that have been most strongly associated with health and wellness—and you will find them reflected in the mastery and wellbeing practices contained in Part 4. However, there are many more personal life values that people hold dear. The following list contains some of them. You might consider posting this list in a place where you will see it frequently, or posting it on your mobile device so that you can refer to it throughout the day. Then observe your emotional experience throughout the day and note when your responses seem to point your attention in the direction of one of these qualities. Feel free to add to the list as you identify other values that are important to you—this is by no means an exhaustive list.

acceptance
appreciation
a sense of belonging
care
healthcare
self-care
connection
cooperation
effective interpersonal communication
a sense of community
companionship
empathy
health
inclusion

intimacy
love
trust
wellbeing
honesty
authenticity
integrity
presence
equality
order
autonomy
choice
independence
challenge
hope
learning

Taking Valued Action

Once you identify your personal life values, how can you start
working with them? Action is the catalyst for change—and for
consciously creating wellbeing. All of the chapters on practices in Part 4 involve taking action of some kind that is centered
on values, so you will have plenty of opportunity to do that
as you progress through that section. Following is a simple
place to start.

Consider two of the options you have if you're with people who are acting in an inauthentic matter. Let's say a person is assuring you that you'll be fine at a time when what
you would most value is empathy and understanding. If this
person is not at all close to you, you could opt to express this
wish, but you may be asking for something that person is unable to give you. Instead, you may want to place your attention on how beautiful it is that you value empathy and understanding—an internal experience of connecting with your
values. If you are with someone who is close to you, on the
other hand, it would be best to express how much you would

like empathy and understanding, and to continue the dialog until you get some satisfaction.

I encourage you to explore all of your personal life values, using your emotional responses as your guide, and develop the habit of noticing them. It will take some time for you to identify everything you value, as there are values that relate to virtually every dimension of your life. For now, though, I suggest you choose just one value you've read about in this chapter that you know is important to you. This is all you need to move on to the next chapter and investigate an extraordinarily empowering next step: living by choice.

11 What Are You Choosing?

The crux of this mindfulness-based system to achieve greater mastery and wellbeing is to recognize and take advantage of a simple fact: that every moment of your day presents you with an opportunity to choose how you will live. These moment-by-moment choices will largely determine the quality of your life—usually far more so than external events can determine it.

The ways you respond to these myriad opportunities to choose—the thought processes and attitudes you employ and the behaviors you select—constitute a daily practice. In this sense, *life is a practice.* Discovering this reality for yourself and acting in accordance with it are immensely freeing. You learn that you have a great deal of room to move despite any limitations or constraints that may accompany your health challenges. We will return to the idea of life as a practice in the next chapter. But first we will take a closer look at choice.

Taking advantage of your freedom to choose entails becoming fully responsible (response-able) for making conscious choices in every moment: making an earnest and repeated effort to choose to behave in ways that are aligned with your personal life values.

Mounting evidence from brain scan research clearly demonstrates that every time you make a fully conscious choice, you *reinforce the neural circuit* for that choice, which makes it easier to make that choice again. So when you begin to recognize and act upon the choices that align with your personal values and promote health and happiness, you have the

opportunity to make use of your own brain circuitry to create wellbeing, consciously enlisting an aspect of your brain's
functioning that usually operates outside of your awareness.

How to Live by Choice

Living by choice is not a mystery; the steps are simple. But
it doesn't come easily, especially at first. If it did, everyone
would drop their old habits and start living with intention
so they could reap all the benefits and live healthier, happier
lives. The challenge of living by choice is to make the commitment to practice the following steps faithfully, and consistently over time.

*Set an intention to make conscious choices
throughout the day, each day.*
The first step is a matter of focus, of deciding how you want to
direct your behavior. Since most of us live quite unconsciously most of the time, setting the intention to make conscious
choices is a necessary step that needs to be revisited again and
again.

*Cultivate an awareness of how often you make
unconscious choices throughout the day.*
For this step, notice those times when you are engaged in doing something you didn't deliberately decide to do: eating a
food that isn't healthy for you, eating until you feel full, or
obsessing over an upcoming medical appointment. You don't
need to change anything with this step; simply notice when
you're doing something you didn't deliberately set out to do.
This can prove very illuminating, and you will get better at it
with practice.

*Notice how often your behavior
is not aligned with your personal values.*
This is where the real power of living by choice lies: discovering the things you think, do, and say that don't line up with
what you value most—those qualities and behaviors you

One of the most profound mindfulness practices is that of going through each day asking yourself the following question: What action am I choosing in this moment?

began to identify in the preceding chapter. This disconnect is the source of great emotional distress and physiological stress, and when you develop the ability to recognize the discord, you gain the opportunity to choose a different, much more health-affirming course.

Make conscious choices as often as you can.
Over time, you will learn to recognize the great variety of decision points you reach throughout the day. When you notice that there is a choice to make—whether to continue ruminating about an upcoming medical procedure, perhaps, or whether or not to call upon a friend for support—you will improve your skills in living according to your personal values. In the preceding examples, the values are peace of mind and support.

Make conscious choices throughout the day
that are in harmony with your personal life values.
With this step you can fulfill the promise of living by choice. If you value self-care, for example, and you find yourself presented with the conscious choice of what to have for lunch when there is little time, you can decide to select something that's nutrient dense, yet light and quick to eat—some leftover tofu, rice, and vegetables, perhaps—and then drive past that fast-food place instead of through it. If you have been practicing loving self-care, you will have prepared such nutritious meals in advance, cooking a little extra food the evening before and setting it aside in order to have a healthy lunch each day instead of eating in a restaurant.

As another example, say you've been avoiding asking for a friend's help for fear of being a burden. But when you consider your personal values, you recognize how much you value support, loving self-care, and authentic self-expression, so you pick up the phone and make the call. Taking valued action not only serves to allow you to live by your personal values, it cultivates a strong sense of mastery: mastery results when you make conscious choices that are in line with your personal life values. It is in such seemingly minor decisions that the promise of living by choice is found, because *all the choices that line up with your values contribute to your health and wellbeing.* And they add up!

A Few Examples of Living by Choice

Here are a few more examples of what it's like to live by choice. All of these emphasize the moment-by-moment nature of life as a practice. Some are very simple, while others demonstrate a thinking process and series of steps.

- When I wake up in the night to pee, because I'm still half asleep, I consciously choose to be aware of my steps to the bathroom in order to avoid bumping into the wall, which could easily happen without that conscious choice.
- When I sit down at my desk, I choose to breathe diaphragmatically and slowly. Normally, without consciously making that mindful, intentional choice, my respiration would automatically become shallow and rapid as I dive into handling dozens of tasks. Healthy breathing improves brain function and physiological functioning in general.
- I realize that a caregiver is providing substandard care. Before confronting the person, I choose to breathe diaphragmatically and slowly, and I choose to clarify my intention in my mind before speaking to that person.
- I'm feeling great frustration, even anguish, in my attempts to get enough exercise. It seems like everything I try exacerbates my pain and disability. I then choose to shift my focus to my values of health and mastery rather

than on what is clearly not working for me. This serves to clarify my intention, thereby creating an environment in which I am considerably more likely to be creative and find a mode of exercise that works for me.

- Upon waking up, I realize I'm thinking that I have to go to an invasive medical appointment. Then I remind myself that I don't actually *have* to go. I remind myself that I *chose* to make the appointment; I choose to go, and I will do this because I value health and living with a sense of being in control of my life.

- I realize that I'm feeling grumpy. I take advantage of that discovery to consciously choose to instead focus on someone or something for which I feel enormous gratitude. This serves to create a healthier state of mind and lifts my spirits.

- I'm feeling deep sadness because I'm losing friends as a result of my illness. They're tired of having me cancel get-togethers at the last minute because of fatigue or malaise. I choose to take action and practice authentic self-expression; I arrange a get-together during which I can express my true feelings and ask for their understanding. Regardless of the outcome, this valued action gives me a sense of being in control of my life once again.

- My wife and I are checking out of a bed and breakfast inn. Two petite women (my wife and the desk clerk) carry all our bags out to the van, where I am already seated. The desk clerk gives me a look that triggers feelings of shame. I recognize that I feel this way because I think I *should* be able to carry the bags myself. I take valued action and choose to practice self-compassion, reminding myself that I did not choose to develop ankylosing spondylitis, and that I am practicing good self-care by not causing further damage to my spine.

Guidelines and Practices for Living by Choice

The essence of living by choice is to practice intention and mindfulness in order to develop an increased sense of control in daily life. That sense of control comes from the skill of being able to live with conscious intention—making conscious choices, moment by moment, throughout the day. The following practices can help:

1. Ask the fundamental question: What am I choosing in this moment?

Examples of possible answers:

I'm choosing self-pity.
I'm choosing anger.
I'm choosing self-criticism.
I'm choosing gratitude.
I'm choosing avoidance.
I'm choosing to reach out to someone.
I'm choosing authentic self-expression.
I'm choosing behavior that is not conducive to health.
I'm choosing behavior that is conducive to health.

2. Ask: Am I making choices that are aligned with my personal life values?
3. Ask: What is my intention in this moment?
4. Ask: What action can I take in this moment to improve my wellbeing?
5. Every time you find yourself saying *have to, need to, must,* or *should,* say instead *I choose to.* The fact is, in each case, you *have* chosen, and if that choice is in alignment with what you value, it's a choice that enhances wellbeing.

It can be a challenge to remember to practice these conscious choice exercises throughout the day; it takes time to develop the habit, and even when you can do it fairly routinely, it's easy to lapse into unconscious thinking and behavior again. Though it may seem like an easy thing to do, in the beginning it is actually very difficult *to remember to ask the question!* Until it becomes a habit, you may find one of these methods helpful:

- Set lots of random alarms on your laptop, iPad, or mobile device to go off throughout the day. Each time you hear one, ask: *What am I choosing?*
- Make use of transition points from one activity to another throughout the day. Whenever you change activities—such as moving from sitting to standing, for example—use that as a reminder to ask: *What am I choosing?*

Another way to remember is to use uncomfortable emotions as signals to ask the fundamental question. For example, if I'm feeling anxious and ask the question, I may find that the answer is that I'm choosing to worry, which is something I usually do unconsciously, since I know it causes emotional and physiological stress and thus would not consciously choose to practice it. Emotional discomfort is often a signal that you have made unconscious choices. As such, it's an invaluable tool for supporting a shift to living by choice.

"I Am Choosing ..." Practice

There is another layer of practice in addition to asking the fundamental question. Once you're comfortable with the idea of asking the question and noticing your answers, you can mentally *declare* your choices to yourself as you go through your day:

> I am choosing to get out of bed.
> I am choosing to put on my exercise clothes.
> I am choosing to exercise.
> I am choosing to blow my nose.

There is no action that is too insignificant to include in this practice. Be sure to include thoughts as well as actions:

I'm choosing to think about my day.
I'm choosing to think about the conversation I had
with the lab tech yesterday.
I'm choosing to complain about the pain in my back.
I'm choosing to focus on the benefits of the invasive
test I *chose* to line up.
I'm choosing to feel grateful for this beautiful day.

The purpose of this practice is to reinforce the realization
that literally *everything* you think and do, you do by choice; it
reinforces the power of choice. Although thoughts automatically pop into your head, you can choose what to do with
them; you can get caught up in them or you can choose to
recognize them as insubstantial and let them pass.

Another reason this can be a powerful, even life-altering
practice is that it keeps you focused on what you value rather
than on what you don't. In fact, it can wake you up to less-con-
scious, automatic habits and addictions that are inconsistent
with your personal values.

Here is an example of how this works: Let's say you're
sitting at a table eating and you say to yourself: *I'm choosing to
eat.* If you're eating a greater quantity of food than you value,
the very simple act of making this statement serves to make
you aware of this. In that instant of awareness, you can say,
I'm choosing to stop eating immediately and *I'm choosing to put
this food away.* Just saying the words *I'm choosing to eat* serves to
put you in full contact with your experience of that moment.

This practice involves making the phrase *I am choosing*
a part of moment-to-moment awareness, and this moment-
to-moment emphasis on choice is a powerful antidote to the
feelings of helplessness and hopelessness that so often plague
those who live with chronic medical conditions and feel lost in
the healthcare system.

Quite often, when you're having a thought that stirs uncomfortable emotions and you're in mid-sentence, you can
interrupt your thinking by saying *I am choosing.* This allows
you to instantly realize that you don't want to be thinking that

The path to living a life of valued action begins with learning to be consciously aware of
as much of your behavior as possible.

particular thought because you know it's not conducive to
your health. At that moment, your newfound awareness allows you to see that the unhealthy thought has to do with
something that happened in the past or that you think might
happen in the future—and neither past nor present exist in
this moment. This realization gives you the option of choosing to focus all your attention on your present-moment experience, which always carries with it the possibility of feeling
vibrant and alive.

Without engaging in this practice, it's all too easy to get
caught up in or fused with your thoughts because you don't
yet realize and appreciate that you have the power to choose
to step back and disengage from them. You don't yet know
from experience that it is truly within your power to get to a
point where you can choose to see thoughts as insubstantial
brain phenomena you need not follow.

Three Applications of I Am Choosing Practice
There are four ways to use this particular mindfulness practice. In describing them, I have used very mundane examples
in order to reinforce that there is no thought or action that is
too insignificant to use as practice.

1. Get clear on the personal life value that is most con-
    nected with any given moment. Then, focus your inten-
    tion on acting in accordance with that value by prefacing
    the chosen action with *I am choosing.* For example, you
    become aware of bladder pressure as you are sitting at
    your desk. You tune in to one of your values: physical
    comfort. You then say, *I am choosing to get up and walk to
    the bathroom.* Then you say, *I am choosing to pee.*

2. Set the intention, as often as possible throughout the day, to silently say to yourself *I am choosing* as a way to bring your awareness to your current thoughts, emotions, and actions. For example, let's say you're engaged in a certain activity—maybe you're doing the dishes—and suddenly you remember the practice. Without having noticed what you've been thinking before now, you say *I am choosing.* Immediately as that phrase appears in your mind, you become aware of your thinking process, which, a moment earlier, was not in your field of awareness.

3. Every time you notice an unhealthy thought or action, immediately say *I am choosing,* followed by naming that thought or action. For example, say you're standing at the sink and you suddenly become aware that you're feeling remorse for something you said to someone months ago. You know that dwelling in the past is not conducive to health—and you value your health! Immediately, say *I am choosing to remind myself of this unpleasant event.* This prompts you to remember that you have the power to change your mind. It's not necessary to find a more pleasant thought; simply becoming self-aware serves to dissolve your fusion with the unpleasant one. Unpleasant thoughts can only plague us when we lack self-awareness and unconsciously go into cognitive fusion.

The most important reason to practice *I am choosing* is to take control of your life and step out of the "poor me," help-less-hopeless, victim-type thinking that is all too common among those of us living with chronic health challenges. You are not helpless; you have a range of choices in virtually every moment of your day. *I am choosing* practice reinforces this truth and helps you take advantage of it so you can live your life with mastery.

CR

As I mentioned in the last chapter on values, action is the catalyst for change. Earlier in this chapter, I introduced the idea that the actions you take throughout your day constitute a daily practice. Armed with your new and expanding awareness of your personal life values, and with developing awareness of the myriad decision points that are available to you moment by moment—your limitless freedom to choose—you are now prepared to take advantage of these skills and live your life engaged in practices that create mastery and wellbeing.

12 What Are You Practicing?

In the previous chapter I introduced the idea that life is practice. And it's true: all habits of thought and behavior add up to the way you practice living your unique life.

Unfortunately, most of us are not fully aware of most of what we practice throughout the day. And if you're not fully aware, it's inevitable that you will inadvertently practice something that's unhealthy or that isn't aligned with your life values.

For example, you may spend a lot of time practicing self-critical thoughts, or ruminating repeatedly over a familiar issue or problem. Your thoughts spin like a hamster in a wheel—running nowhere. And the more you do this, the more you will continue to do it. You will ultimately get very good—expert, even—at something you really wouldn't want to do at all if you were fully aware of how this practice impacts your health and happiness.

When you have a self-critical thought and are not able to recognize it as just meaningless brain activity, you create emotional distress, which then creates physiological stress, and that is not conducive to mastery and wellbeing. Further, each time you have a self-critical thought, unless you are able to immediately disengage from it, it will reinforce the neural pathway for having more such thoughts in the future. And we know that fusion with such thoughts on a daily basis increases the odds of contracting chronic illness and such life-threatening diseases as cancer because of the immunosuppressive nature of stress.

> Everything we do is practice;
> the goal is to consciously
> choose actions that are in har-
> mony with what we value.

We create our own realities through what we choose to practice—whether consciously or unconsciously, and the example I've just given of repetitive self-critical thought is one way we can create an unhealthy reality for ourselves. Another way involves one of the most destructive practices we can engage in, one that people with chronic illnesses can easily lapse into: blaming someone or something else for our state—for our illness itself or for our own internal experience of it. If we go through life blaming other people, corporations, governments, bad luck, or even the weather for whatever it is we don't like about our lives, we are doomed to experience more of the very things we don't like. This is because we have effectively disempowered ourselves, placed someone or something else in charge. We have lost control. When this is what we are practicing, we frame ourselves as helpless victims, which is one of the worst things we can do for our health; it is the polar opposite of mastery.

This is one of the "dark sides" of practice, if you will—the frequently unconscious cycle of blaming and victimhood. But you don't have to practice this way; as you learned in the last chapter, the choice is yours. One of the best ways to increase the odds of maintaining, stabilizing, or improving your health is to elevate what you practice into your conscious awareness and engage in healthful practices with intention.

When you practice living mindfully and making conscious choices, you become increasingly able to practice those things that make you feel happier, stronger, and more alive. Living with *conscious intention* in this way leads to mastery: the felt sense that you are in charge of your life, which can make all the difference in your daily experience.

"What Am I Practicing?"

Just as there is a key question you can use to elevate choice into conscious awareness, there is a simple yet powerful question that will help you shift from destructive practices to healthful ones. Throughout the day, you can ask yourself: *What am I practicing?* The purpose of asking this question is to become aware of what you are thinking, feeling, and doing and to give yourself the opportunity to try something else that's more likely to enhance your health.

Following are some ways you might find yourself responding to this question as your awareness develops and improves:

I'm practicing self-pity.
I'm practicing anger.
I'm practicing self-criticism.
I'm practicing gratitude.
I'm practicing avoidance.
I'm practicing seeing the light side or the bright side.
I'm practicing reaching out to someone.
I'm practicing authentic self-expression.
I'm practicing passivity.
I'm practicing assertiveness.
I'm practicing being the team leader of my healthcare team.

If this list of practices seems familiar, it should. I've added a few items here, but most of these appear in the preceding chapter, What Are You Choosing? as well. In this three-step method, there is actually a *confluence* of choice and practice: if you discover that you have *chosen* self-pity, for example, you will also have found yourself *practicing* it. It's a single mental and emotional process that I'm choosing to describe from two different perspectives: you've made the decision to do it, and as a result, you're doing it.

The reason I've separated choice and practice is that each aspect of your experience is important in its own right.

Practicing this method entails becoming increasingly aware of the *empowering decision points* that present themselves to you moment by moment—your freedom to choose. You must also become aware of the repetitive and self-fulfilling nature of practicing what you have chosen. It's the awareness of the *effects of practice* that helps motivate you to notice those decision points as soon as they arise and learn to make healthier choices more quickly.

As is the case with the key question about choice, it can be all too easy to forget to ask this question about practice too. The methods I described in the last chapter, using alarms and transitions from one activity to the next to prompt you, work here as well. Strong emotions are also cues to access this important tool—and any emotion will do. Here are some examples:

- When you find yourself feeling sad, you can ask: *What am I practicing?* Your answer might help you to see, for example, that the reason you're feeling sad may be that you've been practicing ruminating over an event in your life that makes you feel sad.
- When you find yourself feeling anxious, the answer is usually that you've been practicing assigning negative attributions to future events: *When I go to the doctor today, I bet she'll find my lab values have gotten even further out of range* is one example. You have, in effect, been practicing *inventing unpleasant outcomes* that have no basis in reality.
- When you find yourself feeling lighthearted, you have probably been practicing taking your thoughts lightly— in other words, de-fusing from your thoughts.
- When you find yourself feeling angry, you have probably been practicing blaming someone else.

Keep in mind that all of the particular thought processes in this list are *normal and to be expected,* and are only unhealthy when you are unable to step back from them and recognize that you have been unconsciously practicing something that's not good for you. They are only harmful when you unquestioningly accept them as truths.

> Every time we repeat a behavior, we reinforce the neural circuitry that supports more of that behavior.

Let me offer two more examples. Let's say that while I'm shaving, a memory flashes into mind of a provocative and antagonistic remark I made to someone long ago that resulted in discomfort for both of us. Now, many years later, I'm experiencing shame and regret for having made that comment. Even though those words left my mouth long ago, I'm berating myself today for being so insensitive. My body tightens against my self-criticism. I feel stressed and contracted. Then I remember to ask the question *What am I practicing?* The question wakes me up from my old unhealthy thinking pattern and allows me to feel compassion for myself for having experienced this interaction yet again. And the question and answer bring welcome results: this very simple mental exercise immediately alleviates my tension.

Here's another example: I'm about to go to a medical appointment. As usual, I feel anxiety and dread in advance of this experience. As soon as I realize what I'm feeling, I ask myself: *What am I practicing?* I find that I'm practicing some familiar unhealthy, anxiety-producing thoughts. With that realization comes the awareness of choice. Almost simultaneously, my breathing slows and my anxiety diminishes. I think about how ironic it is that the very stress my body experiences as I anticipate the appointment makes it more likely that I will need even more appointments.

This technique can be applied to thoughts of helplessness or hopelessness as well, which are easy to experience if you have a chronic medical problem. If you get caught up in such thoughts once in a while, they're harmless, but when cognitive fusion represents an entrenched pattern, they become pathogenic; they can lead to depression and become deleterious to your health. Once you learn to identify the pattern by asking,

What am I practicing? your experience becomes *Oh, I'm feeling that way again. I've been here before*—and *I've been able to step back and disentangle from this thought pattern before, just by asking this very helpful question.* With the awareness the question brings, you can develop the ability to change your experience.

Now Ask Two More Questions

Once you've asked yourself this first question, there are two others that can transform your practices from unhealthy ones to those that have been proven to create wellness.

1. Is what I'm practicing in this moment in harmony with my values and goals?
2. And if it isn't: *What action can I take right now that will help me live in accordance with my values and reach my values-based goals?*

Note: Step 2 doesn't mean you have to drop what you're doing and change your behavior that instant. It may simply involve committing to create a plan for doing that as soon as you have the time.

Repeat!

This three-question process—*What am I practicing? Is it in alignment with my values? If not, what action can I take to come into alignment?*—can be applied to the specific behavior we will cover in each of the other upcoming chapters on practices. For example, regarding building relationships, which is so essential to health, I would ask:

1. Step one: *What am I practicing in this moment?*
2. Step two: *Is it in harmony with* my value of relationship building *and* my goal of taking action to expand and improve my relationships?
3. If not, move to step three: *What action can I take right now that will help me live in accordance with my values-based goal of building and strengthening relationships?*

You can apply this method to virtually every aspect of life; the mastery practice of achieving greater social support is just one of an infinite number of applications of this system that will enhance your health and wellbeing.

It is important to maintain your intention, throughout the day, to continually examine what you are practicing in this way, and shifting your practice as necessary to come into alignment with your values and goals. When you do, you will discover that your life is truly your own moment-by-moment creation and that you have tremendous power to shape it. And you will have mastered a skill that gives you the freedom to create ever higher levels of mastery and wellbeing and to live a happier, healthier, more vibrant life.

ᘉ

In the chapters that follow you will apply this basic method to the personal life values that, when consciously engaged, have been scientifically shown to best support and enhance health and wellbeing. You will also learn many other useful practices to help you mine the full potential of living in alignment with your values.

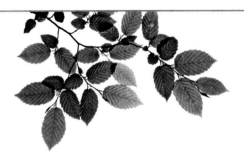

Part IV

Mindfulness-Based Mastery and Wellbeing Practices

By now you have a solid foundation in the nature of illness and suffering and the benefits and practice of mindfulness. And if you have followed any of the suggestions in Part III, Valued-Action Practice, you have begun your mindfulness-based mastery and wellbeing practice. Congratulations! You are probably already experiencing your illness very differently and feeling some relief, and this is just the start. Part IV expands your toolbox with ten more evidence-based practices, which evolved out of epidemiological trials data. By the time you conclude this section, your toolbox will be full and you will always be able to find new opportunities to reinforce your sense of mastery and achieve greater wellbeing.

13 Practice Gratitude

We begin the chapters of Part 4 with one of the simplest mindfulness-based mastery and wellbeing practices of all: gratitude.

Research psychologist Robert Emmons defines gratitude as *a felt sense of wonder, thankfulness, and appreciation for life.* In his studies, Emmons found that when we make gratitude an intentional and frequent practice, we develop the ability to elevate our mood simply by recalling our memories of being grateful.[1] In fact, when grateful people are asked about past events, they tend to exhibit "positive recall bias"—that is, their recollection casts their memories in a rosy light. By contrast, people who are anxious and depressed generally don't live with a grateful outlook, and are prone to negative recall bias; the negative images that proliferate in their minds compound their anxiety and depression.

It's also been shown that "more is better" in terms of using the constructive influence of gratitude to create greater health and wellbeing. Emmons and fellow researcher Michael McCullough demonstrated that the effects of practicing gratitude are "dose-dependent"—the more you practice, the better the results for your health.[2] And this is not unexpected; it's likely that any health-inducing, skill-building practice provides benefits in proportion to the amount of time and level of intention you bring to the practice.

According to Dr. Sonja Lyubomirsky, who has performed rigorous studies on the nature of happiness, expressing gratitude is the single most important skill-building practice to

One of the most evidence-based paths to greater wellbeing is the conscious practice of gratitude.

increase happiness.[3] She found in her studies that the healthiest and happiest people were comfortable expressing their appreciation for all they had. And increased happiness is not the only benefit: Lyubomirsky found that people who were consistently grateful were also more hopeful and more energetic than other people, and they reported experiencing positive emotions more frequently. As if these benefits were not enough, she also found that gratitude actually serves as an antidote to unpleasant emotions such as anger, anxiety, and depression.

Lyubomirsky's research led her to identify a list of eight specific ways in which gratitude increases happiness.[4] Interestingly, as you will see, these ways are all connected with practices discussed in other chapters of this book:

1. Grateful thinking promotes the savoring of positive life experiences.
2. Expressing gratitude bolsters self-worth and self-esteem. It encourages us to consider what we value about our present life.
3. Gratitude helps people cope with stress and trauma. It is an adaptive coping method by which we positively reinterpret stressful or negative life experiences. In those who are regularly grateful, traumatic memories are actually less likely to surface and are less intense when they do surface.
4. Grateful people are more likely to help others because they are more aware of the kind and caring acts of others, and they feel compelled to reciprocate.
5. Gratitude helps build social bonds, strengthening existing relationships and nurturing new ones. When we feel

gratitude toward others, even if we never express it, we experience closer relationships with them. Also, grateful people are seen as being easier to be with than less positive people, and therefore are more likely to make friends.

6. Gratitude reduces comparisons with others, so we experience less envy and jealousy.

7. The practice of gratitude is incompatible with negative emotions. We feel less fear, anger, and defensiveness during times when we are feeling thankful than at other times.

8. Gratitude prevents us from taking the pleasant things in our lives for granted.

Lyubomirsky recommends making a conscious decision to adopt a variety of gratitude practices. Some people may have an affinity for one type of practice, she found, while other people prefer a different kind. For people who enjoy writing, a gratitude journal is very effective. Although the optimal frequency of journaling will vary by individual, her lab research revealed that making weekly entries had greater impact than journaling three times a week. Still, some people enjoy the routine of making daily gratitude journal entries.[5]

Research psychologist Anthony Ong and his team found that experiencing positive emotions helps us disengage from or disidentify with traumatic and other negative events.[6] In this way, the positive emotions we experience in the midst of difficulty help us develop psychophysiological resilience and thereby cope better with the situation. Participation in a skill building–based support group can help those going through a difficult period learn to practice gratitude, as well as mindfulness and other healthy practices, during rough patches in order to better function psychologically and physiologically.

In the studies I cited earlier, Emmons and McCullough discovered that those who consciously practiced feeling more gratitude in their daily lives also *engaged in better self-care*, as evidenced by improving their behavior related to exercise, nutrition, and sleep. They also demonstrated more caring and empathy for those around them.[7] These results indicate that a simple gratitude practice can contribute to a sense of being in control of one's life, thereby increasing health and happiness.

I first became intrigued by the health effects of gratitude when I attended a workshop in the mid-1990s at the Institute for HeartMath, which had just introduced a biofeedback program called the FreezeFramer, recently replaced by the emWave. These devices utilize a photoplethysmograph sensor, attached to a finger, that measures beat-to-beat changes in capillary blood flow. The device then uses this measurement to determine heart rate variability (HRV). On the Freeze-Framer, the user's HRV itself was then used to drive a fun, animated interactive hot-air balloon ride on any computer. As we workshop attendees were told to think of reasons we were grateful to someone, and our feelings of gratitude subsequently increased, the balloon on the monitor rose higher. When we stopped experiencing gratitude, the balloon slowly sank to the ground. Since high HRV is a sign of excellent cardiovascular health, this is still one more reason to develop gratitude.

Biofeedback clinicians commonly use photoplethysmography to help clients increase their HRV. While hooked up, the client is instructed to breathe diaphragmatically. The clinician may then introduce autogenic imagery, which is known to improve physiological functioning. A simple example would be to sit quietly with eyes closed while imagining your limbs getting heavy and warm and your forehead getting cool. Autogenic training such as this can bring about physiologically similar cardiovascular improvements as gratitude practice, and when combined with grateful thoughts, the health benefits are magnified. This focus on gratitude is what's unique about the Institute for HeartMath approach, as reflected in the instructions they give people hooked up to the FreezeFramer or emWave:

> Put your attention on the area around your heart. Put the hand without the sensor on your heart. Imagine your breath going in and out through the area of your heart and breathe slowly and diaphragmatically. Now focus on creating a genuine feeling of appreciation and care for someone or something positive in your life. Really allow yourself to feel deep gratitude.

Simple relaxation techniques don't increase HRV as much as real or imagined experiences of gratitude. In an early Institute for HeartMath study, after one month of practice, subjects evidenced a 23 percent drop in cortisol and a 100 percent increase in dehydroepiandrosterone (DHEA), an endogenous steroid hormone that is produced from cholesterol.[8] This dramatic increase in DHEA is significant because the substance is necessary for the production of sex steroids and plays a role in elevating mood, increasing lean body mass, and improving memory. It also helps protect against cancer and cardiovascular disease. Unfortunately, people spend a fortune taking DHEA supplements, the efficacy and safety of which are controversial, when the DHEA we produce ourselves in our adrenals, gonads, and brain is made in exactly the right formula and dose for each individual.

Gratitude can play an important role in healing, even under circumstances that might seem unlikely. Some cancer patients have related dramatic and wonderful examples of how this works. Terribly sick as a result of their chemotherapy treatment, they have felt gratitude for losing their hair and for being sick to their stomachs. They were able to feel grateful for these horrific side effects because they were proof that the chemotherapy agents were effectively killing the fastest growing cells. Hair and stomach cells are among the fastest growing, yet cancer cells grow even faster. Since the drugs target the fastest growing cells, the awful gastritis and hair loss served as reassurance that the chemotherapy agents were killing cancer cells, which imbued these otherwise miserable experiences with a silver lining.

Gratitude: An Alternative to Medication

New, emerging leaders in the fields of psychiatry and psychology are finding skill-building practices such as gratitude to be a healthier and more efficacious treatment for mild depression than antidepressants, which are now the most commonly prescribed class of drugs.[9] Except for major depressive disorder, where people lack the energy to do any of their daily activities, these drugs can sometimes do more harm than good. Prescribing unnecessary antidepressants is problematic; it puts an enormous drain on an already broken healthcare system and the drugs must be taken for the rest of the person's life. By contrast, offering skill-building tools such as gratitude practice improves people's health and helps them develop a sense of mastery. And once you learn such skills, the endogenous effects are available to you anywhere and anytime, at no charge.

Begin Your Gratitude Practice

There are many ways to practice gratitude. Look for things you can feel grateful for throughout the day—something as big as a loved one in your life or as small as putting on clothing that's still warm from the dryer. Or think of a specific time when you felt thankful, and then compare the feeling of gratitude with feelings of judgment or scorn you can recall. Where thoughts and feelings are concerned, if it feels good, it's health-inducing.

A gratitude journal is a quick and easy way to begin a gratitude practice. I recommend you consider a variety of categories when journaling. For example, you can write down what you're grateful for in this present moment, what you're good at, what you like about where you live, what you do for work, goals you have achieved, opportunities that are available to you, and people who contribute to your health and happiness. Some people prefer to focus on only one object of gratitude each day; others like to routinely list five. Regardless of the approach you take, expressing gratitude in a journal reduces anxiety and depression by focusing on preferences and skill building.

If you dislike journaling altogether, you can practice in other ways. One option is to compose a letter to someone important in your life, expressing your appreciation of him or her. Even if you never actually send it, the act of writing itself opens your heart and has health-inducing effects.

A third method involves no writing at all. From time to time I have practiced by simply thinking of three things I'm grateful for before getting out of bed each morning. I spend a total of no more than a minute at a time on this practice, yet it shines a positive light on my entire day.

Further Suggestions for Gratitude Practice

- Using conscious intention, cultivate a natural sense of wonder, excitement, and appreciation for the newness of every experience.
- Notice how often you take things in your life for granted. Practice feeling appreciation for those experiences instead.
- Even an unpleasant experience, such as going through an invasive medical test, is an opportunity to practice gratitude—in this case gratitude for the technology that allows disease to be diagnosed and treated much earlier.
- Whenever you find yourself thinking *I have to* or *I have no choice,* be grateful that you are able to see that those thoughts are fictional, and that you actually do have choice.
- Throughout the day, recall pleasant events and plan how to have more of them. Then practice feeling grateful for your ability to intentionally create such events.
- Whenever you're feeling anxious or depressed, think of something about the situation for which you can have gratitude. Don't deny the reality of the situation or the reality of your emotions, but if you consciously look for it, you will find something good about the situation, possibly the learning opportunity. Practice gratitude for this.

- When you interact with someone, think of something you appreciate about that person. Just doing that one, simple thing will improve communication and connection. This can be as small and brief as appreciating the efficiency or smile of the checkout clerk at the supermarket.
- Start and end every day by thinking of something or someone for which you feel gratitude. It can sometimes help to do this while holding your hand over your heart.
- Throughout the day, ask yourself whether, in this moment, you're feeling critical or grateful. Then intentionally think of something for which you feel thankful.

◌

As you have learned, though it may be the simplest of all mindfulness-based mastery and wellbeing practices, gratitude is a powerfully transformative one. Interestingly, you may notice that it is also primarily an internal experience, involving awareness of feelings and conscious direction of thought. Just the simple act of intentionally practicing gratitude helps us feel in charge of our lives, and helps us increase our level of resilience. In the next chapter we'll look at a practice that requires translating your internal experience into positive action: loving self-care.

14 Practice Loving Self-Care

"S elf-care" is a straightforward term that encompasses all the actions we take during the day to nurture our health. Finding the right physicians to help us manage our conditions, receiving appropriate treatments, eating a nutrient-dense diet, and getting sufficient rest are all examples of self-care. But what is *loving* self-care?

When we practice loving self-care, we give ourselves the gift of full, mindful presence, moment by moment, while we are engaged in self-care activities. This is especially beneficial for people living with serious or chronic medical conditions, as the ability to be fully present to this experience builds mastery and increases feelings of wellbeing.

Excellent nutrition, adequate sleep and exercise, skilled and knowledgeable medical care, complying with treatments, and dropping unhealthy habits—the typical concerns of behavioral medicine—are all critical in maintaining health. But for people living with such conditions as autoimmune diseases or cancer, they don't go far enough. Of critical importance is to pursue self-care with an attitude of caring for ourselves with the same commitment and focus we would bring to the task of caring for a newborn baby: fully engaged in the activity and acting out of love. Mindfulness practice and the new psychotherapies—Acceptance and Commitment Therapy, Mindfulness-Based Cognitive Therapy, and the practices recommended in this chapter—can help us achieve this kind of enhanced, more meaningful, and more effective self-care.

The analogy of caring for an infant, who isn't yet capable

Loving self-care involves forming the mindfulness habit of asking yourself throughout
the day: What do I need in this moment?

of telling us what it needs, is a very helpful one because of the
degree of attention this requires; we need to continually watch
for signs of what the baby needs to be safe and healthy and
respond to these signs as immediately as we can. Engaging in
loving self-care means frequently asking ourselves what we
need in order to feel better and improve our health. This becomes a valued *way of life*, one that carries with it a sense of
meaning and purpose. Parents often find meaning and purpose in caring for their young children, who are utterly dependent upon them. In much the same way, our own care,
survival, vitality, and quality of life are intrinsically worthy
endeavors.

Unfortunately, most people fall far short of devoting this
level of attention to their own care. They may lovingly attend
to their pets, other people, their gardens, and even their cars
but not turn the same quality of attention toward themselves.
They may receive wonderful advice concerning diet, exercise,
sleep, and changing their habits, only to ignore it because
they haven't yet committed to loving self-care practice. Yet the
benefits of such a practice are many. For the chronically ill, it
not only ensures better self-care, as one might expect; it also
makes for a rewarding mindfulness practice and increased
happiness. And these benefits, in turn, improve health outcomes.

Choosing Self-Care

We make choices about how we care for ourselves all the time,
but we usually make them without conscious awareness. A
commitment to living with presence and intentionality can
change that. For an example of how this works, let's return to
a practice I wrote about in chapter 11, What Are You Choos-

ing? This morning I found myself thinking *I have to go all the way in to San Francisco for another dreaded medical appointment.* Practicing loving self-care, I replaced *have to* with *want to* because, even though it's no fun, it's a productive and meaningful activity for my self-care. Keeping the appointment and recognizing that I was doing so out of choice connected me to its meaning and purpose. And I knew that if I used the whole experience to practice staying present with my inner experiences, I would build mindfulness and mastery skills, contributing in highly effective ways to my own health, happiness, and wellbeing. Following through on the appointment would also mean that I was authentically living my life in accordance with my personal life values—it would be an act of self-care firmly rooted in the Valued-Action Practice I outlined in chapters 10 through 12.

This is the same process I engage when recognizing choices concerning food, exercise, formal sitting meditation, or any other aspect of self-care. I also tune in to intentionality and choice when I go in for an MRI, an endoscopy, or any other unpleasant procedure; this is loving self-care. Recently, I chose to go in for a repeat esophagogastroduodenoscopy and colonoscopy. Drinking the four liters of polyethylene glycol solution the evening before was, as usual, extremely disgusting and very close to being intolerable. However, in practicing loving self-care, I was able to remind myself that I was doing it out of choice, and that every time I choose to take care of myself I am cultivating a sense of mastery and living by my values.

Loving Self-Care in the Hospital

Recently, my wife needed major surgery, and I stayed with her in her hospital room round the clock during her three-day stay. It provided me with an opportunity to practice another kind of loving self-care. Being there to care and advocate for her was the most loving thing I could do for myself because instead of staying home and worrying, I was able to be where I could actually do something whenever she needed help.

Being a patient in a hospital can be very disempowering because your care is completely in the hands of the doctors, nurses, techs, and nurse assistants. Where we normally take care of ourselves and value our independence, as inpatients we are dependent on the care of the hospital staff. The way we can practice loving self-care in this environment is to allow ourselves to accept and appreciate the care we receive from those on whom we are dependent.

Not all doctors, nurses, techs, and nurse assistants deliver good care. Most do—or they would no longer be working in the hospital—but there will be days when you will get a certain nurse or nurse assistant who should be in another line of work. In that situation, the way to practice loving self-care is to treat them and yourself with respect. Try to work with them, but if that doesn't work, request to see the charge nurse. In this way, you are practicing loving self-care.

Loving self-care includes making sure there's a family member, friend, or professional who will stay with you day and night. Many of us have trouble asking for such a big favor from family or friends. It's quite a commitment to stay overnight with someone in the hospital, but making the request is part of practicing loving self-care. Some of us also have trouble receiving the help our friends or family offer; we don't want to inconvenience anyone. But this is a way to take valued action and practice loving self-care. Others of us are knowledgeable enough to know how hospitals work and how to get our needs met in a hospital environment, but when we are sick enough to be in the hospital, we may be too heavily medicated or otherwise altered to be able to advocate for ourselves. For that reason, loving self-care includes acknowledging our vulnerabilities and requesting someone to advocate for us. Even with an advocate with you all the time, it's still important to cultivate a caring relationship with your nurse and nurse assistant each shift. Not only will you get better care if you do, but it will help you to feel safer in what can often be a frightening environment. And it, too, is a way of practicing loving self-care.

Also, despite doctors' and nurses' good care, complications are not unusual. Loving self-care includes monitoring and reporting even the slightest changes in signs and symptoms.

Playing Our Best Hand

Life consists not in holding good cards, but in playing those we do hold well.
—Josh Billings

The meaning and purpose we derive from loving self-care are especially important for those of us who have been dealt a bad hand. Some people are luckier in life than others; some are born with terrible genetics while others inherit outstanding genes. But genetics is only one factor. In most cases, the ways in which we live our lives are exponentially more important than our genes.

When you live with any type of debilitating medical condition, it can often seem like you have to focus far too much on self-care—all day, every day. Many people in support groups I've facilitated have expressed how depressed they feel that so much of their time is spent going to medical appointments: events that often entail fear and discomfort. But when you add the mindfulness component to all of this very necessary self-care activity, you can use it as a means to achieve a sense of mastering your life.

Loving Self-Care, Want, and Need

Often, we can improve our health by acting in accordance with what we need rather than what we want. For example, I often want chocolate, pie, cake, or ice cream when people around me are eating them. But I almost never eat more than one bite because I know I don't *need* any of them. I live with a severe malabsorption syndrome, which means I don't absorb all the nutrients in the food I eat. This is a serious condition because the nutrients in food make adenosine triphosphate (ATP), which allows the mitochondria in our cells to make the energy that keeps all our cells functioning. One of the ways I practice loving self-care is to remind myself that eating more than one bite of any foods that lack nutrients—like sugary treats—is equivalent to scratching an itch for five minutes straight; in both cases, it will do more harm than good. On those very rare occasions when I decide to eat an entire piece of cake or pie and ice cream, I practice loving self-care by eating mindfully, focusing all my attention on savoring every moment.

Without mindfulness, we end up attending to our wants instead of our needs. It's important to learn to clearly discern the difference:

- *Wants* are those things we think will bring us comfort or pleasure.
- *Needs* relate to an inner knowing of what the body requires for health in terms of nutrition, sleep, exercise, and stress management.

It can be a challenge to spend considerable time engaged in self-care—in what we truly need—when we would rather be working or playing or chasing what we want. Unless we use our self-care time to practice mindfulness and lovingkindness toward ourselves, these activities can contribute to a host of unhealthy emotional states: anger, frustration, isolation, sadness, loss of meaning and purpose, lack of joy, guilt, and shame.

Also, in addition to needing to spend more time engaged in self-care activities, many people living with chronic health challenges have to postpone or cancel activities quite regularly and without warning because of fatigue, pain, malaise, flare-ups of various disabilities, or emergency medical appointments. Learning how to infuse all of these situations with loving self-care and presence—to give ourselves what we need instead of fixing on what we want—can serve as an antidote to the common feeling that life is passing us by.

Exercise—Don't Believe Everything You Think
It is vital to know when you are *genuinely* too tired or in too much pain to exercise—needing to rest instead—and when these feelings are really

Loving self-care is about re-placing *have to* with *choose to*.

just thoughts that you can observe with curiosity, and even amusement, reflections of what you want or prefer. I get practice discerning the difference when I'm on the elliptical cross-trainer early in the morning. I often become aware that I want to get off because I'm not enjoying myself and I feel too tired. My mind creates logical, convincing reasons why I could skip exercise this morning. Mindfulness and dedication to loving self-care allow me to enjoy the parade of thoughts that are telling me it would be okay to get off the machine and go have something to eat instead.

Because I can recognize these thoughts for what they are—nothing but transient mental events—I'm able to let them go while I take loving self-care by staying on the machine for the full forty minutes I set aside for daily aerobic exercise. Listening to lively music with a beat helps immensely. Following my forty minutes on the machine, I do thirty minutes of stretching and strengthening of my core muscles. At the end of the exercise period, not only have I done my body an immense favor, I also have reinforced a sense of mastery. When I live by my values, and in this case I value the health benefits of exercise, it is very clear that I am the master of my life. This is very empowering and creates the states of mind that are most likely to enhance health and wellbeing.

If I instead give in to my insubstantial thoughts, stop exercising, and hurry to the breakfast table, I know from experience that I'll feel guilty, weak, and helpless and I'll be letting myself down in terms of self-care. Not only that, but instead of seeing myself as the master of my life, I'm more likely to see myself as an unfortunate victim of circumstances.

Cultivating a Healthy State of Mind through Body Mechanics

I have often been impressed when I see Cesar Millan, TV's *The Dog Whisperer,* teaching dog owners to improve their dog's self-esteem by holding its tail up, whether they're out for walks or just sitting with the dog. We are like dogs in this way. When we walk with good posture, we feel more aware and more awake, and we feel better about ourselves. Walking around with shoulders slouched forward and head down is not conducive to awareness or to healthy self-esteem. Maintaining a downward gaze with our eyes creates a similar result and interferes with being fully awake and alert to our surroundings. Shallow chest breathing is another aspect of body mechanics that diminishes self-esteem, and the resulting hypoxia interferes with our ability to be fully present with our moment-to-moment experience.

Those of us with chronic illness may need to get creative about maintaining body mechanics that are conducive to a healthy state of mind. For example, to retrieve an object from the floor or a low drawer, it would be best to squat. But in my case, because of severe arthritis, I have had to devise other ways to retrieve low objects. Maintaining healthy body mechanics under these circumstances—an immensely valuable act of loving self-care—requires mindfulness and experimentation.

Walking and Self-Care

While we may first think of food, rest, and medical treatments as the mainstays of loving self-care, the simple act of walking with great attention can also be an important loving self-care practice. This is something else I have discovered for myself.

I have very severe osteoporosis. Not long ago I was told that the treatments for this condition were no longer working and I immediately had visions of falling and breaking a hip. But because by then I'd had lots of practice in loving self-care, I asked myself what I could do to care for myself in light of this new information. I realized that I didn't have to passively await an "inevitable" hip fracture. I became empowered to practice mindful walking throughout the day to avoid a fall. I could have gotten angry about needing to be so careful; instead, I have used the severe osteoporosis (and arthritis) as an opportunity to practice mindfulness. This is another way for me to live as the master of my life. I have come to realize that it doesn't matter how many health challenges we live with—as long as we practice making conscious choices regarding how to care for ourselves throughout the day, we can enjoy a rich life.

Walking mindfully has other profound benefits. For example, with aging, it is all too easy to get sloppy with posture, which exacerbates spinal degeneration and results in shallower breathing. This negatively impacts the functioning of various organs in the abdominal cavity as well as the brain. Walking mindfully and erect while breathing diaphragmatically is also associated with a greater sense of presence and connection with the environment. With practice, walking mindfully can become a habit and an act of loving self-care.

Partnerships in Loving Self-Care

One of the best ways to develop loving self-care is to have a life partner and/or close friends with whom you have a mutually caring relationship. (A one-sided caring relationship, in which someone else cares for you with no corresponding effort on your part, doesn't work here, as it can reinforce feelings of powerlessness.) If you don't have such a close relationship, you can gain some of the same benefits by joining a small group: a psychotherapy group, a support group, or any other regular gathering where the members are able to be authentic and caring. The shared experience will serve to make it easier to practice loving self-care.

ᔆ

Here we have explored the meanings of the mindfulness practice of loving self-care, and I have given some examples of how I incorporate this practice into daily living. When you

apply yourself to the practice in your own life, you will discover many more ways in which you can empower yourself
to feel better and find new meaning in the necessary tasks you
engage in to support your health.

Suggestions for Practicing Loving Self-Care

- As you learned to do in chapter 11, eliminate the words
  should and *have to* from your vocabulary. Anytime you
  find yourself dreading going somewhere or doing a
  certain activity in support of your self-care, ask yourself
  how you would feel if you cancelled it; would you have
  regrets? If the activity is something you value, replace
  should with *want to*.
- Also practice saying "No." If an activity you dread isn't
  conducive to health, recognize that you are choosing that
  activity and reject that choice. For example, you may feel
  depressed about an upcoming visit with someone who
  always seems to leave you feeling worse: perhaps you
  only do it out of a sense of guilt or obligation. Recognize
  that this mental state is not consistent with loving self-
  care, and make a different choice.
- Focus all your attention on the activity at hand. This is
  a challenge with routine activities that you can literally
  do with your eyes closed, such as showering. It's less
  of a challenge with activities that require our full attention, such as driving a car on slippery roads or carving a
  turkey.
- As you go through the day, and especially whenever
  you experience an unpleasant sensation or emotion, ask
  yourself what you need in that moment.
- Whenever you are in doubt about how to proceed—even
  concerning really small decisions such as what to eat—
  approach the choice as a loving self-care practice; simply
  choose what is best for you in the same way a good parent would choose what is healthiest for a young child.
- When you become aware of thoughts urging you to do
  something unhealthy, perhaps skipping exercise or eat-

ing unhealthy food or too much food, remind yourself that thoughts are nothing but insubstantial mental constructs: you do not need to obey them.

- When you notice any unpleasant emotions, ask yourself if your thoughts are aligned with your personal life values. If the answer is no, then appreciate that you can let those thoughts just float on by as if they were clouds in the sky.
- Do more activities that leave you feeling better afterward, and do fewer activities that leave you feeling worse.
- Practice self-compassion. Remember how you have felt when you have extended compassion to someone else and give that gift to yourself. When you notice self-critical thoughts, soothe yourself just as you would a dear friend.
- Practice good posture. You will feel better about yourself when you stand tall in good postural alignment. This is one of the most loving ways you can treat yourself.
- Practice conscious breathing; there are many methods. Most of the time, your breathing will be unconscious and that is perfectly okay. But slowing your breathing from time to time throughout the day and making sure you're breathing diaphragmatically can improve your state of mind and physiological functioning. The calming effect is instantaneous. You will soon realize that this practice gives you a sense of control, allowing you to cultivate mastery.
- Remember that every little thing you do to care for yourself in a loving way matters—sometimes enough to create a noticeable improvement in your health and wellbeing.

೦೩

Over the course of this discussion, you may have noticed that one of the "tricks" to loving self-care is accepting the reality that, because you are living with chronic illness, you need to make a deeper commitment to your health and wellbeing than others might have to make. Rather than fight this reality, or get depressed or angry about it, the key is to acknowledge it and find within it myriad opportunities to achieve greater mastery and wellbeing—to take your health into your own hands. In the next chapter, we will delve further into the importance of acceptance by exploring the practice of self-acceptance: mindfully embracing the totality of your experience, including your mental and emotional states.

15 Practice Self-Acceptance

We need to face what we are thinking and experiencing, and to tolerate the initial discomfort of doing so, if we are to make significant change.
—Cancer survivor and psychooncologist Dr. Alistair Cunningham

Ralph Waldo Emerson once complained to his physician that he felt depressed, and the doctor recommended a long sea voyage. Emerson took his advice. At the end of the journey he wrote in his diary: "It didn't work; when I got off the ship in Naples, the first person I met was myself!" As Lawrence LeShan writes, sometimes it's important to change our external circumstances, but without self-acceptance, the external changes we make won't be very useful.[1]

A Modern Epidemic

The lack of self-acceptance is everywhere today—most likely the result of living in cultures that punish people for their undesirable behavior instead of helping them find healthier behaviors. The tragedy of this inability to accept ourselves is that when we are taught that *we* are wrong rather than that our *behavior* is wrong, we develop shame: the belief that we're not okay the way we are. This leads us to behave in ways that are not in harmony with our deepest values and authenticity. Instead, we go to great lengths to avoid thoughts, emotions, and situations that could trigger even more feelings of shame. Doing so strengthens and reinforces shame, leading to further

Self-acceptance is practiced by tuning in to your inner subjective experience as much as possible throughout the day.

inauthentic behavior, still more shame, and self-rejection. It is an endless downward spiral in which far too many people in the world seem to have become hopelessly trapped.

But each of us has the power to consciously intervene through a self-acceptance practice—and break the cycle. The path to health and happiness involves cultivating unconditional acceptance and presence that help us more fully engage with life, living with a sense of mastery.

The Antidote to Experiential Avoidance

This chapter is about a proven antidote to the unhealthy practice I described in chapter 5: experiential avoidance. As we learned in that chapter, the uncomfortable or frightening thoughts, mental images, sensations, or emotions that arise naturally within all of us have the potential to do tremendous harm, *but only if we try to resist or reject them.* When we employ strategies to avoid the discomfort they generate, we risk dissipating our energy to the point of exhaustion.[2] This results in part from the bodily constriction that accompanies our avoidance—we tense up. Clearly, wasting your energy in this way is a drain on your health.

By contrast, when you put the antidote to experiential avoidance into practice, you reduce physiological stress. Each time you let yourself acknowledge and accept your inner subjective experience, you undergo an automatic physiological response of slowing and deepening respiration. This creates healthy heart rhythms.[3] Your entire chest wall relaxes, and this is often connected with a so-called "heart-opening" feeling. Neurofeedback researchers Evgeny and Bronya Vaschillo have found that this response also creates healthier brainwave rhythms.[4]

Research psychologist Jason Luoma has written that acceptance can only be found by looking—
acceptingly—within.[5] Behaviors that distract us from our inner conflicts, no matter how good they make us feel, never
lead to self-acceptance. We can only find self-acceptance when
we are willing to live in full contact with our own inner experience.

It is important to understand that giving up the struggle
to avoid inner states you consider unpleasant is not a nihilistic
acceptance of suffering. On the contrary, a primary reason to
do it is to free up your energy so you can experience a greater
degree of aliveness and joy in life.[6]

It's worth noting that all of the practices in this book help
build acceptance, and this is because they are mindfulness
and mastery based. For example, once you become practiced
at finding meaning and purpose in everyday activities, you
will find it easier to accept all the things in your life that you
cannot change. After you have absorbed the principles contained in this chapter, you will find ample opportunity for
self-acceptance in the other practice chapters as well.

An Empowering Fact: Uncomfortable Inner States Are Inherently Harmless

Luoma writes that uncomfortable thoughts, images, sensations, and emotions are harmless—regardless of how awful or
frightening they may seem.[7] Feelings of shock, terror, anxiety,
sadness, frustration, rage, pain, fatigue, embarrassment, and
shame are all survivable—always! This is not only welcome
news for people who have lived in fear of their inner states;
it is a key understanding in the practice of self-acceptance. As
you learn through practice that this is true, you will become
stronger psychologically and physiologically and increase
your ability to live with mastery and wellbeing.[8]

Mindfulness as a Self-Acceptance Practice
Mindfulness practice is conducive to self-acceptance for a
very good reason: because self-acceptance is a byproduct of

the mindfulness skill of recognizing thoughts as transient mental events or constructs—of repeatedly witnessing their harmlessness. When we develop this understanding of the ephemeral nature of thoughts through practice, we find even the most uncomfortable thoughts far less troubling, and we gain confidence that we can handle them.

The Usefulness of Fears and Aversions

Approaching your fears and aversions mindfully deepens your self-acceptance practice. The key is to view them as interesting growth opportunities rather than as things to reject and avoid. Do this over time, and you will become less and less likely to attempt to reject those parts of yourself.

Interestingly, psychologist and co-creator of Mindfulness-Based Cognitive Therapy (MBCT) Zindel Segal et al found that when we increase our awareness through increased perception, we find fewer things about ourselves that engender aversion and fear in the first place.[9] And when we engage in mindfulness practice over time, we generate fewer of the negative attributions that create aversion and fears.[10]

Because fears and aversions naturally arise when you live with chronic health challenges, these conditions offer you opportunities to learn how to live with greater acceptance of your experiences and yourself. Cancer survivor, psychotherapist, and mindfulness teacher Elana Rosenbaum puts it this way: "It became clear that the more I could let go and accept these limitations the better I felt and the freer I became. The more I lived in the present moment as it was, rather than what I wished it would be, the happier I felt."[11]

Identifying Values and Needs

The greatest value of unpleasant states is that they help you identify your values and needs. For example, anger can serve to inform you that you're fused with the belief that the situation or person that sparked your anger *should be* different in some way. Sadness can let you know that something you value has been lost, or that you have not yet achieved or acquired it. Shame tells you that you are judging yourself as flawed. If you fail to accept all these rich inner-life experiences, you are practicing *self-rejection* rather than acceptance. And in doing so, you disempower yourself, losing rich opportunities to live with mastery and create healthier states.

Avoidance and Medication

Our culture incorrectly informs us that pain and all forms of emotional distress are avoidable and *should be* avoided at all cost, and the pharmaceutical industry spends billions of dollars to introduce and reinforce this unhealthy belief. Perhaps the industry's ultimate disconnect from reality lies in its introduction of a nearly infinite array of "anti-aging" products. But pain, stress, sickness, and aging are a normal part of life, and our attempts to avoid them, bolstered by industry propaganda, cause considerable unnecessary suffering and self-rejection.

Remember, unpleasant states are harmless in and of themselves. But what can be harmful is the behavior we adopt—including taking unnecessary and possibly dangerous medications—in an attempt to avoid experiencing these states. Choosing unnecessary medication is contradictory to mastery and self-acceptance, which reinforce one another. Neither is possible when we rely on drugs to short-circuit the personal skill-building that can actually reduce our suffering.

Accepting Disease

In the *New York Times* bestseller *Blindsided,* author Richard Cohen's courageous transparency reveals what can happen when someone living with a chronic, progressively debilitating disease believes physical health and athletic prowess are prerequisites for living with dignity, mastery, and wellbeing. The extent to which he tried to hide his multiple sclerosis symptoms directly correlated with the degree of his suffering.

In a world where physical attractiveness and strength are mistakenly equated with mastery and wellbeing, it's easy to see why we instinctively try to hide our physical limitations.

However, Christopher Reeve, in his heroic visits to testify before congressional committees in order to educate them in the
need for funding for medical research, demonstrated for us all
that quadriplegia and dignity can go together. Actor Michael
J. Fox has allowed the world to see the face of Parkinson's
disease, and that, even while flailing his limbs—the result of
medication—he is still living with dignity. Both actors fully
accepted their new physical limitations without losing their
sense of mastery and wellbeing.

Self-Acceptance, Ambiguity,
and the Sensations of Respiration
When we live with a chronic illness, we are likely to live with
ambiguity, uncertain about the course of the disease, whether
opportunistic infections may set in, and whether a new treatment protocol will work. We never know when our plans will
have to be changed because of symptom flare-ups. Vidyamala Burch, who teaches mindfulness practices for those living with chronic pain, suggests using the breath to ride these
waves of change: "Living *with* life's continual changes instead
of fighting against them creates strength and stability. And
all the time the practice is held by the kindly breath, soothing
and caressing all of your experience."[12] Her approach of gently living in harmony with the natural processes of respiration
builds acceptance.

Accepting Pain
There is solid science behind the value of accepting pain.
In randomized controlled trials on pain management using
control versus acceptance, university students were divided
into experimental, control-based, and placebo groups. Using a cold pressor task (placing the subjects' hands in ice
water) to produce pain artificially, the participants in the acceptance group—who were instructed to fully acknowledge
their painful sensations—demonstrated significantly greater
tolerance of pain compared to those who were instructed to
try to control or not feel the pain.[13]

Self-acceptance can be practiced by allowing yourself to fully experience your feelings.

Research psychologist Lance McCracken teaches that one of the most helpful aspects of mindfulness-based mastery practices for those with chronic pain is that they lead to an acceptance of pain and disability, an ability to disengage and detach from the pain, and improved overall quality of life.[14] The pain *doesn't even need to diminish* in order to reduce suffering and improve one's quality of life. This is because, as we learned in Part 1 in the chapter on theories of suffering, so much of our suffering is caused by the negative attributions we assign to pain and not from the actual painful sensation. Again, accepting our pain and disability means accepting ourselves and what we cannot change.

Accepting Anxiety

Before I facilitated my first daylong workshop at Spirit Rock Meditation Center, I felt considerable anxiety. One source of it was cognitive fusion with the belief that I had nothing of value to offer the participants. I had attended many such workshops there, but all the presenters were well known in their fields and experienced in appearing before large audiences, whereas I was practically unknown. But the greatest source of my anxiety was not accepting my anxiety and fear.

I continued to experience some anxiety on the day of the workshop. But, applying the lesson I learned when demonstrating my work to an audience of peers a few years earlier (described in chapter 5), in the morning I allowed myself to fully experience it, which dramatically and instantly reduced it. In fact, I was able to use the remaining anxiety to motivate me to keep my heart open to everything I was going through, because I knew it was the best antidote. By the end of the day,

by staying with the anxiety and vulnerability, I had developed
greater self-acceptance and mastery.

Self-Acceptance, Authenticity, and Relationship Building

When you allow yourself to be fully present with your
thoughts and feelings, you grant yourself the possibility to
express them in authentically healthy ways. This lets you pursue meaningful relationships—which is another very healthy
mindfulness-based practice. You give the supportive people
in your life the opportunity to respond to your authenticity.
And when they have that opportunity, you will find that they
are more likely to respond with understanding, empathy, and
connection.

A good "laboratory" for practicing this authentic communication is a support group appropriate to your situation.
When you are with people who validate and accept you as
you are, and recognize you for your contributions, you will
find it easier to accept yourself. This is a tremendous benefit of
support groups. And there is proof that it works. Supportive-
expressive psychoeducational groups for people with cancer
or AIDS, for example, have proven to build self-acceptance
because the authentic self-expression that takes place in such
groups both reduces the intensity of harmful negative emotions and builds acceptance for such emotions.[15]

The meaning and purpose you derive from the relation-
ship-building activities of your self-acceptance practice serve
as strong paths to self-acceptance as well. If you live each day
so that at the end of it you feel good about how you lived
it—if you have a sense of satisfaction that you made someone
else's life better, for example—it's only natural to believe that
your life has meaning. Self-acceptance and mastery are both
benefits of such a way of life.

What We Need Not Accept

The most health-inducing approach is to accept all our experiences, even the distressing ones associated with illness. Yet for

those of us with physical challenges, it is important to distinguish what we need *not* accept as well. This is a key distinction. For example, when an oncologist tells a patient that the cancer is too far gone to treat, and to go home and get his or her affairs in order, the passive, helpless type of acceptance would involve following that injunction. Acceptance, from a mastery perspective, is quite different; it would involve, yes, accepting the diagnosis—*and* repudiating the prognosis and the oncologist's advice. The diagnosis is a fact, demonstrated through measurable tests. The prognosis is an educated guess based on probabilities, not certainties. We have no obligation to accept it any more than we are obligated to accept any other type of thought. One of the biggest predictors of who gets well, in fact, is the degree to which people accept rather than resist their diagnosis *and* then assertively do all they can to get well.[16]

Suggestions for Practicing Self-Acceptance

Unfortunately, if, like most people, you have spent a lifetime rejecting your inner experiences, it's not easy to change. When you've formed long-term habits of responding to internal and environmental stimuli in a certain prescribed way, it can seem like a Sisyphean task to react differently. But experts in the field have found effective ways to accomplish this. Countless people have done it, and with practice, there's no reason you can't break the cycle of self-rejection.

Psychology researcher Michael Twohig teaches that the place to start is to simply agree to be willing to try another way.[17] Then, according to ACT cofounder Steven Hayes the next step is to identify ways in which your usual responses are attempts to reduce suffering by avoiding certain internal experiences.[18]

Next, according to researcher Jonathan Abamowitz, it's important to identify ways in which these entrenched and automatic responses have the paradoxical effect of increasing your suffering.[19] Once you understand this, says Hayes, you have good motivation to practice acceptance.[20]

Following are a few more acceptance practices.

- One very effective way to develop self-acceptance consists of two steps: First, be compassionate with yourself
  each time you become aware of a painful thought or feeling, just as you would extend compassion to a loved one
  who is having a difficult time. Then remind yourself of
  the fundamental tenet of mindfulness: that your painful
  thoughts are just secretions of the brain and that, like the
  secretion of hormones, enzymes, and other information
  molecules, they are a natural human function. You do
  not have to embrace painful thoughts and feelings; you
  merely have to be willing to be present with them instead
  of looking for ways to run away.
- Set an intention to consciously practice acceptance in
  your daily life—acceptance of your thoughts, your
  emotional state, your physical condition, and any other
  aspects of your life you may be tempted to reject.
- When you feel anxiety or are becoming aware of self-
  deprecating thoughts, put your hand over your heart
  area, accept the fact that these thoughts and feelings are
  occurring, and extend compassion to yourself.
- A method that works well for some people is to start a
  journal of negative self-talk. The healing value is in the
  writing; it's not important to ever read the journal.
- Apologize to yourself. We commonly apologize to others
  for any negative, judgmental criticisms we may express;
  doing so helps maintain good relationships. Apologizing
  to ourselves makes for a healthy, nurturing relationship
  with ourselves.
- Make an agreement with yourself to be more accepting,
  appreciative, and understanding of yourself.
- Change your relationship to unpleasant thoughts and
  feelings by learning to see them as clouds floating across
  the sky—completely harmless. This can best be learned
  through a dedicated mindfulness practice, which takes
  time, so until you develop that skill, it's important to
  practice self-compassion by noting your experience. For

example, you might say to yourself, "I'm really suffering right now as a result of being so entangled with that
thought and this feeling."

- Build your mindfulness skills. Practice mindful awareness of thoughts, beliefs, images, feelings, emotions, and
  sensations, including all sensory experiences, regardless
  of whether they are based in the present environment—
  internal or external—or in a memory of a past sensory
  experience.
- Practice mindful awareness of the attributions or interpretations you attach to what you're thinking and
  feeling.
- Self-acceptance is often developed by being in relationships with individuals who are accepting and respectful
  of others. This applies to romantic relationships as well
  as work and play relationships. Make sure your relationships are healthy and supportive.

CR

There is a direct relationship between developing the ability
to accept the fullness of your inner subjective experience and
becoming better able to convey what you are thinking and
feeling to others. The more fully present you are with your
experience, the better able you are to mindfully discern your
state of mind moment by moment and the more opportunity
you have to tell people what is really true for you. This kind of
authentic self-expression builds strong, intimate relationships
as well as mastery and it is the subject of the next chapter.

16 Practice Authentic Self-Expression

It's as if the immune system hears self-expression as an order to start fighting . . .
—Lawrence LeShan, PhD

Psychologists used to believe that people who expressed the most negative emotions were the least healthy. But the work of University of Arizona psychophysiology researcher Dr. Gary Schwartz and others have demonstrated that we are more susceptible to cancer and other diseases if *we are very distressed but report that we are fine.*

Medical researcher George Solomon, MD, who coined the term *psychoimmunology* in the 1960s, reported that auto-immune diseases, infectious diseases, and cancer were associated with the inability to authentically express what we're thinking and feeling.[1] Research psychologists have also consistently found a strong association—after controlling for all potentially confounding variables—between health and emotional self-awareness and expression. Although it is only one determining factor in illness and there isn't a definitive causal link, the ability to express genuine thoughts and feelings has been so closely and consistently correlated with better health that I consider it an essential mindfulness-based mastery practice, particularly for those living with chronic health challenges.

A good way to begin a discussion of the practice of authentic self-expression—recognizing and communicating what we're genuinely thinking and feeling—is to examine some of the research demonstrating its myriad positive impacts on health. In this chapter I include results of studies that examine the topic from several different angles.

We can start with the work of research psychologist Lawrence LeShan, who pioneered the application of psychotherapy to improve longevity in advanced metastatic cancer patients. Over the course of his lengthy career, he consistently observed that the people who went into remission were those who had learned to "sing their own song" in life.

The Power of "No!"

"No" means "I am."
—Lawrence LeShan[2]

During the 1950s, LeShan discovered that he could tell that his psychotherapy sessions with hospitalized patients were getting results when the nursing staff began complaining about those patients; once deemed compliant, his most successful patients were now labeled "difficult" or "noncompliant." Suddenly, for example, when a nurse came in to do a procedure, the patient might say, "No, not right now!" As soon as these so-called difficult patients began to ask for what they wanted and to say "no" to what they didn't want, their health began to improve. LeShan's groundbreaking work provides dramatic examples of the health benefits of self-expression.

Many other researchers have revealed similar findings, including Dr. Solomon. In a retrospective review of early AIDS patient studies, it emerged that the ability to say "no" was the strongest predictor of long-term survival.[3] Solomon's research also found that assertive people had higher-functioning immune systems than nonassertive people; they were better able to resist and easily recover from a wide range of diseases and conditions.[4]

Others working with cancer patients have also found that those with the longest survival times are those who authentically express their true feelings of anger, fear, pain, and

Researchers have demonstrated a strong correlation between emotional suppression and decreased immune cell counts and decreased immune function.

distress, while patients with cancer and other illnesses who are unable to identify and express their authentic emotions have higher rates of morbidity (rate of disease) and mortality.[5]

UCLA psychiatrist and psychooncology researcher Dr. Fawzy Fawzy found that malignant melanoma patients who were the most authentic in their emotional self-expression had thinner, slower-growing tumors, along with greater numbers of lymphocytes traveling to the cancerous site, than did those who were not able to authentically express their feelings.[6] Here is further evidence showing the consistency with which a repressive style of coping has been associated with poorer immune function.

The Hazards of Stoicism
Cancer patients who respond to their diagnosis stoically, or with fatalistic hopelessness and helplessness, have the shortest survival times.[7] They are generally completely out of touch with their authentic feelings, so even when they do express themselves, it doesn't reflect their genuine inner experience. Docility is a form of smoke screen that serves to prevent the expression of anger or other feelings that the patient may have been brought up to believe were unacceptable. But being nice rather than authentic portends poor physiological functioning. In terms of health, the inability or unwillingness to authentically self-express leads to malfunctions in neurotransmitter systems, endocrine disruptions, and down-regulation or over-regulation of the immune system by the nervous system.[8]

Medical researchers Dr. Keith Pettingale and Dr. Steven Greer performed psychological testing at the start of a prospective study of 160 women with breast lumps, prior to

biopsy. The biopsies of sixty-nine of them came back positive for cancer. When Pettingale and Greer cross-referenced
the psychological tests, they discovered that 50 percent of the
women diagnosed with malignant tumors were deemed to
engage in extreme emotional suppression, as determined by
psychological evaluation prior to getting the bad news. *Many
claimed to have never gotten angry in their entire adult lives.* Not
one of the 69 women whose biopsies were positive for cancer had actually expressed anger more than twice in her adult
life.[9]

Dr. Greer and Dr. Tina Morris performed psychological
testing at the start of another prospective study of cancer patients. The women who tested highest in emotional suppression later turned out to have the highest rates of cancerous
tumors, while those who tested lowest on emotional suppression had the highest rate of benign ones. And anger was not
the only emotion the women with cancer suppressed; they
had been suppressing *all* their negative emotions throughout
their adult lives.[10] This important research helps explain the
nature of the connection between emotional suppression and
cancer. It appears suppression per se does not cause disease.
Rather, it may well indicate low self-esteem, shame, lack of
mastery, poor social skills, and alexithymia (inability to express any feelings in words)—all of which have been associated with poorer health.

Dr. Gary Schwartz and his colleague Dr. Larry Jamner interviewed 312 patients, all of whom were tested for immune
function along with a basic endocrine panel. The immune
cell counts and immune function tests of people who unconsciously suppressed their emotions showed dangerously low
levels. Conversely, those who reported high levels of emotional distress had better-functioning immune systems than
people who reported being fine despite the fact that their levels of stress hormones (cortisol and norepinephrine) revealed
they were not healthy.[11] This study in particular offers solid
evidence that emotional repression is immunosuppressive.

Other studies have reached similar findings: In a multivar-

Many people believe that unpleasant emotions are bad for their health, but all the research indicates that authentic expression of those emotions correlates with improved health.

iate analysis of American and European studies by Dr. Lydia Temoshok, it became clear that patients with good emotional self-expression had more natural killer (NK) cells and other T-cells, better immune function, and slower-growing tumors.[12] Dr. Greer replicated Temoshok's original studies.[13] And in a review of cancer studies, Dr. Mogens Jensen discovered a 46 percent greater remission rate among breast cancer patients who scored highest on authentic emotional expression.[14]

Suppression versus Repression
It's worth briefly examining the difference between suppression and repression, as the Schwartz and Jamner study looked at both. Someone who responds to a question with the very commonly heard responses "Let's not go there!" and "Whatever!" is practicing *suppression;* the person knows unpleasant emotions are lurking and deliberately chooses to avoid them. By contrast, someone who unconsciously engages in avoidant behavior is practicing *repression.*

Of the conscious suppressors in this study, those who got defensive evidenced even more immunosuppression than the repressors did. Researchers concluded that although emotional distress is in itself immunosuppressive, denying that distress is much worse. The immune system recovers rapidly from short-duration, acknowledged emotional distress, but the effects of chronically denying feelings are considerably more harmful.

While I wanted to acquaint you with the difference between suppression and repression here, the terms are commonly used interchangeably in many studies, making it hard to know which of these the researchers really measured. But since they both correlate with worse health outcomes, the question may be purely academic. The more important question explores the health differences between authentic self-expression and the lack of it.

Expressing the Negative Is Positive

Many people believe that when they allow themselves to feel unpleasant emotions such as anger, frustration, shame, or sadness, they will feel worse, and that this is bad for their health. But as we have seen throughout this chapter, all the research indicates that authentic expression of those emotions correlates with improved health outcomes. Research psychologist Julie Cobb found that the ability to authentically express and cognitively process negative emotions serves to greatly diminish the suffering associated with so-called negative emotions. In fact, she and her team found that authentic self-expression and cognitive processing of negative emotions make so-called positive emotions such as joy and hope more accessible.[15]

Authentic Expression of Anger versus Hostility and Rage

The kind of anger that is healthy to express is an authentic emotion, expressed assertively but not aggressively. Assertiveness is often mistaken for aggressiveness, but while the former is associated with authenticity, health, and a sense of mastery, the latter is associated with insecurity and experiential avoidance of thoughts, sensations, and emotions—not to mention especially high rates of cardiovascular disease.

Hostility, rage, and aggression are closely related unhealthy states. Research psychologist John Barefoot and his team examined prospective studies of lawyers and physicians. Physicians who scored high on the Cook-Medley Hostility Scale were four to five times more likely to develop coronary artery disease; 14 percent of them were dead before age fifty and only 2 percent of those who scored lower on the hostility scale were dead by that age. Twenty percent of the hostile lawyers were dead from heart disease before age fifty as compared with only 4 percent of the less hostile ones.[16]

The explanation for these findings lies in the physiological ramifications of hostility. According to medical researchers Edward Suarez and James Blumenthal and psychophysiology researchers Jerry Suls and Choi Wan, hostile individuals tend to be hypertensive and have elevated heart rates as well as elevated cortisol and catecholamine (stress hormones) levels.[17] The high levels of these hormones contribute to increased platelet aggregation (which can increase clotting where it is not helpful) and increased deposits of lipids on arterial walls—a combination that strongly contributes to heart blockages. That, says medical psychology researcher Johan Kop, leads in turn to the formation of plaque, which injures the arterial endothelial linings, the main site of atherosclerotic damage.[18]

Psychoneuroimmunology researcher Gregory Fricchione explains that increased catecholamines also lead to increased serum lipids, which are processed into oxidized LDLs (low density lipids).[19] Once plaques begin to form, macrophages and endothelial cells down-regulate nitric oxide, which narrows blood vessels. (Nitric oxide is very important for keeping blood vessels open.)

Dr. Suarez and his team found that hostile individuals also have reduced beta-adrenergic receptor function, which further feeds hostility because beta adrenergic activity serves to inhibit sympathetic (fight or flight) activation.[20] Hostility also reduces heart rate variability (HRV), and many researchers have demonstrated that low HRV is predictive of coronary heart disease as well as increased morbidity and mortality in general.[21] As if all that is not bad enough, the increased sympathetic tone, heart rate, and blood pressure lead to increases in homocysteine, an amino acid that is a strong biomarker of heart disease.

There is no question that expressing anger is healthy. In fact, suppression of or inability to express anger has been associated with higher rates of cancer. But if expressing your-self is healthy and hostile people express themselves loudly and often, why is hostility unhealthy?

My hypothesis is that while expressing *anger* is healthy, expressing *rage* is not. What probably makes the difference between healthy physiological processes and the unhealthy ones I have described is determined by how people feel after expressing themselves. If they feel a calm sense of mastery and loving self-care, or a deepening connection to the person to whom they expressed their feelings, enhanced immune function and improved physiological functioning will follow. An outburst of rage stimulates entirely different feelings, a sense of being out of control and disconnected from the person who is subjected to it, and this is when the harmful physiological effects of hostility manifest.

Expressive Writing and Immune Function

You do not need to express your thoughts and feelings to an-other person to reap the health benefits of authentic self-ex-pression. Writing can serve this purpose very well. Dr. James Pennebaker's research on journaling revealed that the key to improved immune function was not the *catharsis* of expres-sion through writing—the release of tension—but simply a *recognition* of our deepest feelings by means of a healthy way to express them.[22]

Psychophysiology researcher Dr. Carmen Uhlmann did a study in which she wired computer keyboards to bio-feedback instruments. Collaborating with Pennebaker and computer programmer Martha Francis, she measured heart rate and electrical activity of the skin as college students wrote about various traumatic experiences in their lives. The sensors in their keypads went to a central computer that enabled researchers to get readouts of fluctuations in the electrical activity of the students' skin on a word-by-word, phrase-by-phrase basis. This unique biofeedback experiment showed the researchers that specific words were associated with specific physiological changes. Negative descriptors of emotion—words like *scared, hate, hurt, guilt,* and *shame*—correlated with increased autonomic arousal (stress response) as measured by increased heart rate and electrodermal activity. Words associated with positive emotions correlated with reduced stress response.

Perhaps that outcome was to be expected, but a surprising finding of this experiment was that words associated with reflection, insight, and a degree of resolution of a problem—such as *understand, realize, because,* and *reason*—also correlated with increased heart rate and electrodermal activity. Why? The likely answer is that as the students wrote about an event or problem on the way to developing an understanding of it, they felt emotional, which correlated with increased electrical activity. Interestingly, though, when they wrote about an emotional trauma or problem over a period of several days, the autonomic activity associated with it diminished. This last finding is evidence of the power of journaling to improve one's state of mind and sense of mastery, and this could explain the improved immune function of the participants in the Pennebaker psychoneuroimmunology studies.

These researchers followed the student subjects' health over a number of months by tracking visits to the university medical clinic, and found that the students who expressed negative-emotion words experienced better health than those who continually expressed positive-emotion words.

Pennebaker's surprising conclusion was that people who used negative-emotion words experienced a release of emotion that contributed to increased *self-awareness, self-understanding,* and *self-appreciation,* and that this improved mind-state led to improved health—further evidence of the importance of expressing uncomfortable emotional states.[23]

Self-Expression and Meaningful Relationships

In one of the longest-running prospective studies related to self-expression, thirteen hundred medical students at Johns Hopkins were followed for forty years. While at Hopkins, they were given psychological tests exploring their ability to have meaningful relationships. Thirty years later, the researchers discovered those who had shown the least ability to accept authentic emotional expression in themselves as well as in those closest to them developed cancer at *sixteen times the rate* of those who were comfortable with authentic emotional expression.[24]

To Sum Up

The inability or unwillingness to express anger or any other emotion does not cause cancer, but as we have seen in this chapter, there are strong associations between the lack of authentic self-expression and higher rates of cancer.[25] It's important to keep in mind that the lack of authentic self-expression is simply one of many variables, and that although associations reaching statistical significance have been found, there is no direct, one-to-one, cause-and-effect relationship between poor self-expression and cancer. The only thing that is absolutely certain is that chronic emotional distress, such as that created by emotional suppression and repression, leads to physiological stress, thereby making it much more likely we will succumb to diseases to which we are genetically or environmentally predisposed.

A Hypothesis

I have long wondered about the connection between the ability to be aware of our inner subjective experience, the ability to put it into words, and health outcomes. The data coming out of all the studies connecting certain personality styles with cancer, autoimmune, and other disease categories can sound mysterious and even mystical. But I believe the mystery can be explained as follows:

1.   Alexithymia—the inability to identify and describe in words what we are feeling—is a source of emotional distress and if chronic, is a major source of physiological stress.

2. In addition, unexpressed emotion gets expressed in un-
    healthy behavior (drinking, overeating, addictions, risky
    behavior) in an attempt to avoid feeling the uncomfort-
    able emotion: a second cause of physiological stress.
3. The inability to authentically express ourselves interferes
    with relationships, and relationship problems are a third
    source of emotional distress, with its concomitant physi-
    ological stress. Also, isolation is a source of stress.
4. The inability to ask for what we want or to say "no" to
    what we don't want is orthogonal to mastery and leaves
    one feeling helpless—a fourth source of emotional dis-
    tress and physiological stress.
5. Physiological stress, regardless of its etiology, leads to a
    weakened state, which then paves the way for diseases
    to which we are genetically or environmentally predis-
    posed.

The stress created by 1 through 4 leads to 5, which may
explain the appearance of many cases of cancer and other diseases that would ordinarily never manifest despite genetic
predispositions or environmental exposures. Emotional distress is often what makes the difference between illness and
health. However, even chronic emotional distress cannot directly cause cancer or any other disease—there are always
other variables.

Asking for Help: An Important Form of Authentic Self-Expression

Another category of self-expression, one that does not come
easily for many people, is asking for help. Studies have shown
that the ability to do so is associated with better health—even
when the requested help never arrives.[26] While it's not entirely clear why the capacity to ask for help might result in better
health outcomes, it may inversely correlate with certain other
attributes associated with health. For example, people with a
hopeless, helpless, fatalistic attitude—associated with worse

health outcomes—don't ask for what they want because they typically believe nothing will help. On the other hand, taking the risk involved in simply making such a request can actually reduce feelings of hopelessness and helplessness.

Suggestions for Self-Expression Practices That Develop Mastery

There are numerous ways to develop the skill of self-expression. Biofeedback is a simple and effective way to increase the ability to better identify and put words to physiological sensations and emotions. Group psychotherapy is exceptionally effective in helping develop or improve authentic self-expression because its two prime goals are to gain insight into inner, subjective experience and to authentically express that insight in the group; members are coached in how to express their most difficult feelings aloud. Another way to build these skills is through a really good social support circle in which everyone's ideas and feelings matter (see chapter 19, Practice Building Relationships, for more on the value of social support).

Authentic self-expression is best practiced with people who are willing and able to take in what you are expressing. Most of us have had at least one family member who meets authentic self-expression with disinterest, or even with shaming remarks. It's not a good idea to open yourself up to people who respond this way. Unhealthy work situations in which your feelings are not respected aren't good places to practice authentic self-expression either. If your life partner isn't willing or able to hear authentic self-expression, it is essential for your health to see a couples therapist together in order to improve the situation. If it can't be improved, for the sake of your health, you need to get help ending the relationship. It is vital to find at least one individual with whom you can authentically express your deepest feelings and concerns.

Here are a few more suggestions to develop mastery:
- Because you can't express your authentic feelings to others until you can identify them, engage in the funda-

mental mindfulness practice of recognizing all of your thoughts, sensations, and emotions. Don't analyze them; rather, simply acknowledge and honor them.

- Take risks in sharing your authenticity with others. You will quickly learn that some people feel threatened by true authenticity—and you can cross them off your list of those with whom you can share your feelings. Others will open to you in very deep ways.

- Practice assertively asking for what you want. If you're in touch with your true feelings, you'll be seen as assertive and likely to get what you request. But if you try to express yourself before you know what you truly feel, you may be seen as aggressive, abrasive, or ineffectual, and will be less likely to get what you request—and even if you get what you request, it could come at the expense of relationships.

- Although the ultimate goal is to become skilled at authentic self-expression in interpersonal communication, journaling is a valuable practice. It provides an opportunity to be completely honest about all your thoughts and feelings without worrying about reactions from others.

- Notice if you sometimes find yourself being *nice* to someone when you don't feel a genuine positive connection. This behavior is inauthentic and disrespectful to both of you.

- Don't do anything you do not wholeheartedly want to do. Remember the lessons of Valued-Action Practice discussed in chapters 10 through 12. Living with authenticity means taking actions that are in harmony with your values. In this sense, the actions you take are expressions of your authentic self.

- Whenever you are ambivalent about doing something, ask yourself how you will feel if you do it versus if you don't do it; let that be your guide.

- Practice asking for help whenever it is appropriate and practice not being attached to any outcome of that assistance.

- Practice saying "no" whenever it is genuine and appropriate.

- Ask yourself throughout the day: *How authentic am I in this moment? What am I feeling and needing in this moment? Am I being completely authentic in my interpersonal communications in this moment? Am I being* nice *or am I being* real?

- Be on the lookout for feelings of self-pity, hopelessness, or helplessness; these indicate emotional suppression and repression. People who take risks in order to express their authenticity do not experience those feelings, and this holds true no matter how many times they fail in their attempts.

- Be on the lookout for feelings of hostility, which can spark belligerent emotional expression and even rage. Rage is the result of the failure to express authentic anger, and it creates a sense of losing control—the opposite of mastery.

- Find a good psychotherapy group to join. When facilitated by an experienced and skilled group psychotherapist, it will provide an exceptional opportunity to improve authentic self-expression. In fact, it is probably the very best way to improve authenticity as well as self-expression.

- Set the intention to stay in touch with feeling states and authentically express yourself from those authentic states.

- Hang out with people who are very authentic and accepting. That experience will engender those qualities in you.

- Throughout the day, practice recalling an instance when you found authentic self-expression to be particularly satisfying and rewarding, and focus your current-moment attention on how much you value authentic self-expression.

- Think of an instance in your life where you authentically expressed yourself to someone and were respected by the other person. Intentionally recall that incident throughout the day, every day. Doing so will give you confidence to practice that behavior again.

- Look for every opportunity to share how you feel about something with someone you trust. Take risks in expressing to people close to you what you like and don't like regarding their behavior. The resulting mastery will provide meaning and purpose to your life. Cultivating meaning and purpose is an important mindfulness-based mastery and well-being practice in its own right, and is the subject of chapter 17.

17 Practice Cultivating Meaning and Purpose

The terms *meaning* and *purpose* often appear together, and I would frame their relationship this way: when we act with *purpose,* we take actions that are important enough to lend *meaning* to our lives. Meaningful actions are always in accord with our personal life values, whether we value accomplishment, wellbeing, comfort and safety, healthy relationships, artistic expression, or any other quality of life. Living purposefully, engaged in an active search for meaning, is a highly beneficial mastery and wellbeing practice that can have a profound positive impact on physical and emotional health. It is particularly effective in alleviating depression.

Finding Meaning in Illness

Throughout history, when people have fallen ill, they have searched for meaning in their illness. For many, this was because the possibility of being a victim of random bad luck was simply unacceptable. Patients often attributed supernatural causes to their disease and interpreted it as just punishment for unacceptable behavior, or even impure thoughts. Sometimes when a family member got sick, it brought the family together, and this was interpreted as divine intervention. It is still very common to search for some meaning in disease, and it doesn't have to be in the realm of the supernatural. For many people, illness serves to teach them how to have greater appreciation for all the good things in their lives that they previously took for granted.

Sometimes the meaning we ascribe to an illness catalyzes

physical, psychological, and emotional healing. When we view an illness as a chance to examine our lives and take action in line with our authentic life values, it serves as an opportunity rather than as some terrible thing that has victimized us. Imbuing the illness with meaning is self-empowering, enabling us to rearrange our lives to better conform to our life values. In doing so, we not only catalyze all our natural physiological healing mechanisms; we develop that all-important sense of being in control of our lives.

No one can predict the degree to which a debilitating disease will prevent someone else from living a meaningful life. Theoretical physicist and ALS patient Stephen Hawking has found a way to live with meaning and purpose despite unimaginably extreme quadriplegia. Perhaps this is why he is still alive after fifty years of living with a disease that normally kills in a few short years.

Many researchers you have met earlier in this book have observed and studied the phenomenon of finding meaning in illness. Dr. Lawrence LeShan and Dr. Carl Simonton both found that living with a serious disease, especially one that is life threatening, often leads to a renegotiation of life values and priorities, which eventuates in a new search for meaning and purpose—of both the diagnosis and life in general.[1] Behavioral medicine researcher Roger Katz discovered that an active search for the benefits of having a disease—the proverbial silver lining—leads to greater compassion for others and a greater willingness to openly express feelings.[2] And psychooncology researcher Dr. Sharon Manne and her team discovered that this search often results in a greater appreciation of one's own inner strengths as well as the greater possibilities in life—all of which add up to living more vibrantly and with greater enthusiasm.[3]

What Studies Reveal about Meaning and Health

Again we turn to psychoneuroimmunology researcher George Solomon, this time to learn what science can teach us about

In older Americans, one of the best predictors of happiness, health, and longevity is whether or not they think their lives have purpose.

meaning and health. In his studies, he found that the healthiest elders are those who stay busy, volunteering or engaged in other activities that keep their minds alert. The healthiest among these tend to engage in a variety of activities they find personally meaningful.[4]

Solomon also revealed the surprising finding that, historically, cancer rates have been much higher among soldiers in peacetime than during wartime. He discovered that being challenged and stressed can actually be good for one's health, and that an easier life without challenge is deleterious to it.[5] During the stress and chaos of wartime, there is always plenty to achieve; fighting to save the world or to defend one's country can be profoundly life altering. During peacetime, soldiers spend less time doing the various things they find important—mostly they just take orders and don't get to see the results of their actions.

Gerontology researcher and physician Robert Butler performed an eleven-year study of highly functional people between the ages of sixty-five and ninety-two. He, too, found that in older Americans, one of the best predictors of happiness, health, and longevity is whether or not they think their lives have purpose. If they didn't, seven out of ten felt unsettled about their lives, and if they did, the same proportion felt satisfied.[6]

These same statistics have also been found among college students, so this pattern is not the sole province of older people. Those students who enjoyed their studies found purpose in them, and were happier than those who didn't.

If you recall the work of Dr. James Pennebaker on journaling as a means of self-expression from chapter 16, you may

remember that those who used the words understand, realize, or see in their journaling enjoyed improvements in their
health. Pennebaker and his team hypothesized that when our
experiences have structure and meaning, they seem considerably more manageable than when they're associated with
meaningless chaos. This argues persuasively for an active
practice of seeking meaning in the events of life. Lawrence Le-
Shan also developed insights about meaning and purpose in
his work, noting that his cancer patients who discovered and
then pursued what gave their lives meaning—who had something to live for—had much higher rates of survival than those
who didn't.[7]

Dr. LeShan found that he could help people reclaim the will
to live by helping them identify something they were willing
to fight for—as if their survival depended on it. In the 1950s,
when he switched from traditional Freudian psychotherapy
to his own method, the mortality rates of his advanced, metastatic, end-stage, hospitalized cancer patients went from 100
percent (as would be expected) to 50 percent; half went into
long-term remission from the end-stage cancer that had been
predicted to kill them. Some lived a year beyond what had
been expected while others lived ten to twenty years or more.
The common variable in all these remissions was the patients'
newly discovered sense of meaning and purpose. Sometimes
this change of heart was the result of taking up a musical instrument they had always dreamt of playing. Other times it
came from finding a way to help make life better for others.
Many of the case studies in his book *Cancer as a Turning Point*
relate to finding meaningful work.

Despite making significant changes in their lives, many of
the people Dr. LeShan worked with still died as predicted by
their oncologists. But they lived much more fully in the time
they had remaining, and often even their dying process became a meaningful experience.

The Importance of Setting Goals

Dr. Carl Simonton always impressed upon participants at Simonton Cancer Center retreats that energy is essential to healing and that the act of pursuing goals is itself energizing.[8] Setting goals helps us conceptualize our reasons for living. Once we have a purpose for being, we are more motivated to do whatever it takes to get well. The future and the present appear more positive when we set goals, and doing so also helps many people commit to engaging in healthy behaviors. Goals provide a sense of control over our lives and create mastery. Going after what we want means we believe our lives have value. Ultimately, goals help us live with vitality, presence, and intentionality.

Neuropsychology researcher Dr. Richard Davidson reports that working hard toward a goal and making progress to the point of expecting it to be realized serve to activate positive experiences and diminish anxiety and depression—and this is true even without actually achieving the goal.[9]

Research psychologist Laura King found a positive correlation between journaling and goals. After just a few weeks, people in her study who spent twenty minutes a day journaling about their most deeply held goals reported less depression and fewer medical complaints than people who spent twenty minutes a day simply recording the details of their daily lives in a diary.[10]

Further demonstrating the value of setting goals, research psychologist Dr. Sonja Lyubomirsky and her team found that the happiest and healthiest people are deeply committed to lifelong goals.[11] But there is a cautionary note to parents. Psychology researchers Andrew Elliot and Kennon Sheldon point out that when children aim for goals that are set by their parents, and pursue those goals only to please them, they find no meaning, purpose, or joy in the activities they undertake to achieve those goals.[12] Goals that result in health benefits must be connected to personal aspirations.

A key understanding about the health benefits of goals,

one that may seem surprising, is that reaching them is unimportant. The value lies in having goals and pursuing them.

Finding Meaning in the Loss of Loved Ones

When psychoneuroimmunology researchers Dr. Julienne Bower and Dr. Margaret Kemeny studied HIV-positive men who had lost partners or close friends to AIDS at the peak of the AIDS crisis, they discovered that the survivors who were able to find meaning in the death of partners or friends had healthier immune systems and better longevity over the following three years than those who found none. And they became committed to living life more fully than they had before their loss.[13]

Candy Lightner provides a dramatic example of this. After her daughter was killed by a repeat drunk driver, she channeled her pain and despair into taking action in harmony with what she valued. She became determined to find a way to take drunk drivers off the road and, with enormous resolve, founded Mothers Against Drunk Driving (MADD). Thanks to her and many others sharing her purpose, MADD has improved DUI (aka DWI) laws and enforcement.

Psychiatrist Dr. Viktor Frankl discovered that of the small percentage in the Nazi death camps who were not murdered, those who survived the longest were often not the most physically fit; they were the most connected to a purpose in life. Most of these survivors got the meaning they needed to continue from the image of reuniting with their families. Almost all of them eventually learned that everyone else in their family had been murdered, and soon after being liberated from the camps and learning this news, many lost the will to go on and perished. Their immune systems and physiological functioning in general simply shut down when their lives lost meaning. A few survivors, like Dr. Frankl, found meaning in living to create a more peaceful and sane world.[14]

Finding Meaning and Purpose
When Death Is Near

Dr. LeShan (1989) writes about two very different ways of working with people living with advanced metastatic cancer, depending on the stage they are in: As long as they have reason to hope for recovery, they can find meaning and purpose in fighting for their lives, and LeShan made use of that in his work. But here's what he says about dealing with the later stage, when recovery is impossible:

> The "dying mode" is about finding meaning to the life one has led. What is left for that person to do in order to die peacefully? It may involve working with unresolved relationships. Questions are asked of someone in the dying mode in order to create meaning even in this period such as: "What was the most important decision you ever made?" "And why?" "What was the period in your life when you were most really you?" "What would you like to have changed in your life?"[15]

In answering these questions one can gain new understanding and acceptance of why she or he did certain things. In sharing this with children and grandchildren, one gains meaning and purpose. In other words, it is never too late to search for meaning and purpose.

Suggestions for Cultivating
Meaning and Purpose

- Find activities or projects that leave you with the sense that you're doing something important. It can be related to work or play—anything that leaves you feeling that you're doing a good thing. And you don't have to set out to change the world; many retired people, for example, find meaning in gardening, cleaning the house, or even improving their golf game.
- Every night, just before going to sleep, think of what you did during the day that provided you with a sense

of accomplishment. This allows you to connect with what you find meaningful.

- Similarly, before getting out of bed each morning, think of what you will be doing today that feels meaningful.
- Throughout the day, set the intention of asking yourself what you are practicing in that moment. Are you practicing something that gives you a sense of accomplishment, something that you feel good about, something that can make life better for others or for yourself, something in harmony with your personal values and goals? These are the meaningful practices.
- If tragedy has struck you, emulate Candy Lightner; find a cause you believe in that will give meaning to the tragic event.
- Redefine even the simplest of events in terms of accomplishment. For example, as I'm cleaning pots and pans in the kitchen, I can find meaning and purpose in my chore by recognizing that I am creating a clean, neat, ordered environment.
- Reflect on what gives your life meaning and purpose. Think of instances from the past as well as upcoming events and opportunities.

18

Practice Connection and Service to Others

I n this chapter we examine a particularly effective mindfulness-based mastery and wellbeing practice: finding ways to be helpful and generous to others. In numerous studies, researchers have determined that connecting with others in order to be of service to them is strongly associated with superior health. Here I will share some of those studies with you, touch on a few related topics, describe some of the physiology at work, and offer suggestions for practice.

What I refer to as connection and service practice is often called *altruism,* and I use that term here as a kind of shorthand. I'm primarily emphasizing connection, though, because it is the aspect of altruism that actually improves health. The nature of an altruistic act—whether you're preparing a meal for someone in need, running errands for someone with mobility challenges, or simply holding open a door—is far less important than the connection that takes place between you and the other person. Especially in my work in biofeedback, I have found that contact itself has the effect of physiologically opening the heart, and this is where health benefits are to be found. And when you experience this feeling of connectedness, you will probably be motivated to reach out and serve others whenever you see an opportunity, so this is a practice that builds upon itself. Reaching out contributes to a sense of belonging, community, and participation in contributing to the greater good. And this creates a state that enhances wellbeing—psychological, emotional, and physiological.

Many studies have shown that the healthiest and

Those who did volunteer work once a
week had a tenfold health advantage over
those who volunteered once a year.

happiest people are commonly the first to offer helping hands,
in particular to coworkers and strangers. In her extensive
study of happiness, research psychologist Dr. Sonja Lyubomirsky found many reasons altruism is associated with health.[1] It
fosters a sense of mastery, which often creates healthy physiological changes. Focusing on others who seem to be worse
off than we are allows us to see ourselves as healthier than we
had previously thought. And while we are involved in helping others, we focus less on our own problems.

A large study by Howard Andrews, a psychology professor at Columbia University, yielded a wealth of information
that clearly demonstrates the health advantages we experience when we help others. If you're seeking confirmation that
altruism can benefit you, you need look no further than some
of these impressive numbers. In his study, 3,296 people who
were engaged in volunteer work at more than twenty volunteer organizations filled out a survey. Here are some of Andrews's findings:

- *Ninety-five percent* of participants said they experienced
  a sense of physical and emotional wellbeing during and
  immediately following their helping activities.
- *Seventy-eight percent* said they experienced this again
  during the following week, even though they were not
  serving others.
- *Ninety percent* said they believed their health was better
  than that of others their age.
- Those who volunteered weekly throughout the year had
  a *tenfold* health advantage over those who volunteered
  once a year.

- Those who got the greatest psychological and emotional benefit also got the greatest health benefit.
- A very interesting finding was that volunteers who primarily helped strangers reported the best health, as opposed to those who primarily helped family or friends. The researchers on the Andrews team hypothesized that the reason for this was that those who helped family or friends were often motivated by obligation, guilt, or economic necessity. The people who helped strangers did so because it helped them feel like they were part of something larger than themselves; they felt an openhearted connection or oneness with other people in general.[2]

The Andrews study also revealed that many who volunteered to help friends or family experienced emotional distress, not feelings of wellbeing, because they were invested in a positive outcome. By contrast, people who helped strangers were less invested in results and helped others primarily because of the joy it brought them.

Although I have not seen any research on the health benefits of being in the helping professions, such as psychotherapy or medicine, those clinicians whose service takes place in an environment of time pressures and claim forms and documentation may possibly not gain the same health benefits due to the stressful work environment.

Another finding supports the idea that the act of connecting itself, not the particular generous act you perform, carries the health benefits. The volunteers who had personal contact with the people being served received greater health benefits than those who did administrative volunteer work, and the study documented numerous specifics including relief from chronic headaches, backaches, bellyaches, asthma, arthritis, lupus, and insomnia. Volunteers who had direct contact also got fewer colds. This correlates with what I've heard anecdotally. Several people in top management positions in nonprofit, service-based organizations have told me that if they had it to do over again, they would work more directly with the people their organizations help because it is more heartfelt work—an interesting term to use in light of the healthy effects of serving others on cardiovascular functioning, which you will read about a little further on.

Further Studies of Connection and Service to Others

In another study, research psychologist Stephanie Brown tracked 423 older couples over five years. She found that couples who reported helping someone without pay, even as infrequently as once a year, were between 40 and 60 percent less likely to die during the five-year period than those who reported not helping anyone. And their service to others was pretty straightforward: volunteering, babysitting for grand-children, or assisting family members in other ways.[3]

In the famous Tecumseh study of almost three thousand people by psychology researcher James House at the Univer-sity of Michigan, an interesting tidbit of information emerged. While this study focused on a different topic—the health ben-efits of social support—one of the variables they uncovered was that volunteer activities were among the most powerful predictors of reduced morbidity and mortality in men. In fact, they discovered that, more than any other single activity, do-ing regular volunteer work correlated with better health and longevity. The men who did no volunteer work were two and a half times as likely to die during the time period of the study as the men who did volunteer work, even just a couple of hours a week.[4]

Research by Dr. Allan Luks, reported and interpreted by Howard Andrews, indicates that being part of an organized effort seems to be the best path to follow in doing volunteer work. However, Andrews also hypothesized that small, every-day acts of kindness, such as holding the door for a stranger or helping someone cross the street, produce the same health benefits as organized volunteer work: giving meaning to life and catalyzing a sense of openhearted connectedness to the world.[5] If we are all members of the global community, then

Inherent in helping others is a dramatic increase in optimistic attitudes and a sense of meaning and purpose, as well as an increase in feelings of belonging and community.

every time we do something as simple as reach down to pick up an item a stranger has dropped, we strengthen our sense of belonging in that larger community.

Harvard psychiatrist George Vaillant has spent his entire career running a prospective study of the health of former Harvard students over the course of their lifetimes, looking for connections between their health and the ways they live. One of his most consistent findings (after controlling for confounding variables) has been that those who are involved in volunteer work are healthiest and live longest.[6]

Psychologist Ute Schulz and her team discovered that inherent in helping others is a dramatic increase in optimistic attitudes and a sense of meaning and purpose, as well as an increase in feelings of belonging and community.[7] This is clearly a complex topic because many of the ingredients of service to others, such as belonging to a community, social support, optimism, and meaning and purpose—all of which have been identified as components of volunteer work—have been discovered to be independent variables that are strongly associated with better health.

Some researchers have found that when people train themselves to think and behave in ways that center around service to others, they actually develop a more optimistic personality; this is referred to as learned optimism. Psychologist Martin Seligman found that one common element among such people is the belief that things can change for the better.[8] In fact, altruism scholars Samuel and Pearl Oliner discovered that altruists generally share a healthy belief system.[9]

The Oliners also discovered the following about the most altruistic people:

- Becoming an altruist starts with turning your focus away from egocentric self-involvement. Once you break that habit and learn to focus on others, you naturally begin to develop an altruistic mind state.
- Real altruists believe in the humanity of all people. Their commitment to helping others extends beyond the bounds of nationality, race, religion, and culture.
- Altruists tend to view themselves as part of something greater than themselves. They think of community and they value the needs of everyone on the planet equally.
- Altruists tend to be very connected to diverse people and groups.
- Altruists feel a strong sense of inner control, but they do not try to control others. They believe they can control their destinies, are willing to risk failure, and do not spend time mourning their failures.
- Altruists are optimists, believing they can succeed.
- Altruists perform altruistic deeds without ulterior motives. This particular point could explain why those who work in the helping professions for pay have not been found to receive the same health benefits as those doing volunteer work.
- Altruists are conscious of their life values and are not afraid to take action that is in harmony with those values.[10]

The Health Benefits of Caregiving

New research suggests that caregivers often derive health benefits from taking care of a loved one who is disabled or very ill. While earlier studies by Stephanie Brown had documented just the opposite—negative health effects of caregiving—more recent research has shown that elder spouses who helped their partners fourteen or more hours a week with activities related to eating, dressing, and preparing meals lived longer than those who did these activities for less than fourteen hours a week or not at all.[11] Perhaps the caregivers tracked in earlier studies whose health deteriorated had put in closer to fourteen hours a day rather than fourteen hours a week.

A Caregiving Caveat
Not all caregivers benefit from improved health; there are certain qualifiers. Lyubomirsky discovered that caregivers of spouses with Alzheimer's disease experienced declines in their own health and wellbeing.[12] In the case of this disease, or any condition that includes serious neurological impairment, it is quite possible that any caregiving health benefit is negated by grieving the loss of the spouse's intellect and personality. Someone with Alzheimer's gradually becomes a different person, and this can be profoundly traumatic for the healthy partner.

Service to Others and Unusual Longevity
A disproportionately large number of centenarians exhibit a strong sense of service to their extended families and others. The Nicoyans, a community in Costa Rica, are known for having one of the largest proportions of centenarians in the world. Individuals in this culture have a deep-seated feeling of belonging and connection, and they value caring for one another. They refer to their sense of service as *plan de vida*, or life plan.

Okinawans also have one of the world's largest proportions of centenarians. They refer to the sense of service as *iki-gai*, or reason for living. It results in part from being revered by younger generations. *Plan de vida* and *ikigai* both relate to feeling needed and an abiding desire to contribute to the greater good. Feeling needed is associated with feeling connected.

Although people in these cultures would say that they help family members because it is their obligation to do so, their interpretation of "obligation" is different from the way we usually think of it. For them, being able to help out in their families and communities allows them to feel needed, valued, and appreciated.

The Physiology of Openheartedness

I recall psychiatrist Dr. James S. Gordon hypothesizing at a 2009 behavioral medicine training in San Diego that love is what makes the difference in inspiring caring behavior in service to others, as well as in how well the help is received.[13] It may also be that the feeling of love improves the health of the person offering help. This is a physiological phenomenon: when you experience love as an authentic emotion, you also experience an actual dilation in the blood vessels throughout the body, including the heart. The physiology adds yet another variable to the complexity of the question of why helping others is so healthy for the helper.

When we set an intention to connect with others, our hearts are open—metaphorically and physiologically. Almost universally, when we are engaged in service, we experience a warmth and openness in the area of our heart, so this behavior is most likely very healing for ischemic forms of cardiovascular diseases. These pleasant sensations are the result of endorphins and a cascade of neuroendocrine and immune hormones, enzymes, immune complement, and peptides that support life. The warmth in the chest also tends to correlate with diaphragmatic breathing, which can be very healing for heart rhythm abnormalities. The practice of feeling connected to others and opening our hearts to them can automatically slow and deepen respiration, dilate vessels, and regulate some cardiac dysrhythmias.

At the other extreme, when we criticize, judge, and fail to help others, regardless of whether we do it overtly or just in our thoughts, breathing becomes shallower and we experience a cascade of stress hormones, platelet activation, and vasoconstriction. The vasoconstriction in turn leads to higher blood pressure and a greater chance of cardiovascular problems. In other words, just thinking well of others confers a number of health benefits.

Volunteer Work and Depression

Throughout history, and in all cultures, volunteer work has been proven to increase optimism. Depression is often associated with a loss of meaning and purpose in life, which can be restored by donating time to a worthy cause. As we have seen, helping others, purely for the sake of helping, is extremely rewarding and meaningful. It also serves to build a sense of mastery, purpose, and connection—all of which are sorely lacking when people feel depressed.

Although many people suffer terribly with Major Depressive Disorder and require antidepressants in order to function in the world, the vast majority of people using antidepressants have milder forms of depression and would be better served by performing satisfying and rewarding generous acts that give them the sense of joy they lack in isolation. I believe that if doctors prescribed volunteer work instead of antidepressants, people with milder forms of depression would feel more optimistic and more in control of their lives.

Medical Appointments Are Opportunities for Connection and Service

I have discovered that when it comes to dealing well with the many medical appointments that are a necessary part of my life, the intention to connect and serve can be invaluable.

When I was younger, I used to get frustrated with bureaucratic inefficiencies and I didn't hesitate to express it. My irritation never helped resolve the problem. Then one day I decided to adopt the attitude that the people I was dealing with and I were on the same team. I decided that I was there to connect with them. The result was that both sides ended up feeling satisfied that we had handled the situation well, and I think we both felt good about working together to resolve the problem. In fact, I discovered that when I complained with a

respectful and collaborative attitude, those to whom I'd addressed my complaint were willing to spend as much time as
necessary to resolve the problem. It actually began to seem
to me as if they were acting like they worked for me. An
atmosphere of mutual respect and caring changed potentially
tense situations into rewarding interactions for all involved.

My new attitude not only helps both parties reach a mutually satisfactory resolution to the matter at hand; it surely
contributes to our mutual health and wellbeing. I have actually been told by nurses that I have a nice bedside manner—a
comment usually reserved for their favorite physicians. I am
not a physician, but because of my change in attitude, nurses
and others see me as someone who works with them in a supportive way, for the good of everyone.

Now, instead of dreading a discussion with a clinic or hospital worker about something that's not going as smoothly as
either of us would like, I look forward to contributing to a
resolution. I ask pertinent questions that are intended to help
both of us explore what we may not previously have considered. And my attitude of wanting to work together for the
common good contributes to the best possible results. I invite
you to try this "appointment connection" practice yourself
and see what it can do for you.

Suggestions for Practicing
Connection and Service

The essence of this practice involves intentionally changing the way you view yourself in relation to others: you set
a conscious intention to see yourself as being one with the
people of the world. This alone can improve your physiological functioning enough that you could even experience actual
improvement in your health.

Beyond that, the practice of caring about and caring for
others is very simple: look for opportunities to do so throughout the day. The smallest of things can have a profound effect
on you, those you help, and society as a whole.

Here are a few more ideas about tapping into the healing power of this practice.

- View your work and as many of your other activities as possible in terms of how the things you do can help the world. Steve Jobs, for example, was motivated by his firm belief that the world was a better place because people used his Apple products.
- Imagine a situation in your life in which you find yourself feeling self-conscious and embarrassed. Now imagine feeling connected to those around you and wanting to serve them. How does this change your emotional state? Typically, focusing on connecting and serving will lead you to feel much more comfortable with others in an uncomfortable moment. It's much harder to feel self-conscious or embarrassed when your heart is open.
- When you find yourself negatively judging someone, imagine yourself as that person and try to accept that his or her behavior makes sense according to that person's life experience. Then imagine helping that person. It may not be appropriate to offer actual help at that moment, but you might find a way to be of service, and you can definitely help yourself by thinking about that person with empathy and understanding.
- When you find yourself considering skipping your daily exercise or you realize you are about to engage in unhealthy behavior, think of how important it is to your family that you remain as healthy as you can. Take care of yourself so that you can be there to take care of others.
- Get involved in an organized volunteer effort for a cause you believe in, and keep in mind that it's healthiest to work alongside whomever the cause benefits rather than behind the scenes.
- Ask yourself throughout the day, *Does my behavior contribute in any way to the suffering of others or of myself?* This question serves as a mind-training practice to help us to

live in full contact with the present moment, to be fully awake to our impact on those around us, and to live in a healthy, openhearted state of mind.

- Look for opportunities to do simple things for strangers, such as holding open a door or giving up your seat on the bus. Notice how uplifting this is for you.
- If you notice that you're doing something helpful in order to get something in return, remember that this does not contribute to your wellbeing.
- Whenever you think of it, focus your mind on ways you can serve others. You will discover that this will generate more such thoughts and will likely increase both your helping behavior and the good feelings that result.
- Think "we" rather than "I." Instead of thinking of yourself as an individual against the world, remind yourself throughout the day of how connected you are to those around you.

Voices for Serving Others

Before I close this chapter, I'd like to offer the thoughts of some of the most respected minds who have expressed the value of serving others. My hope is that they will help inspire you to take up or expand this valuable practice of connecting with others and serving them.

> You must give something to your fellow men even if it's a little thing. Do something for those who have need of help, something for which you get no pay but the privilege of giving. The only ones among you who are really happy are those who have sought and found how to serve.
> —Albert Schweitzer

> Life's most persistent and urging question is "What are you doing for others?"
> —Martin Luther King Jr.

The best way to find yourself is to lose yourself in the service of others.
—Gandhi

Ask not what your country can do for you; ask what you can do for your country.
—John F. Kennedy

People who want to live a more fulfilling life should quit reading self-help books and start helping others.
—Laura King

Here's the secret of happiness: Find something more important than yourself and dedicate your life to it.
—Daniel Dennett

This is the true joy in life, the being used up for a purpose recognized by yourself as a mighty one, the being a force of nature instead of a feverish selfish little clod of alienation and grievances complaining that the world will not devote itself to making you happy. I'm of the opinion that my life belongs to the community and as long as I live, it's my privilege to do for it whatever I can. I want to be thoroughly used up when I die, for the harder I work, the more I live. I rejoice in life for its own sake. Life is no brief candle to me. It's sort of a splendid torch, which I got hold of for the moment. I want to make it burn as brightly as possible before handing it on to the future generations.
—George Bernard Shaw, from his play *Man and Superman*

My own hypothesis is that volunteer work attracts people who already have an openhearted sense of connectedness with people in general; this is what motivates them to volunteer in the first place. But this doesn't mean that if you haven't felt very connected before, it's beyond your reach. A connec-

tion and service practice can begin at any time and will bear
fruit right away. When more people engage in this practice,
opening their hearts to the global community and those in
need, the world will be a better place.

ଔ

There are two sides to the equation of human connection:
giving and receiving. In this chapter we have looked at the
health-giving effects of serving others. In the next one we
will explore the value of connecting in order to receive social
support. You will experience equally powerful benefits from
reaching out and accepting the help and encouragement of
others.

19

Practice Building Relationships

As you have just discovered in reading chapter 18, there is ample and compelling evidence that serving others is a health-enhancing practice. The evidence for the health benefits of building supportive relationships is even more remarkable, and in this chapter I present a host of studies that demonstrate this. The fundamental message is that humans are meant to be in community, and the degree of community we experience directly correlates to the degree of health we experience.[1]

A healthy network of supportive relationships is essential for the health of all people, and especially for those of us living with chronic or life-threatening illness. It provides a sense that we can trust and count on other people for friendship, emotional and problem-solving support, help with tasks, and physical or material assistance. An essential element of healthy social support is mutuality. We strengthen our sense of mastery when we can offer support to others and feel comfortable asking for it.

Around the world and in all cultures, the healthiest people belong to some kind of community, have close friends, and, as is the case with altruism as well, feel connected with the whole of humanity. In fact, all forms of chronic and life-threatening health challenges are more prevalent where there is the least social support. In parts of the world where multigenerational families remain together living in tight communities that are closed to outsiders—communities in which every member is known and valued—disease rates of all types are dramatically lower than in countries like the US, where a large segment of the population lives alone and in relative isolation. (Living alone can be perfectly healthy, however, if you have a close circle of friends or family nearby, or work in a tightly knit community.)

Kenneth Pelletier, a world-renowned researcher at the Stanford Center for Research in Disease Prevention, sums it up well when he concludes, "A sense of belonging and connection to other people appears to be a basic human need, as basic as food and shelter. In fact, social support may be one of the critical elements distinguishing those who remain healthy from those who become ill."

What the Research Shows

The studies I will briefly encapsulate demonstrate our common need for support in community and the extent to which our health outcomes are associated with the quality and quantity of such support.

Studies of General Morbidity and Mortality

In a very famous epidemiology study, one of the most referenced of its kind because of its impressive sample size, researchers Dr. Lisa Berkman and Dr. Leonard Syme studied seven thousand residents of Alameda County, California. All of them were observed for a nine-year period in order to discover all the common denominators among the healthiest residents. The researchers controlled for gender, race, ethnicity, socioeconomic status, alcohol, tobacco, obesity, depression, and medical care. The study showed conclusively that the healthiest people were the ones with the greatest quantity and quality of social support. And conversely, the most socially isolated people had the greatest morbidity and mortality. A large social support network and high frequency of contact directly correlated with health and made all the difference between health and illness.[2]

In an eight-year follow-up of the Alameda County study with 6,848 of the initial seven thousand subjects, the researchers found results consistent with the first study: a very strong correlation between the amount and quality of social support and reduced morbidity and mortality of all causes. Those who lived fairly isolated lives had a mortality rate that was three times greater than that of those who had family or friends. It also found a very robust inverse correlation between the quantity and quality of social support and cancer. Those who were most socially isolated had a significantly greater chance of developing cancer and dying from it.[3]

In another famous study, epidemiology researcher Dr. James House and his team conducted a prospective study of 2,754 residents of Tecumseh, Michigan, observing their social ties and group activities for ten years. This was a very rigorous study in that residents with any medical or psychiatric condition that could possibly interfere with their ability to be active in a social community were excluded. Over time it became clear that people with the greatest participation in a social support network or group were the healthiest. Those who initially had great support but who, because of various life circumstances, lost their connection to community were found to develop a variety of health problems. Those with the least social support were found to have *four times the mortality rate* of those with the most support.[4]

Remarkable Findings among the Elderly

Some of the most intriguing studies of the value of social support have tracked elderly people, and some of these have indicated that social support can actually counteract what we might consider "normal" deterioration as a result of aging.

One study conducted over a ten-year period in Australia, for example, revealed that older people with a large circle of friends were 22 percent less likely to die over the period of the study. And in 2007, Harvard researchers found a strong association between social support and neurological health in older people.

In a study by psychologist Bert Uchino, thirty-eight residents of a retirement community received visits from volunteers three times a week for a month. Immune function tests were performed on all the residents at the beginning, during, and at the end of the month.[5] At month's end, immunoglobulin (antibody) levels as well as natural killer (NK) cell activity were increased. NK cells attack and destroy cancer cells and virus-infected cells.

In another study conducted by psychoneuroimmunology researcher Dr. Janice Kiecolt-Glaser and her team, volunteers visited thirty elderly retirement home residents three times a week for one month. The residents agreed to allow the researchers to draw blood multiple times throughout the study, and they found a very significant increase in NK cells. They chose a three-times-a-week schedule for this study because they had previously noticed that residents who had visitors three times or more each week had significantly stronger immune systems than those residents who had fewer visitors.

A surprising result of this study was that although the residents of the retirement home knew the visitors were strangers who were only visiting them as part of an experiment, they still received a boost in their immune systems. Under the circumstances, these visits would barely seem to qualify as social support, yet they still had a positive effect. Presumably, visits from people close to them would have produced an even greater effect.[6]

Physician and psychophysiology researcher Dr. Bengt Arnetz and his team ran a prospective, randomized, controlled study of sixty retirement community residents. They discovered that the residents who received the most social support *evidenced increased levels of DHEA and stable levels of growth hormones*, both of which were unheard-of in elderly populations.[7]

Neurobiologist Dr. Robert Ornstein and physician Dr. David Sobel performed a study involving twenty-five hundred elderly men and women in order to determine the effect of social support on health—a very impressive sample size. At the start of the study, the subjects were interviewed to determine the level of social support each was receiving. The researchers observed those subjects who were hospitalized following heart attacks. They had controlled for co-morbid conditions (multiple illnesses) and severity of the heart attack. Of the patients who had two or more sources of social support, mortality was 12 percent. The patients with no social support had a 38 percent mortality rate.[8]

The Karolinska Institute in Stockholm conducted a six-month study to determine the benefit of social support among the elderly and whether it can improve health outcomes. The study involved sixty residents of a local retirement community. The staff involved thirty of the residents in a six-month "social activation program." At the start of the program, a complete blood count and levels of testosterone, dehydroepiandrosterone, and estradiol were recorded for all sixty subjects. Psychosocial tests were also administered to everyone. Both groups were then tested again at three months and at the end of the study. One of the findings included statistically significant hormonal increases in the treatment group but none in the controls. The thirty subjects in the control group evidenced a decrease in hemoglobin levels, while these levels were unchanged in the treatment group. (This is significant because hemoglobin levels are ordinarily on a steady decline in old age.) In addition, height decreased in the controls but not in the treatment group. The thirty treatment subjects were engaged in group physical activity and group skill building to improve self-efficacy and self-empowerment.[9]

One of the attributes of the healthiest centenarians throughout the world, as we learned in the preceding chapter, is that they maintain strong social networks. In addition, their lives have traditionally revolved around family life. Multigenerational families commonly live together. And despite having so much family around, they also make time each day for friends.[10]

Social support at its best includes the opportunity for everyone to experience the deep joy of giving to others in the group. Research psychologists Charlene Depner and Berit Ingersoll-Dayton studied seven hundred elderly adults and discovered that the degree of health and vitality among the

> When we set an intention to connect with others, our hearts are open—metaphorically and physiologically.

elders was directly associated with the personal contributions they made to their social network; it was not based on what they took out of it.[11] This finding further reinforces the conclusions reached in the preceding chapter on serving others.

Social Support and Heart Disease

The evidence of a connection between social support and heart disease is compelling. One Swedish study, for example, tracked 736 men over six years and found that those with close friendships had less heart disease.[12] We have all experienced heartwarming feelings when we were with close friends. As we saw briefly in the last chapter, such feelings have physiological correlates. They have been traced to relaxation of the smooth muscle in the cardiac arteries, which then triggers other healthy physiological responses including vasodilation (the widening of blood vessels). This allows arteries that may be lined with plaque to open and carry more blood and oxygen to the heart, resulting in fewer and milder cardiac events. The heartwarming feeling itself is the literal result of increased blood flow to the center of the chest. This is probably one of the physiological mechanisms at work in the effects of social support on cardiac health.

Most behavioral medicine studies involving heart patients focus on the efficacy of lifestyle changes to reduce atherosclerosis (hardening of the arteries) and reverse ischemic heart disease (reduced blood supply to the heart muscle). World-renowned cardiologist Dr. Dean Ornish's behavioral medicine program includes weekly psychoeducational group participation, which he initially instigated as a way to promote the healthy lifestyle changes he advocates, especially adherence to a very strict low-fat diet. Doctor Ornish reported that although the researchers in his studies had not previously controlled for the effects of participation in the group, it was his personal belief that the social support aspect of these gatherings might be the single most powerful intervention of the entire program.

When research psychologist Ute Schulz and her team studied the efficacy of the Ornish program, they found the social support aspect to be one of the ingredients that made it a lifesaver for cardiology patients who had failed with previous behavioral medicine interventions.[13]

Prior to the establishment in their city of American fast food outlets and other unhealthy American influences, the residents of Tokyo and other major Japanese cities had one of the lowest rates of heart disease in the world. It was generally accepted in the early 1970s that the differences between US and Japanese incidents of heart disease could be accounted for in two ways: Americans ate a red-meat-based diet and the Japanese ate a fish-based diet, and Japanese had a much stronger sense of connectedness to family, friends, and even work associates than Americans.

Despite the exceptional cardiac health of the Japanese in their home country at that time, researchers discovered that Japanese immigrants to San Francisco in the early 1970s were even healthier than their already healthy Tokyo counterparts. These immigrants often ate American food, smoked cigarettes, and had cholesterol levels as high as their American counterparts. The most dramatic finding was that despite their new, unhealthy American lifestyle habits, their cardiac health was not only superior to that of Americans but was even better than the Japanese back home, all of whom at that time were eating a much healthier diet.

Epidemiology researcher Dr. Michael Marmot and his team studied these immigrants, controlling for every imaginable variable. They concluded that the reason for this very surprising finding was that the immigrants had become even more involved in the tightly-knit Japanese cultural community of San Francisco than the average Japanese was in Japan. It was social support that allowed them to be so healthy despite eating unhealthy American food, smoking, and not exercising.[14]

In a study of several hundred cardiac patients in Sweden, Dr. Bertil Hanson and his team wanted to know why some patients had better health outcomes than others. After controlling for potentially confounding variables, they discovered that hospitalized people with the best outcomes were those whose teams of physicians and nurses were always close by and who had the most human contact. After returning home, the patients with the best outcomes, again controlling for variables, were the ones with the most social support.[15]

Although the psychophysiological mechanisms at work are still a medical mystery, it is now clear that social support not only correlates with lower rates of all-cause morbidity and mortality, but can cure existing disease. In a prospective study from Sweden, physician and medical researcher Dr. Kristina Orth-Gomer and her assistant Dr. Anna-Lena Unden divided 150 men into three groups. One group was made up of post-MI (myocardial infarct) patients. Men in the second group were relatively healthy except they had risk factors for ischemic cardiovascular (CV) disease. Men in a third group were healthy and had no risk factors for any CV disease. The men in all three groups received identical psychological testing as well as a complete physical at the start of the study. Variables for which the researchers controlled included socioeconomic status, marital status, education, occupation, social class, smoking, alcohol consumption, Type A behavior, social activities, and social integration. All the men in all three groups were then observed for ten years. At the end of that period, thirty-seven of the men had died—twenty of them from ischemic heart disease. After all the data were processed these associations became clear:

- The men with the most disease or the most risk factors ten years earlier were not necessarily the ones with the highest mortality rates.

- Social isolation was the single factor above all others that contributed to the highest mortality rates.
- The men with existing heart disease ten years earlier who had the greatest social support *outlived the healthiest men* who were the most socially isolated.[16]

Social Support and the Immune System

Psychoneuroimmunology researchers have consistently found a positive correlation between social support and the immune system.

Dr. Janice Kiecolt-Glaser and her team proved that social support improves immune function and can reverse the damaging physiological effects of emotional distress. She found that social support improved leukocyte cell counts and immune function.[17]

College students are under enormous emotional distress during exam periods. At Ohio State College of Medicine, students were interviewed prior to a period of final exams to determine their baseline emotional distress levels as well as their level of social support. Researchers collected saliva samples before, during, and after the exam period. (Researchers often use salivary immunoglobulin A (s-IgA) because it is one of the few lab measures they can collect noninvasively.) Researcher Dr. Susan Kennedy, working in Dr. Kiecolt-Glaser's lab, found that s-IgA was significantly diminished in the emotionally distressed students who lacked good social support, making them more vulnerable to both bacterial and viral respiratory diseases. The students with good social support had far less diminution of their s-IgA as well as higher levels of s-IgA during all three collections.[18]

In other studies by these Ohio State researchers, they measured NK cells during stressful periods. Reductions in NK cells correlated with lower levels of social support. The significance of this finding is that people without social support are more likely to develop cancer because NK cells attack and

> In a study of three thousand breast cancer patients, researchers found that women without close friends had a mortality rate of four times that of women with a close circle of friends.

destroy cancer cells after the cancer cells are flagged by CD-4 (T-Helper) cells.

Dr. Kiecolt-Glaser's husband, Dr. Ronald Glaser, is also a psychoneuroimmunology researcher. In one of his studies, forty-eight medical students at Ohio State Medical School received inoculations of the standard series of three injections of hepatitis B vaccine on days that coincided with a very stressful exam period. His remarkable finding was that *the students who reported having the most social support produced the most antibodies in response to the vaccine.* These same students also manifested the most robust T-cell responses to the hepatitis B surface antigen.[19] (Antigens are the substances that initially provoke the immune response. Antibodies are the proteins that are secreted as a result of the antigen-triggered immune response.)

Social Support and Cancer

In a substantial study of three thousand breast cancer patients, all of whom were nurses, completed in 2006, researchers found that women without close friends had a mortality rate of four times that of women with a close circle of friends.

In another study of 514 women, 239 were diagnosed with breast cancer. One of the results of this study was that those with the least social support were *nine times* as likely to develop cancer following a stressful life event. In fact, most psychooncology studies have found a positive correlation between survival time after cancer diagnosis and the amount and quality of social support.[20]

One reason social support is so valued in psychooncology

and behavioral medicine is that medical patients who have the most social support tend to be the most engaged in self-care (for more on the benefits of self-care see chapter 14). They are also more knowledgeable about their conditions and their treatments and have better recovery rates than those without good social support.[21]

Epidemiology researcher Elizabeth Maunsell and her team interviewed 244 breast cancer patients, asking them how many people they had confided in during the three months post surgery. They followed up with the patients for several years, and these were the results:

- The seven-year survival rate for the patients who had not confided in anyone during that three-month post-surgery period was 56 percent.
- The survival rate for those who had confided in one person was 66 percent.
- Those who had confided in two or more people had a 76 percent survival rate.[22]

POW Reports
Further evidence for the essentialness of social support can be found even in the extremity of war. Tortured POWs have reported that being separated and isolated from their trusted comrades could be even worse than the physical torture inflicted on them. This is why it is standard practice for torturers to separate all the members of a captured platoon. It is common knowledge that keeping captured soldiers together can empower them, whereas isolating them has the reverse effect.

The Lesson of Roseto
Roseto, Pennsylvania, was a small community made up exclusively of Italian immigrants. Physician Stewart Wolf studied this town in the late 1950s and again in the 1970s. In the 1950s, Roseto residents' health habits were awful. They chain-smoked cigarettes, drank, did not exercise, and ate a red meat diet that was even higher in fat and cholesterol than the typical

American diet of that era. They worked in mines, breathing filthy air all day, and lived in an environmentally unhealthy area. Their incidence of obesity and hypertension was equal to those in surrounding towns. Despite their abysmal health habits, the Roseto men had one-sixth the incidence of heart disease compared to other American men.

A generation later in the mid-1970s, Dr. Wolf and his original research team again looked closely at the residents of Roseto and discovered that they now had the same morbidity and mortality rates as the people of the surrounding towns. Referring to the 1950s study, here is what the researchers concluded:

> More than any other town we studied, Roseto's social structure reflected old-world values and traditions. There was a remarkable cohesiveness and sense of unconditional support within the community. Family ties were very strong. And what impressed us most was the attitude toward the elderly. In Roseto, the older residents weren't put on the shelf; they were promoted to "supreme court." No one was ever abandoned.[23]

The Sense of Belonging

As with Okinawan and other cultures around the world that enjoy exceptional health, in the Roseto of the 1950s there was a very strong sense of community and everyone had a well-defined social role in their family and in the community. In the interim between the 1950s and 1970s the younger generation had married and worked outside the community.

By the 1970s, the younger generations had lost the close cultural and community identity, but their health habits were now excellent. They smoked and drank less and ate a much healthier diet. They had higher rates of daily exercise. Yet despite all these dramatically improved health habits, their rates of heart disease, cancer, and other diseases were now as high as in all the surrounding towns. The researchers' conclusion was this: "This experience clearly demonstrates that the most important factors in health are the intangibles—things like trust, honesty, loyalty, team spirit. In terms of preventing disease, it's just possible that morale is more important than jogging or not eating butter."[24]

Research psychologist Christopher Peterson has found that trusted personal relationships serve as a buffer against life's adverse events. Having a sense of belonging to some type of community has consistently been correlated with better health, although the research indicates that *the quality of our relationships in our social networks is more important than the quantity of social contacts.*[25]

Social Support and Love

Social support at its best includes mutual feelings of love, as the experience of love is physiologically regenerative. There is an expression: *Love heals all.* And it has been shown that people in loving relationships are healthier than people in contentious ones.

Well-known Harvard University Health Service physician and researcher Dr. David McClelland tested immune function on students who were shown films that triggered loving feelings. He found that the films resulted in increased NK cells, increased IgA, and overall improvements in immune cell numbers as well as function.[26]

Similar studies by James McKay found that people who are open and friendly to strangers had half the rate of major illnesses of those who kept a cold and distant attitude toward strangers. These "affiliator types" (people who value relationships) had stronger defenses against viruses and cancer cells and their CD-4/CD8 ratios were better.[27] (CD stands for "clusters of differentiation," and the immune cells that have the CD8 marker on the membrane kill invaders such as viruses. The cells with CD4 markers on their membranes are necessary to help the CD8s work. For that reason, CD4s are known as T-helper cells.)

The Example of Karmu

In the 1970s, David McClelland noticed over a period of time
that people in Cambridge, Massachusetts, who went to a local
healer named Karmu were recovering not only from flu but
even from cancers and a multitude of serious illnesses at better
rates than those treated by the Harvard Health Service.

Karmu was of African descent. His father was a famous
Ethiopian rabbi and his mother was West Indian. He was highly educated and came from a fairly well-to-do family, yet he
lived in a poor section of Cambridge because he liked being
"a man of the people." His real name was Edgar Warner; he
had been given the name Karmu by a Tibetan monk who pro-
nounced him a healer of the highest magnitude.

Karmu was very charismatic in the way he made people
feel better. One time when Dr. McClelland developed the
typical early symptoms of flu with high fever, he went to see
Karmu instead of going to the Harvard Health Service. Here
is his account:

> He had a big crowd waiting for him. He saw me, and
> right away knew I was very sick. He was intuitive that
> way. Karmu put aside his other patients, took me into
> his office, and basically held me in his arms for thirty
> minutes. Now, grown-ups just don't get held like that.
> He's a big man, I'm a big man, but he held me like a
> baby the whole time. When I left his office, I didn't
> feel any different—I was still very sick. So I went home
> and got into bed. The next morning I was fine, which
> never happens otherwise with influenza.[28]

It is impossible to know with certainty what healed Mc-
Clelland, but as he said, waking up fine the day after the onset
of the flu simply never happens. There were no confounding
variables, as the only treatment he received was thirty minutes
of being held like a baby—an experience of love and affection.
Maybe it is true that love heals all.

McClelland's experience with Karmu led him to conduct

studies on the nature of health and healing. The association of social support to health had already been established, but he discovered that people who were affiliators were healthier. They had fewer and less severe illnesses. Interestingly, people motivated by status and power rather than human connections had weaker immune function than individuals who were motivated by human connections but had smaller social support networks. This finding points to the strong association between intrapsychic motivations and health outcomes. However, research shows that the quantity and quality of social support per se is strongly correlated with health outcomes.

In one of Dr. McClelland's studies, half of a large group of students with the earliest signs of a cold went to Karmu for treatment and the other half to the Harvard Health Service. Most of those who were treated at Harvard developed severe colds. *None* of the Karmu-treated patients developed colds. None of the Harvard-treated students mounted an immune response as evidenced by increased salivary IgA. All of the Karmu-treated patients did.[29]

After Roseto

There are not many communities like 1950s Roseto still left in the twenty-first century. Most of us in the world of today must create our own social support community. But the actual feeling of belonging, which was so healing to residents of Roseto, cannot be acquired simply by joining organizations. Thomas Moore expressed it this way:

> Loneliness can be the result of an attitude that community is something into which one is received. Many people wait for members of a community to invite them in, and until that happens they are lonely. There may be something of the child here who expects to be taken care of by the family. But a community is not a family. It is a group of people held together

by feelings of belonging, and those feelings are not a birthright. Belonging is an active verb, something we do positively.[30]

The Importance of Genuine Support

Social psychology researcher Dr. Karen Rook found that if the people with whom we seek social support are not empathic, we may derive no health benefit; in fact, we may experience a negative health impact.[31] Not surprisingly, people who are in conflictual or contentious relationships with their partners or others close to them commonly suffer worsening of their health.

Emotional support is essential, and it is important for us to be around people who are empathic and understanding. Unfortunately, oftentimes the source of the greatest stress in people's lives is their relationship with their partner or spouse. It is essential to get professional help with this primary relationship because that potent stressor is not conducive to mastery or health. To recover from cancer or other serious disease, in addition to getting good medical care, it is important to resolve major conflicts because chronic emotional distress impairs immune function.

Being around people who say things like "poor you" serves to disempower us. It is best to be around people who appreciate the seriousness of our condition and comprehend what we are going through. It is critical to have people in our lives who provide a type of emotional support that leaves us feeling better. Life is too short to spend it in stressful relationships or dysfunctional communities.

Support Groups

When one is not feeling well, it is very difficult to view a disappointment as an opportunity and a challenge. The support of a group helps participants avoid going into a hopeless, helpless frame of mind. Shared inspirational stories can help group members develop the courage to appreciate undesirable events as opportunities and challenges rather than as defeats.

Studies on the effects of being in a support group show that *the best support groups include skill building.*[32] When I trained at the Simonton Cancer Center, we divided everyone into small groups of six to eight each. The groups met for two hours every morning and every afternoon all week, and every group session was focused on skill building of some type. When I spent a week at a retreat that Dr. Lawrence LeShan led, we met in a supportive group format the entire time, and most of that time was also spent in some form of skill building. The most important skills we taught patients were how to practice distancing themselves from their unhealthy thought patterns and how to identify and pursue what mattered most to them in their lives.

I believe that one of the reasons social support is so strongly correlated with health is that at its best, it serves to empower people. Self-empowerment serves as a potent catalyst to healing and maintaining health. Being a member of a well-facilitated, skill building–based support group should result in an increased sense of mastery.

છ

You can improve your social support and strengthen your ties to community through many of the recommendations found elsewhere in this book. For example, we often do volunteer work in community with other volunteers and those they serve. We most often learn and practice mindfulness in community with other meditators. Social support is so absolutely essential for health that it is important to be diligent and creative about finding a community of some type to join, and make new friends. Following are a few more specific ideas.

Suggestions for Building Social Support

- Talk to strangers. Support takes place even in casual, one-time interactions. All relationships are important opportunities for us to meet our universal need for connection.
- Ask yourself throughout the day if your need for social support is being met; if not, take some immediate action to meet that need.
- Find an appropriate psychotherapy group to join. This can serve at least five functions. First, group psychotherapy is far more cost effective than individual psychotherapy. Second, it offers a much greater opportunity for personal growth because group members are in a therapeutic relationship with six to eight other members and up to two group leaders. The group doubles as a source of social support. It gives the group members the experience of being in a functional community. And finally, the long-term physical health benefits of group therapy can be profound as a result of all its mental health benefits.
- If you are experiencing problems in any close relationships, find a psychotherapist or counselor who specializes in couples therapy or family therapy.
- Get involved in activities that are performed in groups. Examples are book clubs, bridge clubs, and any type of activity involving interpersonal interactions.
- Take up a hobby that involves being with other people.
- Engage in humanitarian work that involves working on a team.
- Look for opportunities at work to be engaged in team efforts.
- If you don't already have someone in whom you can confide, find someone. Your health and your life depend on it.

20 Practice Finding Humor

F or those of us living with chronic health problems, it's important that we don't take ourselves and our medical situation too seriously. Worrying or agonizing about our health challenges isn't helpful—in fact it's deleterious to our health—so it's highly beneficial to learn to see the humor in our day-to-day life. This means learning to take our thoughts more lightly, which hinges on the core ability we develop through mindfulness practice: the ability to see even our most troubling thoughts as nothing but passing brain phenomena.

In the Words of a Flustered Researcher . . .

At a 1998 professional conference I attended, Dr. Joe Kamiya, a pioneer psychophysiology researcher who was then probably in his late seventies, did a PowerPoint presentation before a large audience. PowerPoint technology at that time posed a challenge even for younger presenters. At a certain point in his talk, the program on his laptop malfunctioned. He gasped at first, but then quickly laughed, remarking to the audience, "You have to have a sense of humor about these things *or you will surely die prematurely.*" Dr. Kamiya remained calm, accepting the reality of the computer malfunction and refusing to worry about the implications. This was an expert's opinion— albeit demonstrated accidentally—of the importance to health of disengaging from troubling thoughts.

The Tonic of Finding Humor

Seeing the humor in the events of the day has great healing properties. In my three-year training at the Simonton Cancer Center, I noticed that Dr. Simonton and his colleague Dr. Mariusz Wirga routinely cultivated their ability to look for the funny things in life. Whenever something failed to go as planned during one of the residential cancer retreats, rather than becoming irritated or distressed, their automatic strategy seemed to be to look for what was funny about the situation. They usually found it, took a moment to laugh about it, and freed themselves of the burden of taking themselves too seriously.

University of California–Berkeley research psychologists Dacher Keltner and George Bonanno have performed studies examining the effects of laughter on health. In their words: "Laughter facilitates the adaptive response to stress by increasing the psychological distance from unhealthy thought patterns and by enhancing social relations."[1] So when Drs. Kamiya, Simonton, and Wirga laughed at problems in their presentations, their laughter played a dual role: it allowed them to disentangle from their thoughts about what went wrong; and by laughing in front of their audiences, they enhanced their connection with those watching what otherwise could have been a very stressful experience.

Public health researchers Lee Berk and Stanley Tan at Loma Linda School of Medicine and Public Health found that laughter reduces stress hormones, increases immune cell counts, improves immune function tests, and increases beta-endorphins as well as human growth hormone. They also found that even *the anticipation of laughter* improves regulation of neuropeptides, neurotransmitters, and neuroendocrine hormones. In one study, men who anticipated watching one of their favorite funny videos tested 27 percent higher in beta-endorphin and 87 percent higher in human growth hormone than the control group. These improvements in physiological functioning occurred merely through recollecting the pleasur-

---

Laughter reduces stress hormones, increases immune cell counts, improves immune function test results, and increases beta-endorphins as well as human growth hormone.

---

able experience of laughter and looking forward to laughing again.[2]

Laughter in the Fast Lane
One summer evening long ago, my wife and I were sitting in traffic on the freeway, not moving an inch, late for a dinner engagement in San Francisco and feeling frustrated and angry. Both of us were busy telling ourselves a story: the freeway would not be at a standstill if they hadn't turned the breakdown lanes into traffic lanes, which results in no place to move damaged vehicles out of the flow of traffic! This was before cell phones, so we had no way of calling our friends to tell them why we weren't there, which added to our emotional distress. Suddenly, the passenger in the next car leaned out the window and spoke to us, imitating a well-known TV commercial for mustard at the time with a very proper British accent: "Pardon me, but do you have any Grey Poupon?"

We cracked up, of course, and his joke served as a wake-up call to presence. It allowed us to realize that cognitive fusion with our thinking was causing us to suffer. We had become entangled with our brain secretions, with thoughts of assigning blame for our plight, and were missing everything about the present moment, including the possibility of laughter.

Laughter Clubs
You don't need to wait to see or hear something funny to have an opportunity to laugh. "Laughing clubs" originated in India and can now be found around the world. How do they work? People get together and start laughing artificially, and very

soon, their laughter becomes genuine. At first, the laughter seems inauthentic, which could paradoxically increase emotional distress. But, as people begin to feel more comfortable laughing for no reason, the laughter starts to feel more authentic and spontaneous; that's what catalyzes healthy physiological effects.

I've offered this in workshops and skill-building groups I've led. With a very serious expression, I direct participants to try repeating after me: *hee, hee, hee, ha, ha, ha, ho, ho, ho.* Then I say, again unsmiling: "Make sure you don't make a mistake. Okay, are we ready to start?" At that point, the laughter usually becomes genuine and quite infectious.

In these groups, I always set an intention to look for opportunities for people to laugh. I have never done stand-up comedy, but I've found that setting an intention to take thoughts lightly is a very powerful mindfulness practice that is quite life-enhancing.

> *I venture to say that no person is in good health unless he can laugh at himself, quietly and privately.*
> —Gordon Allport

> *Never underestimate the unimportance of everything.*
> —Steve Allen Jr.

> *He who laughs last, lasts.*
> —Steve Allen Jr.

Suggestions for Humor Practice

- Two questions can be helpful reminders to take your thoughts lightly when things appear to be going wrong, or not as planned. Ask yourself: *Is anyone's life in danger? Am I at risk of ending up homeless?* This can help you put life's more minor difficulties in perspective and make it possible to find humor in the situation.
- Follow Michael J. Fox's example and learn to see your physical challenges as funny stories. You might even

want to write about them as he did. In his book *Always Looking Up,* he describes how he brushes his teeth: "Grasping the toothpaste is nothing compared to the effort it takes to coordinate the two-handed task of wrangling the toothbrush and strangling out a line of paste onto the bristles. By now, my right hand has started up again, rotating at the wrist in a circular motion, perfect for what I'm about to do. My left hand guides my right hand up to my mouth, and once the back of the Oral-B touches the inside of my upper lip, I let go. It's like releasing the tension on a slingshot and compares favorably to the most powerful state-of-the-art electric toothbrush on the market. With no off-switch, stopping means seizing my right wrist with my left hand, forcing it down to the sink basin, and shaking the brush loose as though disarming a knife-wielding attacker." See if you can think of a way to turn a challenging physical moment into a funny scene.

- Live with conscious intention to surf the big waves that come at you throughout life. The people who are most in control of their lives are not the ones who stay out of the surf; they're the ones who learn to ride the waves. Learn how to ride the unavoidable challenges that are part of life. This is a good image to use when you know you need to increase "your psychological distance from stress" in Keltner and Bonanno's words, and find something to make you laugh.

- Although my best recommendation is to take your thoughts lightly, and this results from cultivating life skills, it can also be very therapeutic to sit back and watch funny movies and read anything that makes you laugh, especially when you're not feeling well. Before discounting the enormous power of this passive method to improve how you feel, remember that Norman Cousins recovered from a life-threatening disease by spending his days watching *Candid Camera* and Laurel and Hardy movies. In this case, medicine had nothing to offer, but

Cousins realized that in laughing all day, he reduced
emotional distress, which reduced physiological stress,
which could then improve physiological functioning.
This laughing treatment, like all the recommendations in
this book, should never be used instead of recommended
medical treatment.

- When you realize you're entangled with unpleasant
thoughts, experiment with smiling. Giving yourself this
physical cue to take a lighter approach may be enough
to help you disentangle. Part of why this is effective is
that when the smile muscles are engaged—especially the
orbicularis oculi, the facial muscle that causes the crows-
feet squint beside the eyes, which is only apparent in
genuine smiles—the brain gets a message that results in
the release of beta-endorphin, dopamine, and serotonin.
In other words, although the smile may seem artificial at
first, within seconds it often becomes genuine because
you have tricked your brain into thinking something
pleasant has happened.

Try one of these suggestions the next time you notice that
you're taking yourself, your illness, the state of the world, or
anything else so seriously that you can feel negative feelings
welling up. Interrupt them with a reality check and a smile.

21 Practice in the Eye of the Hurricane

Mindfulness, Distraction, Dissociation, and Conscious Breathing

Growing up in New England, I was fascinated by the phenomenon of the eye of a hurricane—the peaceful realm at the center of a rampaging storm. When a hurricane hit our area, its destructive winds and heavy rain passed through, and then there was a period of calm and quiet before the violent weather returned.

Being outdoors at this time was a mystical experience for me. As the intense energy of the storm raged outside the eye, within the eye there was calm. It was silent, windless, aromatic, and tranquil. There was something otherworldly about the experience. I enjoyed a wonderful sense of being completely isolated from the rest of the world because I knew that, except in emergencies, people wouldn't dare travel in or out of the area surrounding the eye; it was too dangerous. And so, for a time, I had this otherworldly realm all to myself.

When we find ourselves in situations that seem tumultuous—as an inpatient in the hospital, perhaps, or in the midst of an intense argument—it is important to be able to find the eye of the hurricane. During the most chaotic experiences of our lives, we can find the eye in a variety of ways: through mindfulness, distraction, dissociation, imagining a sense of control, or by doing a yogic or other form of conscious breathing.

The extreme anxiety or fear that we experience in a meta-

As long as we are fully engaged in
the activity at hand, fully aware in the
peaceful eye of the present moment,
we are unflappable—and can cultivate
mastery—when things go wrong.

phorical hurricane is often the result of unhealthy images or constructs conjured up in the brain and has little to do with the facts. Mindfulness practice trains us to stay fully present with those very upsetting situations, which in turn allows us to find the tranquil space amid the storm. When we are in full contact with whatever is occurring now, we are less overwhelmed and the situation we are in becomes much simpler to manage. Think of Kwai Chang Caine, the fictional character of the 1970s TV series *Kung Fu*. In the midst of a violent bar room brawl, he occupied the eye of the storm, perfectly calm and safe, because he had the skills to be able to remain fully aware of all the chaos swirling all around him without getting entangled with it. Importantly, cowboys discovered that they couldn't hurt Kwai Chang Caine with their words or their fists because he was unfazed by both.

Research psychologist Lizbeth Nielsen of the National Institute on Aging and colleague Alfred Kaszniak discovered that long-term mindfulness practitioners are able to *discern and identify emotions* much more effectively than others. They also found that these practitioners were less physiologically reactive to ambiguous stimuli, as measured by biofeedback instrumentation.[1] This provides further insight into how mindfulness practice allows us to create an eye within which we can thrive amid the hurricanes of life. It teaches us how to live in harmony with all that is happening in and around us from moment to moment.

As long as we are fully engaged in the activity at hand, fully aware in the peaceful eye of the present moment, we are unflappable—and can cultivate mastery—when things go wrong. We accomplish this by training ourselves to develop and practice mindfulness of present-moment thoughts, images, emotions, and sensations and by maintaining an open and curious attitude toward all of our inner experiences— both pleasant and unpleasant. Through practice, and by living with intentionality, we develop the ability to bring full awareness to our present experiences and to welcome them all.

Alternatives to Mindfulness

If our situation is too terrifying to permit us to practice mindfulness in the eye of the hurricane, distraction, dissociation, imagining a sense of control, and conscious breathing are four healthy alternatives. These four methods can provide a healthy and necessary refuge from an experience that is simply too powerful to withstand in the present moment. Distraction simply means busying the mind with any activity that takes our minds off whatever it is that is disturbing us. It is antithetical to mindfulness, but it does have utility in situations where aversive stimuli are simply too intense—such as extreme acute pain. In the most extreme and terrifying situations, however, dissociation often becomes a refuge. Dissociation involves actually escaping to a safer place in our minds. Unlike distraction, dissociation involves losing awareness of the stressor. For example, when children are sexually abused, especially in ritual abuse, they commonly find themselves somewhere else in their minds—such as up on the ceiling or in a tree outside the house in which the abuse is occurring. Unlike distraction, we don't usually consciously choose to dissociate—it just happens. However, with hypnosis training, the skill can be cultivated.

To further explicate these concepts, *distraction* is engagement in an alternative activity in order to take the mind off the activity at hand; this can be done in the mind exclusively or by doing something physical. *Dissociation* is different; it is where thoughts, sensations, or emotions are split off from consciousness. *Compartmentalization* is a form of dissociation in which consciousness of specific life activities is kept separate from the rest of the person's life.

Although these escape mechanisms are healthy in terrifying or dangerous situations from which there is no possible escape, normal, everyday, run-of-the-mill stressors are best faced by making full contact with the present moment through mindfulness practice—consciously and intentionally staying within the hurricane's eye.

An Example of Helpful Distraction: Imagined Control

Let me offer an example of a time when I used distraction myself, quite unconsciously, in a highly stressful situation.

I was about to undergo an MRI. It was the first time I had been given gadolinium (the contrast material, administered by IV, used in MRI scans). I anticipated experiencing claustrophobia, due to my fear of being trapped in the scanner. I recall hearing myself ask the tech which brand of gadolinium I was being given. I don't know who was more surprised by this question—the tech or myself. I quickly realized that I had no real interest in the brand, that I had no idea whether there was any difference among brands, and that, in fact, I didn't even know if more than one company made gadolinium. I had unconsciously asked the question for one purpose only: as a way to *gain a sense of control* because I was so distressed about going into the narrow scanner. This is still another way of handling emotionally distressing situations.

I had already discovered that the more involved I became in my own tests and treatments, the more in control I felt. It doesn't matter that I didn't *actually* have control under such circumstances; in terms of minimizing emotional distress, what mattered was the *sense* of being in control. Though this kind of control is imaginary, I nonetheless found it both calming and empowering.

Imagining I am in control is a method of distraction that works for me. Some people are just the opposite: the more details they're given about what's being done to them, the more likely they are to panic. There are different pathways to the eye of the hurricane, and we all have to learn those that are best suited to us and how to choose the appropriate one for the circumstances in which we find ourselves.

About Control

When a hurricane is raging around you, you may find yourself searching for ways to regain control. Although many researchers use the term *control*, it can be confusing because it is often misinterpreted as an attempt to control *the outcome* of events. For example, in one type of lab experiment, one group of rats are foot-shocked and they are powerless to control the electric shock. A second group of rats is provided with a lever that turns off the current. A third group is provided a lever to depress when they are shocked but it doesn't turn off the current; this third group gains a sense of control even though their lever only provides the illusion of control. Similarly, with my own human experience of inquiring about the brand of gadolinium being used, asking the question had no real effect on what would happen to me, but seeking the answer provided me with a sense that I was in charge of my experience, and that illusion of control dramatically reduced both my emotional distress and my physiological stress.

Here's another example: In the beginning of World War II, the copilots on American bombers experienced distress because the pilot not only controlled the plane but had the only gun with which to fire at enemy aircraft. These copilots were eventually given a gun they could fire. It was completely useless because of its poor placement, but it gave them a sense of control.

Chronic Pain and Other Symptoms

Although my primary personal practice is mindfulness, sometimes my experience of pain is such that the most helpful thing I can do for myself is to use dissociation—going away somewhere in my mind. When I was in private practice specializing in chronic illness and chronic pain, one way I helped people was to help them learn how to dissociate from pain. Typically, they limped into my office in the throes of severe pain, and at the end of the session, their self-rating of their level of pain was often unchanged. But they consistently reported (with a very genuine and relaxed smile) that although the pain was unchanged in intensity, it was no longer bothering them.

The three methods I have just described—distraction, dissociation, and imagining a sense of control—have somewhat similar physiological effects. They reduce the secretion of catecholamines, the chemicals that prepare us for fight or flight. As we reduce the levels of cortisol, norepinephrine, and other agents that cause vasoconstriction and sympathetic arousal, we simultaneously activate endorphins and other health-inducing agents. Ordinarily, these methods have no place in mindfulness practice with its focus on everything that is truly happening—all our inner and outer experiences. However, when we are feeling completely overwhelmed emotionally or physically, these three methods can allow us to get centered enough to be able to return to mindfulness practice.

Intentional Breathing in the Eye of the Hurricane

Another key to practicing in the eye of the hurricane is to experientially understand your respiration and learn how to alter it intentionally to experience healthy effects. Being a neutral observer of the sensations of respiration is the most common mindfulness practice, and this relates directly to breathing's unique status as an automatic process that can also be altered with conscious intention. Breathing is the only automatically regulated visceral function that can also be very easily regulated through volition. There are other visceral functions that can be indirectly regulated with the conscious mind, but they require extra steps such as using mental imagery or biofeedback.

From a mindfulness perspective, by observing natural changes in the rate, depth, and rhythm of respiration, we can gain insights into our thoughts and feelings at any given moment. For example, when we suddenly get agitated, respiration automatically becomes shallow. When we suddenly relax, we're more likely to breathe diaphragmatically.

In order for an intentional breathing practice to be effective, it is important to understand the basic history and foundations upon which it is built. First, I'd like to clarify that the conscious breathing method used in mindfulness practice most often involves paying close attention to the sensations of respiration, such as the sensations of expansion and contraction of the chest and abdomen, which could also be interpreted as increased and decreased abdominal pressure. This is a passive form involving simply observing respiration without trying to alter it. The other conscious breathing methods described here involve actively altering the rate, depth, and rhythm of our breathing for the purpose of calming the nervous system.

Self-regulation of respiration has been integral to all forms of yoga and a component of European as well as Asian forms of meditation for millennia. In addition, most forms of the martial arts include some form of conscious, intentional breathing. Some form of practiced breathing is also central to professional dance, singing, and athletics.

It is helpful to understand something of the mechanics of breathing. The diaphragm is a muscle in the form of a large sheet that separates the chest cavity from the abdominal cavity. In contraction of the diaphragm on the inhalation, the downward flattening creates negative pressure in the lungs. This inflates the lungs from the bottom to the top. In relaxation of the diaphragm on the exhalation, the large muscle returns to its natural, upwardly curved position. The resulting positive pressure deflates the lungs.

There are many healthy ways to breathe, most of them involving slow, relaxed (without effort), natural (not forced) diaphragmatic breathing. Some yogic forms of breathing are quite rapid, but these are not intended to be used all the time. There is also controversy related to the ideal breathing rate, varying between six and twelve breaths per minute.[2] Although shallow chest breathing is unhealthy, deep breathing, involving complete inflation and deflation of the lungs, is also unhealthy. The best known method for breath training is a pranayama technique found in Hatha yoga that involves slowing the exhalation, through resistance, to half the rate of the inhalation and increasing the involvement of the diaphragm.

Stop-Breathe-Feel
Duke research psychologist Ruth Quillian-Wolever has devised one of the simplest, fastest, and most effective ways to become calm and centered in the eye of a storm. She calls it Stop-Breathe-Feel, and the name itself contains the three-step instructions for the practice. Although she initially offered it as a tool for people with eating disorders, it can be a very helpful way to identify and be fully present to emotions in any given moment.[3]

Because the rate, rhythm, and depth of respiration are exquisitely sensitive to changes in states of mind, we can gain great insight into our mental states simply by paying attention to these subtle changes. Stop-Breathe-Feel is a quick way to simultaneously tune in to and step back from our thinking and behavior so we can view them objectively, as opposed to being unconsciously fused with our experience. For example, regardless of how fast an argument is developing, you can intentionally pause, take a deep breath, and tune in to your feeling state with complete acceptance of your full inner experience. Ideally, stay with the sensations of respiration. This process allows you to gain enough emotional calmness to be able to observe your thoughts, emotions, and sensations with full acceptance, and this will allow you to more effectively resolve the conflict.

Another way to use intentional breathing to reduce emotional distress and physiological stress is a powerful, science-based method known as respiratory sinus arrhythmia (RSA), which causes rapid and dramatic physiological and psychophysiological alterations in our biochemistry. For an explanation of the science behind the method described next, see appendix B, Respiration and Health.

Respiratory Sinus Arrhythmia

Although many breathing techniques have been used to optimize mental states, gas exchange, and physiological functioning in general, the one shown by psychophysiology researchers to have the greatest efficacy is RSA. This in no way means that RSA is superior to any of the ancient yogic forms of breathing; it has simply been exposed to the most scientific scrutiny. Simply put, RSA refers to a naturally occurring variation in heart rate, and is directly related to the rate and depth of respiration. For example, rapid, shallow breathing decreases RSA and slow, diaphragmatic breathing improves it.

RSA breathing increases your heart rate variability (HRV) (described in the respiration appendix), and increased HRV is a strong predictor of heart health. World-class athletes, for example, have very high HRV.

The fastest way to learn RSA is by getting a couple of sessions with a professional biofeedback clinician, but it is not the only way.

RSA Without Biofeedback Instrumentation

Applied psychophysiology expert Ira Rosenberg has written extensively about learning RSA breathing without biofeedback instrumentation.

1. To start, practice taking your pulse until you can do it comfortably.
2. Then, get comfortable following your natural breathing pattern while taking your pulse.
3. Once steps 1 and 2 have become familiar, pay attention to how your heart rate slows as you exhale and speeds up as you inhale.
4. Now you are ready to do RSA breathing. At the end of each exhale, do not inhale immediately. Instead, wait until you can feel your pulse rate increasing.[4]

I have used this technique with exceptional results to treat insomnia. However, learning RSA in this manner, without biofeedback instrumentation, requires considerable practice. I recommend initially learning this technique from a professional biofeedback clinician.

A Second Way to Practice RSA Without Biofeedback Instrumentation

Cognitive neuroscience researcher Evgeny Vaschillo suggests this method:

1. Exhale to the count of eight.
2. Inhale to the count of four.[5]

Watch the second hand on a clock so you can time your breathing at approximately six breaths per minute.

Home Biofeedback Programs

There are several home biofeedback programs that can help you learn and practice RSA breathing. The three types I have tried and can personally recommend are emWave, Journey to Wild Divine, and StressEraser. They are all fun and very easy to use, and you don't need to know anything about physiology. However, these methods are not as good as getting a couple of sessions with a biofeedback expert.

A Personal Experience with RSA

Mitral valve prolapse with regurgitation, atrial fibrillation, and preventricular contractions—all conditions affecting the heart that are associated with my chronic health challenges—are considered beyond our ability to manage or correct without medication or surgery. But RSA has helped me eliminate atrial fibrillation and dramatically reduce my preventricular contractions. Although mitral valve prolapse with regurgitation is a structural problem, RSA is such an extremely heart-healthy practice that it can actually improve conduction within the heart. No breathing method can actually fix structural defects, but I believe RSA breathing may slow the progression of mitral valve prolapse and regurgitation, allowing me to maintain a healthy ejection fraction (the percentage of blood pumped out of the heart with each heartbeat).

୧

In this chapter, we have looked at several ways to find the eye of the hurricane when we face chaotic or frightening circumstances. Upheaval and surging emotions are inevitable human experiences, whether the situation we are in relates to our chronic health challenges or to some other dimension of our lives. Distraction, dissociation, imagining a sense of control, mindfulness, and various yogic and other forms of intentional breathing are all effective ways to cope when the hurricane winds start to blow, and using these tools when you need them is one of the best ways to build mastery.

22   **Practice Something Different**

All healing takes place in an altered state of consciousness. This means that the state of consciousness in which the illness began must somehow be distanced from in order for the person to get well.
—Jeanne Achterberg, PhD

When something we're doing to improve our health isn't producing the desired results, the wisest thing to do is change the treatment or self-treatment plan. Changing course is probably the single most efficacious path to the development of mastery.

Though mindfulness is foundational to the mastery and wellbeing methods in this book, the need for the flexibility to change course still applies. This could involve trying a new teacher, registering for a residential retreat, reading mindfulness books, or possibly even switching to a very different mindfulness practice, such as from vipassana to Zen, or from a Tibetan practice to a Theravada practice. You may not even want to do any sitting meditation practice at all, but instead switch to physical practices such as hatha yoga or chi gung. These methods all produce different results, but they are all very valuable and each can be ideally suited for certain people at certain times.

Doing something different can involve inner mind-training practices such as these or something external and as simple as spending more time with people around whom you feel loved, appreciated, energized, and fulfilled.

When I had a psychotherapy practice dedicated exclusively to people who had chronic medical conditions or were cancer survivors, my goal was to help my clients develop skills
that would help them live with greater conscious intention
and psychological flexibility. With the exception of unhealthy
behaviors such as drug abuse or unprotected sex, any behavior that results in feeling more upbeat, joyful, optimistic, and
hopeful is healthy behavior; all of these and other positive
emotions serve to improve physiological functioning. To master mindfulness practice, it is important to allow yourself to
fully experience all painful, unpleasant emotions. However,
if you are living with cancer or some other serious disease,
it is best to change whatever you are doing that is resulting
in those unpleasant emotions, because from a purely physical
health perspective, feeling good is good for you and feeling
stressed can be immunosuppressive.

For example, despite being a long-term mindfulness practitioner, there are times when I go into the den to listen to music or watch an upbeat movie because enjoying these things
improves my symptoms for a brief time. Then, after perhaps
an hour, I'm often rejuvenated enough to go back to my work.
At other times I garden, meditate, do mental imagery, or nap
in order to feel better. These are all activities I know will improve my physiological functioning because they have helped
me in the past. But when any one of them isn't improving my
state of mind or physical symptoms, I change to a different
activity.

Become a Symptom Sleuth

When it comes to practicing something different, we need to
become private investigators of our own symptomatology.
This may include keeping meticulous notes about the effects
of medical treatments on our symptoms. It may mean continually changing how we treat the symptom until we find
the best solution through experimentation. In my own case, I
have run a few studies with "an n of one" (a study with just
one participant). For example, I have spent years trying new

> Discomfort and new signs or symptoms are often warnings that something needs to change.

self-administered treatments for migraines, fatigue, cardiac dysrhythmias, severe malabsorption, and other symptoms, continually changing whatever failed to work.

As a result of this experimentation, here are a few things I've learned about altering my own practices. I begin my exercise routine every morning around six o'clock. My symptoms determine the type of exercise on any given morning. If I'm in an arthritis flare, I use the elliptical cross-trainer. If certain other symptoms are present, I wait and do my exercise later in the day. Another adjustment concerns the significant fatigue I live with. If I've already had a nap and still can't keep my eyes open, I go out back and do a little gardening, or if I'm not up to that, I use the elliptical cross-trainer for fifteen minutes. It's important to keep trying something different until your results improve. Never give up!

The same idea that works for physical states applies to psychological ones. Often, when I'm with people older than I am who are able to do all the things I haven't been able to do in many years, I find myself engaging in self-pity. Physiologically, this is very unhealthy, so I immediately call to mind people I know who are even more limited. If that fails to get me out of my self-pity, I allow myself to fully experience the self-pity and come to realize that I can choose to take those thoughts more lightly. There are many techniques, but the most important thing is to recognize the opportunities we have to do something different from whatever it is that we can clearly see is not working.

Change in Response to Discomfort
Discomfort and new signs or symptoms are often warnings that something needs to change. The reason for this is that

all pathological conditions, no matter how minor, come into existence in a very specific physiological environment. It is often difficult to uncover the cause of a new symptom or condition, but identifying the cause is not always necessary. By changing the internal milieu, we can often change the course of the symptom or condition anyway. Of course, if we do discover the cause, we will want to eliminate it whenever possible.

What follows are a few examples of uncomfortable symptoms that clearly indicate the need for changes. Unfortunately, what you need to change will not always be as clear as it is in these scenarios, but these are simple solutions to simple problems that improve the odds of living with greater health and wellbeing, and they can give you the general idea of approaches to change.

Symptom: During the night, you experience a cramp in your calf.

Change: You roll onto your back and place your calf on a warm spot in the bed while relaxing your leg. The muscle spasm immediately quiets down.

Symptom: You experience abdominal cramping.

Change: You lie down in a certain position that has worked in the past, and the cramping abates.

Symptom: You feel a serious headache coming on.

Change: You sit quietly and imagine your feet getting very warm and your head getting cool. The headache abates before it has a chance to become severe.

Symptom: You become aware of sadness beginning to descend.

Change: You sit quietly and allow yourself to fully experience all your thoughts, sensations, and emotions. The sadness does not develop into depression, as it might if you tried to push the feelings away. However, if that doesn't work, and you're living with cancer, try something else.

Symptom: You become aware that you are feeling anxious.

Change: You take a minute to tune in to your breathing in order to slow it down, and you make sure you are breathing diaphragmatically. Your anxiety begins to dissolve.

Symptom: You become aware that you are engaging in a certain anxious habit. Each time you give in to it, you reinforce it.

Change: By allowing yourself to fully experience the uncomfortable impulses that normally drive you to act, you practice observing them without acting upon them. The urge to practice the anxious habit diminishes.

Symptom: Lethargy

Change: Exercise. As important as it is to do an hour of exercise each day, it's been five hours since you worked out, you've been sitting at a desk since then, and now you feel very lethargic. You get up and go for a fast walk around the block. This is healthier than reaching for the caffeine, it re-energizes you, and it builds mastery. Relying on a drug—even one as seemingly benign as caffeine—builds dependence rather than mastery. Mastery results from the cultivation of skills rather than pills and increases psychological flexibility and resilience.

Symptom: If you are working on a project and begin to feel stuck, frustrated, or sleepy, or you are experiencing some other symptom that you know isn't caused by lack of sleep or insufficient exercise, it may be time for distraction.

Change: Do something that completely takes your mind off whatever project you have been working on. One possibility may be a project you had planned to start after finishing the current one—especially if it's radically different. In my own case, when I find myself nodding off while writing or while doing an Internet search, I sometimes get up from my desk and vacuum the house or work in the garden. Usually, after only about twenty minutes or less, I feel refreshed and look forward to returning to the task in an energized and enthusiastic state of mind. It's remarkable how thoroughly I can alter my state of mind just by doing something different.

Symptom: You're experiencing a troubling symptom and realize you are obsessing about it.

Change: Use your imagination. One of the fastest-acting remedies is to go somewhere else in your mind. Imagine a change of scene. Most people who practice mental imagery do so in a quiet place where they can be free of interruptions and external stimuli. Although it's important to practice in a quiet environment in the beginning so you can learn how to go to a deep state, it's also valuable to practice in a noisy environment. That way, when you find yourself in a very anxiety-provoking situation, you'll be better equipped to go to a deep place in spite of it. Intentionally allowing your mind to go somewhere other than the present is orthogonal to mindfulness practice, but from a purely physical health perspective, it is often a good practice.

Instead of the Medicine Cabinet

These are all various ways in which practicing something different, and something that is entirely within your control, can offer relief from some very common ailments. Yet symptoms like these—cramping, headaches, sadness, depression, anxiety, pain, malaise, and lethargy—are typically treated with medications. This ignores the value of these symptoms as red flags that tell you something needs to change. If you take a medication to eliminate a symptom, it's like disconnecting a warning light in the car because you find its persistent glow annoying.

In situations where a symptom could be a prodrome, or early warning, of a possible impending medical condition, it is best to see your primary care physician to explore the cause.

> One of our greatest mistakes is to continue doing something that doesn't work in the hope that it will start working.

Simply treating the symptom with medication instead effectively destroys the clues that may help prevent a more serious problem later. If it's determined that the symptom isn't associated with a condition that requires medical treatment, then it's fine to treat the symptom yourself, provided that the treatment you choose does not cause any adverse physiological, psychological, or emotional effects.

Simple Behavioral Changes and Physiological Functioning
Even the simplest of behavioral changes serve to alter cognition, emotion, and physiological functioning. One of these is varying your posture. For example, when you stand tall, you feel better than if you slump, but it is important to *intentionally practice* maintaining good posture—this can serve as part of your mindfulness practice. One reason you feel better when standing tall is that proprioceptors throughout the body effect healthy neurochemical changes, many of which are related to the triggering of state-dependent healthy memories from times when you automatically held that posture in the past. Have you ever wondered, for example, why a certain memory popped into your head when you weren't doing anything related to it? Sometimes this can happen simply because you're holding your head in a particular position.

When you practice standing tall, smiling, and breathing consciously, you send a positive message to people around you, and they are then more likely to respond in a healthy way. This in turn serves as a feedback mechanism to create further changes as well as to reinforce your new behavior.

Another simple, healthy behavioral change is to smile. As we saw in an earlier chapter, smiling and laughing can be healing even when you aren't feeling amused because smiling increases blood flow to certain parts of the brain. By putting the facial muscles in the form of a smile, a somatic memory signals the brain to synthesize endorphins, and this triggers state-dependent memories of actual past events when you smiled and laughed.[1]

Take a Cue from the Acting Profession

UCLA research psychologist Ann Futterman performed psychophysiological and psychoneuroimmunological studies of actors, testing them as they expressed varied mood states. When actors behaved as if they were happy and energized, even when they hadn't been feeling that way, the new behavior catalyzed healthy psychophysiological changes. The product of those changes was an up-regulation of affect (increase in positive feelings).[2]

The researchers also discovered the reverse: acting as if one was sad caused depressed affect and immune function. The importance of using trained actors as experimental subjects for this study was that unlike most of us, when the actors pretended to feel a certain way, they actually believed it and measurable physiological indicators revealed that they were actually able to change their authentic emotional state.

The psychophysiology of actors can be better understood when we realize that virtually all thoughts, sensations, and emotions lead to a synthesis of neuropeptides. Every time there is an event in the mind, there is a corresponding event in these protein-like molecules that mediate and modulate neurons. Neuropeptidergic changes catalyze cognitive and emotional changes.[3]

The Labile Personality

People living with schizophrenia as well as people living with dissociative identity disorder (DID), formerly known as multiple personality disorder, have one-third the amount of cancer of the general population.[4] It has been hypothesized that this could be because the labile personality (one that continually changes) is physiologically healthier than a steady, constant, durable personality that happens to be chronically anxious or chronically depressed. Conceivably, the labile personality is inhospitable to the laying down of unhealthy neural pathways because of the constant changes in the brain.

Shifting into a Different State: Lessons from Spontaneous Remissions

In *Spontaneous Remission*, researchers Brendan O'Regan and Caryle Hirshberg describe their years of exhaustive research and their meta-analysis of the literature on the topic. They explored more than thirty-five hundred cases of unexpected remission from more than eight hundred peer-reviewed journals from around the world and concluded that every instance is a case of the individual having found—usually unconsciously—a way to activate the ability to self-heal. There is a clear explanation for every so-called spontaneous remission, which is usually the result of something the patient did differently to get well.

As we learned early in the book in chapter 2, all medical conditions begin because of a particular pathophysiological milieu. A causal relationship, however, is not often easy to establish. Just to give you a sense of the power of the mind in this regard, in people who have DID, different personalities can have different eye color, vision prescriptions, autoimmune diseases, allergies, immunity to various diseases, left- or right-handedness, and many other differences.[5] This is a potent illustration of some of the extreme alterations in physiological functioning catalyzed by the mind.

Regardless of the etiology of the disease, however, or the life-threatening nature of the diagnosis, many unexpected recoveries have been reported. The reasons for these are usually as elusive as the reasons people got sick in the first place, but patterns can be found. There are thousands of case studies, for example, of people who made remarkable and unexpected recoveries from life-threatening diseases following a radical positive change in their mental state.[6] These case studies have little in common except that the person began living differently, adopting some of the practices recommended in this book, especially those related to finding hope in the possibility of recovery, and finding meaning and purpose. Any behavioral change that increases happiness and a sense of wellbeing will improve physiological functioning, thereby increasing the odds of experiencing some improvement in health.

In most unexplained and unexpected recoveries from serious illness, patients were absolutely convinced of their ability to recover. It is important to note that they were not convinced they would recover; such a belief reflects "positive thinking," which could also be referred to as delusional thinking. Rather, they were convinced that recovery was simply a very real possibility. This is a critical distinction. When patients are convinced that they absolutely will recover and instead get worse or relapse, they become devastated and deeply depressed.[7] If someone has no hope, it is crucial to find a way to change that very unhealthy line of thinking. Inspirational stories may suffice for some people, whereas mindfulness training may be necessary for others, so that the person can begin to see the unhealthy thinking as just transient, unimportant products of the brain. One way or another, the person must find a way to disengage from unhealthy thoughts of doom and gloom in order to effect a potent shift in state of mind.

Remission and Alternative Treatments

It can be very helpful to read about those who beat the odds. In an earlier chapter, I introduced you to Ian Gawler, who was told he had two weeks to live.[8] No one had ever survived an osteosarcoma as widely metastasized as his, and being a veterinarian, he knew enough medicine and statistics to know that he was in trouble. But despite his awareness that his odds of recovering were not good, he somehow knew that he *could* recover—that it was possible. He knew that there were outliers on the bell curve, and that he could be one of the lucky few to go into a complete remission. When he was told that no one had ever fully recovered from the form of cancer he had, his response was "Great—that means I can be the first." He was determined to commit to doing whatever it took to recover. He then began to radically change his life from being a full-time doctor of veterinary medicine to meditating five hours a day. Most people aren't willing or even able to make that level of major life change, but change is absolutely necessary.

Having rejected the prognosis, Dr. Gawler took charge of his recovery and did everything possible to overcome the disease, including engaging in some "weird," completely un-proven treatments. There is still no evidence that the alter-native treatments he used could have cured or even slowed his cancer. Possibly, it was his deep, unshakable belief in his ability to recover that somehow improved his immune func-tion, enabling him to beat the odds—there is evidence in that arena. We will never know. We do know that he had already been living a healthy lifestyle at the time he was diagnosed, and that even so, he immediately proceeded to make radical shifts in the way he lived his life. Even though much of what he did was not based on scientific evidence, he believed in the possibility that each of those treatments had the potential to cure him. The source of his cure may well have been his very unscientific beliefs.

Shift Your Consciousness

People who have recovered when no one expected them to survive have usually come to believe that they can use their diagnosis as a turning point—an opportunity to explore how they can change and improve their lives.[9] The ability to see the diagnosis as an opportunity is the type of change that can improve the odds.

During the three years I trained at the Simonton Can-cer Center, I often got to sit in on Dr. Simonton's individual sessions. He continually observed that those who identified something meaningful to them that they had previously ig-nored, and decided to finally pursue it, had better rates of re-covery.[10] Sometimes the changes they made in their lives re-lated to work or to a long-term, unhealthy relationship. Other times it had to do with simpler things, such as making time

> Almost every unexpected recovery from a life-threatening illness has been shown to be preceded by a major shift in consciousness, resulting in the creation of a life that was engaging and purposeful.

each day to do some activity that adds enormous joy to life, such as gardening, art, playing with a grandchild, or anything involving passionate creativity. These are important for virtually everyone in order to maintain a healthy, happy life, but following a frightening diagnosis, changing one's life to accommodate these joys becomes essential.

Almost every unexpected recovery from a life-threatening illness that has been studied has been shown to be preceded by a major shift in consciousness, the result of which was the creation of a life that was engaging and purposeful.[11] Sometimes what has the best chance of shifting consciousness is very simple, but it always has to do with moving toward change.

Not unlike people with DID, we all act differently at different times; behavior is shaped by consciousness, which can be fluid. Each time we shift our consciousness, we have the ability to change our physiology. We can change it intentionally by doing something as simple as tuning in to our breathing or switching to a different activity. Small, subtle shifts such as these can enable us, for example, to behave in ways that create more receptive and less critical states of mind.

People with dissociative identity disorder perfect their different selves through the lifetime practice of different roles, and in so doing develop extraordinary psychophysiological plasticity. It can help to be willing and able to practice living differently in order to gain some of the advantage that is normally held by people with that disorder. Sometimes, in cases of unexplained recoveries from incurable conditions, patients report suddenly remembering a long-forgotten memory in great detail, with an actual re-experiencing of that past event. Other reports describe auditory, visual, olfactory, or other hallucinations, none of them drug-induced. In all these cases, the commonality is a change to a euphoric, or at least happy, state of mind marked by a lack of anxiety and a sense of well-being. An experience of very deep love and openness is also commonly reported. This includes openness to other people and different ideas from our own and a natural trust in humanity.[12] Even when the change is unintentional and unconscious, practicing something different can improve the odds.

A Message from Pluto
I will leave the topic of practicing something different with an illustrative story. A few years ago, the air conditioner in the motel room in Blythe, California, where my wife and I were staying made a very loud noise whenever the compressor came on. Despite resorting to ear plugs and a white noise machine, we both awoke every time this happened. So we devised a plan. There was nothing we could do about fixing the air conditioner in the middle of the night, and we knew changing rooms would disrupt our sleep even further, so instead we shifted ourselves. We anthropomorphized the air conditioner. We named it Pluto and decided to think of it as a beloved pet. Now, instead of feeling angry and frustrated when Pluto made the noise, we enjoyed our new pet's company and more easily fell back to sleep each time it woke us up. The changes we usually think of first have to do with our external circumstances — in this case doing something about the air conditioner. But internal changes in the mind can sometimes be the most life altering of all.

A Second Opinion
Sometimes, when you go in for medical treatment, the first physician you see is able to come up with the right diagnosis and treatment. But if you have reason to question his or her treatment plan, getting a second opinion is an important way to practice something different.

CR

All the practices I have described in this book—mindfulness, finding meaning and purpose, building relationships, developing authentic self-expression, and all the rest—share something in common: they are all ways to practice something different. All of them are readily available to you, and any one of them, or even several in combination, could be the change that makes the difference for you. Any time you realize that what you are doing to support your health is not achieving the results you would like to see, I invite you to open the book again, refresh your memory, and try something you haven't practiced for a while. Explore what is possible when you recommit to placing mastery and wellbeing in your own hands.

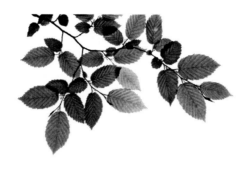

Part V

Medical and Home
Healthcare Self-Efficacy

This part stands apart from the rest of the book, yet is an invaluable adjunct to it. It contains two chapters, the first written for those living with chronic illness and the second for those caring for them at home. Uniting the two is a central aim: to give you evidence-based tools to increase mastery and wellbeing as you collaborate with a healthcare team and manage a medical condition in the home.

Here you will learn ways to

- Cultivate medical and home healthcare self-efficacy
- Advocate for yourself or a loved one in a medical setting
- Care for a loved one without abandoning yourself
- Collaborate effectively with doctors

Whether you are caring for yourself or for a loved one, it is very easy to fall into feeling powerless and lost. These chapters will help you manage this demanding stage of your life in such a way that you can use medical challenges for personal growth. In my psychotherapy practice, my facilitation of numerous chronic illness support groups, my teaching, and my own life, I have observed firsthand the difficulties of managing a life that revolves around going to medical appointments; it is no easy task. Fortunately, I have also seen that the same mindfulness-based techniques you have explored earlier in this book can be applied to these day-to-day challenges. Whether the patient is yourself or someone you love, if you adopt even a few of the tips I offer here, you will give yourself the gifts of feeling less overwhelmed, having more energy for yourself, and living a more vibrant, fulfilling life.

23

Medical Self-Efficacy and Advocacy: An Essential Aspect of Self-Care Mastery

I created the term *self-care mastery* primarily to describe a lifestyle that involves planning every day in such a way as to optimize your health and wellbeing. Managing your healthcare is an essential aspect of that way of life. The actions I recommend in this section serve to build self-efficacy and a sense of mastery while simultaneously improving your odds of receiving better healthcare. Remember: anything you do that gives you a sense that you are in control of your life serves to build self-efficacy, which in turn improves wellbeing. If most people lived with this level of self-responsibility and self-management, there would be no healthcare crisis.

Aside from getting better and safer medical care, people who practice self-care mastery have healthier self-esteem and are less depressed—even if they are physically dependent on others for management of their activities of daily living.[1]

It is important to understand that medical self-efficacy does not mean you must shoulder every task involved in taking charge of your healthcare all by yourself. In some situations, self-care mastery means taking charge of your life by hiring home healthcare workers, visiting nurses, and professional advocates.

Getting the Best Treatment

If you have a rare disease or an unusual medical condition, it is best to find out about studies being done on your diagnosis; this could determine where you get treated. In addition to getting into a clinical trial, it is also recommended that you find a doctor who is well known for treating your condition. In some situations, this may even mean traveling to another part of the country.[2]

Volume Equals Safety

In interviewing potential surgeons or any physician for an invasive procedure, ask how many he or she does *per week.* Older doctors may have done an impressive number over the course of a career, but that does not mean they are up to date and still on top of their game. Therefore, the question should generate information that reveals his or her weekly volume. In his book *Understanding Patient Safety,* Dr. Robert Wachter demonstrates that volume is equated with better results. It's important to go to a high-volume hospital and a surgeon who performs a very high volume of the specific procedure you need.[3]

When I needed rotator cuff surgery several years ago, I first went to a highly recommended surgeon who works out of our local community hospital. I asked him how many of that procedure he did per week. Then I went to a surgeon at one of the large medical centers in San Francisco, forty minutes away. It turned out that he did more than twice as many per week as the local guy, which made the decision easy. High volume usually predicts a better outcome.

In *Confessions of a Surgeon,* Dr. Paul Ruggieri describes all the mistakes he made in his first year of medical residency. For example, working in the emergency department he "accidently punctured a guy's femoral artery while trying to draw some blood." This is a good illustration of why you should never let any doctor or nurse perform any procedure on you with which she or he has little or no inexperience.[4]

Seek Medical Treatment Early

Medical self-efficacy and self-care mastery mean getting care when you need it—early. Whenever you have a new troubling sign or symptom or you think something needs attention, if you request help early, it will be easier to treat the problem. Most disease states are most effectively treated early, yet most patients tend not to go rushing off to the doctor until symptoms become more serious. Ideally, whenever you call your primary care doctor's office with a new symptom that may need attention, someone from the office will return your call within a couple of hours and get you in that day to see a doctor, nurse practitioner, or physician assistant (PA). If your doctor's office doesn't do that, you could go to an urgent care center, sometimes referred to as an acute care clinic. Obviously, if you think the symptom could possibly be life threatening, you would bypass those two options and immediately call 911.

The Emergency Department

Never go to the emergency department (ED) unless you are having a life-threatening emergency. If your symptoms need immediate evaluation or treatment but are not life threatening, go to an urgent care center. However, in a truly life-threatening emergency, as I just mentioned, immediately call 911.

Emergency departments are often overcrowded and, despite triage, not everyone always gets timely care. This is a time when self-care mastery and self-efficacy include knowing how to go up the chain of command. This shouldn't be necessary, but if it is, you will hopefully have someone with you who can advocate for you. For example, if you don't receive necessary care in the ED, especially if you are getting worse, your advocate will need to speak up. When the ED is overcrowded, it sometimes happens that a triage nurse fails to appreciate certain subtle conditions. If you don't get enough priority even after discussing your concerns with the triage nurse, you or your advocate can talk to the charge nurse, nurse manager, shift supervisor, or the ED's director. Although it's highly unlikely, if even that doesn't work, your advocate can locate and pick up the house phone, dial 0, and ask for the hospital administrator or the hospital administrator on call or have that person paged. Your advocate could say, "The patient has an emergency medical condition that should be evaluated right away."[5]

Make note of the names of everyone who treats you. You or your advocate should strive for honest, respectful communication with everyone you come in contact with on that shift. Do not blame individuals; they're doing the best they can, and when things go wrong, it is usually a systems problem.

If you have a complex medical history or a serious chronic medical condition, keep your most important medical records, including medications and other treatments, in your mobile device so that you can always easily provide it in emergencies and even at scheduled medical appointments. I keep mine on Word documents, which I use with the Pages app for my iPhone.

Do Your Own Differential Diagnosis

How can you be sure you have a problem that needs treatment? Another aspect of medical self-efficacy and mastery is self-diagnosis.

Physicians looking for the cause of symptoms perform what is known as a differential diagnosis, a systematic method that uses the process of elimination in cases where multiple factors may be at work. If you are so inclined, you can sometimes obviate the need to seek medical care by doing your own differential. However, if your symptoms could possibly signal anything life threatening, abandon this exercise and call 911.

You can do your own differential diagnosis this way:

1. List all your signs and symptoms. (A *symptom* is something you subjectively experience, such as anxiety or abdominal pain, whereas a corresponding *sign* is measurable, such as an elevated heart rate.)

2. List all possible causes. For example, if you are sud-
    denly feeling anxious soon after eating a big piece of
    chocolate cake, one possible cause could be the caffeine
    in chocolate.
3. Prioritize your list with the most potentially dangerous
    items at the top. If heart attack or stroke is at the top of
    your list, abandon this process and immediately call 911.
4. Starting at the top of the list, rule out all possible causes.
    Let's say you have epigastric pain or discomfort: you can
    sometimes rule out heart attack by taking antacids, but if
    there's no immediate relief, then without hesitation call
    911.

I seek medical care whenever my differential diagnosis
doesn't resolve the problem. Sometimes I figure out what's
happening but need a prescription to treat it, or a lab order
to confirm it, both of which necessitate seeing a doctor. Other
times, I have no clue about the etiology of the problem and
seek medical attention to rule out something potentially serious. However, I can often think about when the problem first
started and what new behavior may have contributed to the
new symptom. Sometimes changing my behavior can resolve
the new symptom. This requires looking at any changes in
diet, exercise, sleep, and other behaviors.

Self-care mastery and medical self-efficacy include always
making sure you get the care you need. Never ignore new
subtle signs and symptoms. If you can resolve them through
your own detective work, great! If not, make an appointment
with your primary care physician (PCP) or a specialist who
has already been treating you.

The Need for More Biomarkers
and Other Early Diagnostic Tests

Unfortunately, we are still living in a time of very few biomarkers for most deadly diseases. For example, pancreatic cancer
is one of myriad diseases that are usually diagnosed too late
to save the patient. Thousands of diseases are asymptomatic

until late-stage. A hundred years from now, biomarkers and other inexpensive, easily available tests will allow doctors to diagnose diseases like pancreatic cancers or glioblastomas at a very early and treatable—even curable—stage. We currently have various scanners that can detect early-stage pancreatic tumors or glioblastomas, but they are far too expensive to use for routine annual exams. Biomarkers will be able to accomplish the same feat very inexpensively.

Economics Determines Screening Recommendations

At the time of this writing, one of my family members has just been diagnosed with early-stage colon cancer. Although it is curable at this stage, it does require major surgery and hospitalization. If colonoscopies were recommended every eight years instead of every ten, a certain subset of patients who had no adenomatous polyps ten years earlier could be cured by outpatient endoscopic polypectomy rather than major surgery in the hospital. Economics is what determines most screening guidelines for most diseases. As another example, MRI picks up early-stage breast cancer long before mammography. The substantial difference in cost between these two tests is the reason women get annual mammograms rather than periodic MRIs. However, nothing is written in stone. Many insurance benefits can be negotiated to a certain degree. By going up the chain of command to a case manager at your insurance provider, you may find that a previously denied claim may be covered. However, you will need to build a case to support your request.

Get a Second Opinion

An important part of looking out for your own wellbeing in the medical environment involves being assertive about getting a second opinion whenever you are uncertain about your diagnosis or proposed treatment. There are several factors to consider here.

When we seek medical help, for various reasons at least four types of errors are all too common.[6]

1. The doctor fails to ask the right questions that could lead to the correct diagnosis.
2. The doctor fails to order the right tests that could lead to the correct diagnosis.
3. The doctor fails to diagnose the problem early enough to effectively treat the patient.
4. The doctor treats the patient based on evidence that applies to *most* patients. He or she does not take into account that a particular patient may have a preexisting condition that would contraindicate that particular treatment.

I once knew a nurse who suspected she may have developed congestive heart failure (CHF). She correctly went to a cardiologist with symptoms that are common to influenza as well as CHF. The cardiologist took one quick look at her and told her to go home, telling her she just had the flu. Because that particular cardiologist (who just happened to be the same one I was seeing at the time) was respected at our local community hospital where she worked, she ignored her nursing experience and her intuition and followed his advice. The result was catastrophic. She had performed her own differential and correctly diagnosed herself, but she didn't follow through. Eventually, she suffered so much damage to her heart that she needed a pacer and a defibrillator implanted. Upon hearing what had happened to her, I switched cardiologists.

We need to question everything our healthcare providers tell us and get a second opinion at a different institution when there is doubt, in order to avoid falling victim to that type of situation, which is all too common. If it can happen to an experienced RN, it is even more likely to happen to a layperson. Her cardiologist was correct insofar as he did not jump ahead and treat her for CHF just because she suspected she had it; his mistake was in not running various tests that would have confirmed his patient's suspicion. Like many doctors, he had little respect for a nurse's diagnostic acumen and believed that patients should simply listen to their all-knowing doctors. But she was also at fault. Her mistake was in not immediately seeking a second opinion.

Decision Analysis, Algorithms, and Probabilities

In the *New York Times* bestseller *How Doctors Think,* author and Harvard physician Jerome Groopman describes cases in which emergency medicine physicians failed to correctly diagnose a patient because the patient didn't fit the diagnostic algorithms. In other words, they tended to choose a diagnosis that was statistically logical but ultimately incorrect. Newer generations of doctors tend to think in terms of algorithms and probabilities, and in doing so, miss some of the outliers. Some patients have very atypical presentations that result in a missed diagnosis. Other patients have a symptom that is almost always associated with a different population or a different diagnosis.[7]

For example, when I was about fifty-four, I requested a dual-energy X-ray absorptiometry (DEXA), used to diagnose osteoporosis (OP), to assess my bone mass. The physiatrist I was consulting looked at me and told me with absolute confidence that I didn't have OP. I managed to get the DEXA anyway, which revealed that not only did I have OP; it was much more advanced than would be found not only in other fifty-four-year-old men, but even in the average ninety-five-year-old woman. It was inconceivable to this doctor that a healthy-looking fifty-four-year-old man could have a disease usually found in elderly women. But I knew enough about physiology to know that the malabsorption syndrome I'd recently been diagnosed with could easily cause OP, which was what prompted me to request the DEXA. Though I had told this doctor about the malabsorption, he still could not see the connection.

Usually, if you are able to present a scientifically valid, evidence-based argument for a specific diagnosis, test, or treatment, physicians give it serious consideration. However, there is a subset of physicians who expect patients to show deference to them and these physicians will sometimes ignore the knowledge, wisdom, and training of any patient who is not a fellow physician, even when the patient is an RN or a biochemist. Clinical trials data are often the most convincing type of information that can give you credibility in conversations with your physicians.

If clinical trials data for your disease are lacking or show wide variability in outcomes across a diverse patient population, you must work with your doctors to formulate a plan for getting the most appropriate treatment for your specific situation. Keep in mind that there is actually no such thing as an average patient; no one is an algorithm.

Three Empowering Questions to Ask
You can actually help your doctor make a correct diagnosis by asking the right key questions.

What Else Could It Be?[8]
If you find yourself in a situation where your doctor is suggesting a diagnosis that, based on what you know, does not seem right, there is one question that often helps remove the blinders: simply ask, *"What else could it be?"* This question may seem too simple to be significant, but it can make a profound difference in getting correctly diagnosed.

In the case of my osteoporosis diagnosis, because I was somewhat knowledgeable about pathophysiological processes and diagnostics, I was able to ask that question and then build a case for doing particular tests that could reveal a hidden diagnosis. Of course, one would hope this kind of flexible thinking would come from the doctor, but I have outlined the reasons this is so often not the case.

Is There Anything That Doesn't Fit?[9]
Groopman's book recommends this follow-up question because it can prompt the physician to pause and think outside

the box. Doubt can be a good stimulus to investigate further. This is another seemingly simple and insignificant question that can dramatically increase your chances of getting correctly diagnosed. Obviously, you would only ask this question when your doctor seems unclear about the diagnosis or when you have medical knowledge that leads you to question the initial diagnosis. These questions are critical because the diagnosis is critical. If you are diagnosed incorrectly, you will receive treatment for the wrong disease.

Ockham's Razor

Still another question to ask is this: *Is it possible I have more than one problem?*[10] Most of the time, all of a patient's signs and symptoms can be explained by one unifying diagnosis, consistent with the notion of Ockham's razor—that nature favors the simplest cause. However, posing this question is another way to help your doctor cast a wider net and look beyond initial impressions. On occasion, some patients will actually have two diagnoses that produce similar signs and symptoms; although it's not the norm, it does happen. Don't be afraid to bring up Ockham's razor when you have knowledge that could possibly cast some doubt on the initial diagnosis.

More on Second Opinions

When you ask those questions and your doctor is stumped, it is time to get a second opinion at a different institution, or from a different type of specialist at the same institution. For example, when gastroenterologists at two large medical centers couldn't explain my intestinal malabsorption, I found that an endocrinologist offered a new, previously unexplored hypothesis. Finally, it was an immunologist who put various pieces together and arrived at the most likely explanation. If your doctor doesn't suggest it, which would be ideal, you should still pursue the second opinion on your own. When your condition has not yet been sufficiently treated, brainstorm with your PCP to determine what additional type of specialist may be able to shed new light on your condition.

Beware of Conflicts of Interest

Never get a second opinion from a doctor who is connected in any way to the pharmaceutical company making one of the drugs under consideration for your treatment or who is involved in a study of one of those drugs. Approximately 80 percent of the funding for medical research now comes from the pharmaceutical and medical devices industries.

Be a Savvy and Empowered Patient

You need to know when you could benefit from a second opinion. In the earlier incident I mentioned in which I asked a physiatrist to order a DEXA, when the results came in the doctor never even called me to notify me that I had this very dangerous condition. When I showed my primary care physician the results, she referred me to an endocrinologist, who correctly started me on a bisphosphonate. However, the endocrinologist also blurted out as she was walking out the door of the exam room that I also had fibromyalgia (which I knew I did not have!) so I never returned to her. In fact, I soon switched PCPs too because of a potentially dangerous mistake in prescribing a medication that I happened to know was contraindicated for me. If you fail to be knowledgeable about your various medical conditions, sooner or later you will be harmed by one of your doctors. The next PCP I went to failed to appreciate the significance of an inflammation on my foot. I immediately self-referred to a dermatologist, who diagnosed it as cellulitis. Those were just a few of the many red flags that eventually motivated me to switch all my care over to one of the large, high-volume tertiary referral medical centers in San Francisco. The physicians at centers such as these are able to recognize the more unusual conditions that doctors connected with a small community hospital would never see.

At another time, still another internist I was seeing told me that some of my lab values were way off. Suspecting a lab error, he correctly reordered the same labs to be immediately redrawn. When I got the results (which I always request), they were still way out of reference range for that lab, but he never even called to tell me. After a few additional incidents of falling through the cracks, being incorrectly diagnosed, and having contraindicated medications prescribed for me, I realized that, as patients, our health is truly in our own hands. Patients who never question their doctors often get inferior care, and patients who fail to learn all they can about their various medical conditions are unable to even determine the quality of the care they are receiving.

Protocols Are for Average Patients

Protocols are developed in order to standardize the most efficacious evidence-based treatments. However, many patients have unusual circumstances, and the standard procedure may not be the best method for any particular individual.[11] Whenever you suspect that you are in that situation, you must speak up and ask if there's an alternative way of doing that particular procedure. If you think of an alternative way of doing something, suggest it; just be sure you can provide a good argument to support your reason for suggesting it. In *The Patient from Hell,* mantle-cell lymphoma patient Stephen Schneider did this throughout his entire course of treatment. In his book, he presents convincing evidence that his recovery was largely due to the probing questions he posed to his doctors.

Following is an example of unusual circumstances from my own life. My cardiologist once called to tell me that after looking at my most recent heart rhythm recordings, he was concerned that I may have developed paroxysmal atrial fibrillation (AF), based on my long runs of pre-atrial contractions. Although I had not been in AF when the last reading was taken, he wanted me to start taking a baby aspirin each day, as there is a stroke risk associated with AF and there is no way to know from day to day whether I am in AF. I reminded him of my mild ITP (bleeding disorder); he then recommended I first consult with my hematologist.

At this point, most compliant patients would simply follow through with their cardiologist's recommendations.

However, a truly empowered patient can think outside the box and consider other options.

The day after I spoke with this doctor, it suddenly occurred to me that there is now in fact a new, very simple way I can know with certainty when I am in AF, and it will save me the risk of taking a daily baby aspirin. I immediately ordered the AliveCore EKG app for my iPhone. You don't need to be a doctor or nurse to learn to interpret AF; if you have not had a course in physiology, you simply need some basic instruction from a doctor or nurse.

Medical self-efficacy means partnering with your doctors and complying with their recommendations. However, the truly empowered patient becomes an expert on his or her particular diagnoses in order to explore all possible treatments. When discovering a new treatment that your doctor is not familiar with, always first discuss the new treatment with the doctor treating you for that particular condition. If your doctor doesn't approve of the new treatment, I recommend getting a second opinion. As I've mentioned before, always present evidence of efficacy in order to be taken seriously.

More Isn't Always Better

Some doctors are known to treat disease quickly and very aggressively while others are more likely to want to do more tests before starting treatment and recommend "watch and wait." Both types of approaches have successes and failures, depending on the specifics of the diagnosis and the age and history of the patient. However, if the aggressive treatment being recommended is high risk, it's important to get a second opinion from an expert at a different medical center. Obviously, there are times when there really is no time to wait before deciding on a high-risk treatment, but usually there is time to get another opinion. If you are at all in doubt about either approach, get a second opinion.

Don't Settle for "Idiopathic"

When doctors use the term idiopathic, it means they're satisfied that there is simply no known cause and there's no reason to continue looking for one. Sometimes, even after a second, third, or fourth opinion from experts at the best medical centers, the correct diagnosis remains elusive and the etiology idiopathic. However, don't accept anything as idiopathic without getting a second and possibly third opinion from an expert at a different institution. Another expert may think of some obscure diagnostic test that reveals new information.

I know this from personal experience. For many years, I had several lab values that were way out of reference range and were considered idiopathic. Eventually my immunologist was able to put various pieces of information together, which provided a possible explanation for all the seemingly unrelated diagnoses, some of which were only tangentially related to the immune system. Although his ability to see the big picture didn't result in any cures, at least the new information may help guide us with future treatments.

Be Vigilant

Vigilance is at the heart of medical self-efficacy. The time and attention you invest in monitoring all aspects of your healthcare will afford you the best chance of receiving top-quality medical care.

Walking Through a Minefield

In my own psychophysiological work with hundreds of medical patients, I was continually horrified by countless stories of patients being given the wrong drug or wrong dose, experiencing a botched or wrong procedure, having an adverse reaction to a diagnostic or treatment procedure, and many other things going wrong. I was especially appalled by the number of patients who had slipped through the cracks. I eventually realized that navigating one's medical care is like walking through a minefield. The minefield is unavoidable, which is why you must learn to discern the quality of care you are receiving and advocate for yourself. This is why it is essential to have a medically savvy advocate with you at all times whenever you need to be hospitalized. For a thorough education on how to survive your hospital stay, visit http://empoweredpatientcoalition.org/ and read the book *The Empowered Patient* by Dr. Julia Hallisy.[12]

Be a Squeaky Wheel
Failure to follow through is another big concern. I, too, have experienced a lack of follow-through by physicians who failed to order necessary procedures and ordered unnecessary ones, prescribed contraindicated drugs, and overlooked or didn't follow up on dangerous lab values. I learned to pay careful attention to every detail of diagnosis and treatment and to speak up immediately if anything did not seem right—to be the proverbial squeaky wheel. Staying on top of things to this extent requires a lot of time and energy, but it can make the difference between not only quality of life, but even life or death.

Talk to the Lab
Having medical self-efficacy means taking the initiative to discuss any ambiguous results with your doctor and, if necessary, asking your doctor to let you talk to someone in the lab. Normally, lab techs only speak directly to doctors, but they will talk to you if the ordering physician approves. Quite often, important new information becomes available from this conversation that could inform a better treatment protocol, although without large data sets, this information is sometimes too ambiguous to use in changing a treatment protocol.[13]

In Diagnostic and Treatment Procedures, Less Invasive Is Safer
Talk to your doctors about your options whenever you need an invasive procedure. Ask if you can choose the least invasive procedure available, unless it is clearly inferior to a more invasive one. At one time a gastroenterologist wanted to order

a diagnostic ERCP (endoscopic retrograde cholangiopancrea-tography) for me, but due to the high risk of post-ERCP pan-creatitis, I requested and received MRCP (magnetic resonance cholangiopancreatography). Another time, I had a choice be-tween capsule endoscopy or push enteroscopy; in this case, my gastroenterologist was the one who recommended the less invasive test and ordered the capsule.

If a certain drug holds less promise of controlling a par-ticular symptom than a drug that is more likely to control the symptom but also more likely to cause adverse events, ask your doctor if you can start with the safer one and then switch to the riskier one only if the safer one fails to work.

Also, know what drugs to avoid given your particular profile. For example, Fentynl is a great analgesic, but because I live with a primary immunodeficiency condition, I would avoid chronic use of it since it is very immunosuppressive. Don't blindly trust your doctors to have that information on their minds when they order a drug for you; they are only human and make mistakes. You must learn what drugs are contraindicated for your medical conditions and add that in-formation to your medication notes. I recommend maintain-ing these in a Word document on your mobile device, because you want to be able to easily update the information.

Be Prepared!

One important way to advocate for yourself is to go to every office appointment fully prepared with a well-thought-out list of questions. I create a list of questions before each medi-cal appointment and maintain that list on the Notes app on my iPhone. At some appointments, I pull out my iPhone and record the entire conversation; then I take notes from the re-cording once I'm home. I always ask permission to record and have never been refused. I start the recording and then leave the Notes app open for easy reference while the iPhone con-tinues to record without interruption.

If you record the conversation with your doctor and listen to it at home, you will find yourself coming up with additional questions at that time. Another reason to see doctors who are directly connected to a large tertiary referral medical center is because increasingly, such centers now have patient portals to the medical center's intranet, allowing you to easily send your questions to your doctor and receive answers, access the results of your various medical tests, and even schedule appointments. This is a giant leap forward in helping patients partner with their doctors.

Be an Equal Partner with Your Doctor

The best way to advocate for yourself is to develop relationships with your doctors based on equality. I consider myself an equal partner with my doctors because, while they are the medical experts, I am the owner of my body and the expert on me.

Most good doctors will spend as much time as necessary with patients who are well informed, respectful, and compliant. When patients ask pertinent questions and can maintain an intelligent dialogue, good doctors won't end the office visit until both parties clearly understand all the issues. If you are not comfortable informing yourself and engaging in a dialogue between equals, it is essential that you bring someone with you to your office appointments who can act as your advocate, ask all the right questions, and take detailed notes.

Have a frank discussion with your doctors to get further clarity about your diagnoses, test results, treatments, and anything else you don't fully understand. It may not seem important on the face of it, but don't do this while you are dressed in a hospital gown. You will feel more like an equal when you are fully dressed, and that makes it easier to be your own advocate.

Educated, savvy patients sometimes read about a new treatment that their doctors may not have mentioned. If you become aware of a treatment your doctor has not considered and you want him or her to look into it, you must become very knowledgeable in order to build a credible case; then approach your doctor as a colleague rather than as a demanding patient. For example, you could say you'd like to get his or her opinion on a treatment you found in a medical journal. Hand your doctor a copy of the article you found in the peer-reviewed journal. Don't just provide the abstract. Pay for the download of the entire article or go to your nearest medical library and photocopy the entire article for free. You can now go into a medical library, find journal articles, take rapid-fire photos of each page with an iPhone, and then drag each photo (page) onto Word documents.

Is There a Chance You'll Receive a Frightening Diagnosis?

Even if you are very skilled at asking all the right questions, medical self-efficacy includes taking someone else with you to your appointment if there is a chance you may get a frightening diagnosis. Even doctors and nurses commonly panic and lose their rational, cognitive acumen when they are given a diagnosis of metastatic cancer or some other deadly or debilitating disease.

If you've just been diagnosed with a very aggressive cancer, unless you and/or a person close to you are very medically savvy, you may want to consider hiring a professional advocate to find the best place for your treatment, the best surgical and radiation oncologists, the best oncologist, and the best treatment for your specific cancer. Professional advocates can sometimes open doors that get you in to see specialists who may ordinarily be booked up for months in advance.[14] If the diagnosis is one that doesn't require immediate treatment, you'll have plenty of time to do that information gathering yourself, possibly obviating the need to hire someone to do it for you.

The Importance of Respectful Communication

Being diagnosed with a life-threatening or debilitating chronic condition can be terrifying. For this reason, it is very common for patients to get angry or impatient with staff at the office, clinic, or hospital where they get their care. Although this reaction is natural and quite understandable, it will not serve you. You will get the best care by being respectful *and* very assertive. If you don't get quality care from an office clerk or other staff member, rather than get upset about it, go up the chain of command. I have only had to do this once, and because I was respectful and assertive, that person's supervisor took good care of me.

Research and Documentation

A great way to place your healthcare in your own hands is to become your own research librarian and to document everything relevant you learn. In addition to maintaining all the personal and general information on each of my medical conditions, I am also very quick to look up anything I don't know.

I carry a medical calculator app on my iPhone so I can double-check medication protocols. A good medical dictionary can also be very helpful. I used to carry one, along with a few medical reference texts on my old PDA, but today everything can be found online, obviating the need to purchase any texts (see recommended sites further on). Be advised, though, that in searching the most recent research literature, you will read about very exciting new research discoveries that, unfortunately, will almost always take many more years to go from bench to bedside than first predicted.

Knowledge Is Power

To a certain extent, the degree of your medical knowledge will be commensurate with the quality of care you receive. That's why when doctors are patients, they tend to get at least the standard of care. Little things you learn along the way can make a difference, such as requesting an IV antiemetic (anti-nausea drug) before the insertion of an NG (nasogastric) tube.

Know Where to Look for Reliable Information

In searching for new treatments, stick with websites that end in ".gov" or ".edu" because they are the two most trusted categories. Four of the best are www.medlineplus.gov, www.PubMed.gov, www.google.com/scholar, and the Cochrane Database at http://www.thecochranelibrary.com/view/0/index.html. Also, go to the site for the medical society that represents the particular specialists who treat your diagnosis. Look up abstracts being presented at recent or upcoming annual conferences because researchers generally present their work in advance this way, up to a year before the treatment is published in medical journals. It's important to differentiate between patient support associations, such as the Immune Deficiency Foundation, and the corresponding professional associations (American Academy of Allergy Asthma & Immunology or the American College of Allergy, Asthma & Immunology). Searching abstracts will provide not only information on cutting-edge treatments but also the names of the leaders in the field whom you can then email.

Patient Support Associations
Once you have a clear diagnosis, get involved with the patient support association that represents patients with that disease or condition. You will get ideas by connecting with other patients. For example, my hematologist referred me to an immunologist in the immunology clinic where I was getting my care, but a patient who was a member of the Immunodeficiency Foundation (IDF) patient support association gave me the name of a different immunologist at that same clinic who specialized in my specific condition. Although the first immunologist was amply qualified to care for me, I would not have known about the subspecialist had I not spoken to people at the IDF.

Maintain Your Own Medical Records
As I mentioned earlier, it's important to keep a record of all your medical information, as well as any questions or observations you may have. I keep everything in Word documents on my laptop and a smaller segment of them on my iPhone.
    Using whatever system works best for you, following are

all the categories of information you should track. Doing so will allow your doctors to provide better care, and if you have to be admitted to the hospital, your records will help you get better care there as well. Creating these various documents can seem overwhelming, but once you have them, they are easy to maintain, provided you keep up with them.

- **Consults (office visits):** Audio-record the session and then take notes from the recording in the comfort of your home. I have often thought of questions for my doctors, only to find that I already had the answers, which I had recorded from a previous office visit.
- **Medications:** If you are on a lot of medications, maintain a document for all those medications, listing both adverse side effects (including allergies) and positive effects you've experienced.
- **Procedures:** Keep a document listing all treatment procedures including surgeries. Note the positive and negative effects of each surgery or other interventional procedure.
- **Pathology reports:** Maintain results of all lab tests and other diagnostic procedures such as biopsies, x-rays, and scans. This document will make it easy for you and all your doctors to track all abnormal lab values and to see any trending. Get a CD or flash drive in DICOM (Digital Imaging and Communications in Medicine) format of all your MRI (magnetic resonance imaging), CT (computed tomography), US (ultrasound), and other scans. This information will be useful when you go for second opinions at other institutions.[15]
- **Doctor's notes:** Request copies of all comments, management notes, consultant reports, and surgical notes from your doctors.
- **Your personal notes:** Still another document can contain any useful information you have run across that is related to your various conditions. This will include any information you download from reliable websites.

Treatment Guidelines
Read the latest treatment guidelines for your diagnosis. You can always find the guidelines at the association representing the specialty that treats your condition. For example, for urological problems it would be the American Urological Association. However, keep in mind that guidelines are often slow to change and that new information may make an official guideline obsolete. Nevertheless, it is good to become familiar with the guidelines for standard of care.

Finding the Right Clinical Trial
Years ago, my immunologist helped me get into a clinical trial at NIH because my immune profile is so unusual that he wanted me to have access to cutting-edge researchers. If you are accepted into a trial at NIH, you will get state-of-the-art care from world-class clinical researchers and will have access to the very latest treatments. As if that isn't enough to convince you, if you are a participant in a study at NIH and you need medical care, they will provide it at no cost to you. Here are some ways to find out about clinical trials:
• Ask your specialist.
• Check with the organization that advocates for your particular diagnosis.
• For new medications in development, go to http://www.phrma.org/innovation/meds-in-development.
• Contact NIH, NIAID, NCI, or other divisions of NIH: http://www.centerwatch.com.
• Go to http://www.nih.gov/health/clinicaltrials/index.htm.

Advance Directives
It is essential that you plan for the future with advance directives in order to assure that your wishes are followed if you are no longer well enough to make your own medical decisions.
    There are three general types:
• *Living Will:* Also known as a healthcare directive or advance directive, this legal document describes the types

of life-sustaining measures you desire.

- *Durable Power of Attorney for Healthcare:* Also known as medical or healthcare power of attorney, or healthcare proxy, this legal document designates someone you want to make medical decisions for you when you are not conscious or are too sick to do so. This is absolutely essential to have in place before you are admitted to a hospital.

- *DNR:* This is ordered by your doctor upon request and must be signed by you. It allows you to refuse cardiac or respiratory resuscitation if at some point your heart or respiration stops. Although it may be in your chart when hospitalized, it should also be available for paramedics and other emergency responders to your residence.

∞

I hope you will find this part of the book useful in your mindfulness-based mastery and wellbeing journey. I cannot overemphasize the importance of medical self-efficacy for those of us who live with chronic illness and other physically debilitating conditions. It can mean the difference between feelings of helplessness and gaining a sense of control over your own health.

24 Mastery and Wellbeing Practices for Family Caregivers

Life consists not in holding good cards, but in playing those we do hold well.
—Josh Billings

E ven the most assertive, confident, brilliant, and self-suffi-cient people can become extremely distressed when sud-denly confronted with caring for a loved one who has been struck down by a chronic, debilitating medical condition and now depends on them for help on a daily basis. It is easy to spiral into feelings of hopelessness and helplessness. Fol-lowing is a look at some of the challenges common to both the ill person and the family caregiver.

Loss of Identity

One of the most difficult life changes we may confront is a loss of identity. We often tend to view ourselves in relation to our work and family roles and the way we imagine others see us. When our life circumstances change dramatically, so can our self-image. When we go from healthy and active to chroni-cally sick or physically disabled, or from carefree to caregiver, we lose the self-image with which we previously identified.

Grieving

The abrupt shift in identity usually involves a degree of griev-ing for what has been lost, and both patient and caregiver need empathic understanding as well as practical support as they grieve. Both people may need to mourn the loss of a

> Things that mattered to you before may now seem superficial and unimportant. Things that you never considered before may take on new meaning.

career, favorite activities, and their relationship as they have known it. These feelings of loss must be embraced, accepted, and expressed.

You may fear burdening your friends with the grief you feel, and some friends will in fact distance themselves from you when you express it. You will learn that some of the people you have thought of as good friends find it too frightening to be around you and your loved one now. Other people to whom you have felt less close will surprise you when they offer emotional as well as practical support.

Reevaluation

Caring for a family member can be an opportunity for personal growth. Things you never considered before may take on new meaning, and things that mattered to you before may now seem superficial and unimportant. It is common to experience a reevaluation of life priorities, and you may develop a need to be around people who truly understand, often because they've been through similar experiences.

Because the things that previously gave your life meaning may now be out of reach or no longer seem important—for both of you—it is absolutely essential that you and your ill family member find new meaning in the illness or disability.

As a caregiver, finding ways to improve your loved one's quality of life can provide you with a reason to go on.[1] Your loved one must also find a reason to persevere. Inspirational people who know the two of you can also contribute, helping you keep your hopes up. This is important because losing hope severely weakens immune function and physiological functioning in general.[2]

Personality Changes

Personality changes in the ill person are common; fortunately, they are usually slight. Various types of medications can cause wide mood swings, including anxiety, depression, or angry outbursts.[3] Medications aside, the daily frustrations inherent in not being able to perform once-normal physical or mental activities often result in attitudinal changes that may negatively impact interactions with you and the rest of your family.

Although some neurodegenerative diseases and traumatic brain injuries result in major personality changes, the vast majority of diseases and medication side effects are associated with only minor changes.[4]

A Note for Spouses

Caring for a spouse is different from caring for a parent or child. The life the two of you have known may be forever lost due to cognitive, emotional, and physical losses. This upheaval can lead to the end of the relationship — or to a deeper, more intimate one.

Children may drift away emotionally from the ill parent, and as the well spouse, you may find yourself disconnecting emotionally if your sick partner pushes you away. This distancing can happen for a number of reasons: fear of expressing sadness or rage or of being misunderstood, or feelings of self-loathing and shame, which are common when body parts are removed or certain conditions result in unpleasant odors or accidents. All the causes of distancing can be successfully addressed with the help of an experienced family therapist, who will focus on improving understanding and communication among family members. A support group for family caregivers can also be very helpful.

Your partner may have been the primary breadwinner or may have been the one doing most of the caring for the children, and now lacks the energy to do that. Changes from the illness are likely to affect your sex life, emotional life, recreational activities, and friendships.

If you are now facing any or all of these circumstances, you are probably—and understandably—distressed. However, when you commit to being fully present with your new circumstances and engage in mindfulness-based mastery practices, you will find new opportunities for personal growth and may even develop greater wellbeing in your life.

Caregiving Can Be Good for Your Health

Numerous studies have revealed that caring for a loved one actually improves the health and wellbeing of the person providing the care.[5] There are some exceptions to this health benefit, however. For example, if you have more to do than you can handle by yourself or if you feel a lot of resentment for all you are doing, your health and wellbeing may suffer. For more on this subject, see Essential Caregiver Practice #2: Practice Loving Self-Care.

Proactive Caregiving: Know Your Roles

You have the power to be the master of your own life, and the decisions you make on a moment-by-moment basis influence your health and wellbeing. Approach life proactively, including your life as a caregiver. What does being proactive mean in your role as your loved one's caregiver? If your patient is mentally alert, you can follow these key guidelines together:

- You must become the leader of the healthcare team. Your loved one may have been his or her own advocate with doctors, nurses, and others providing medical and other skilled care, but as long as your patient is very sick or debilitated, you may have to manage all of his or her care.
- Understand that you know the patient better than anyone else on the healthcare team. As you work closely with medical professionals, there will be many times when it is important for you to assertively express your patient's specific needs. Because you are a close family member, you may in fact be the foremost expert on the patient's overall state of health. Make sure you are heard.

And make sure you can affirmatively answer these two questions related to caring for the person you know so well:

1. Is my immediate behavior helping me care for my loved one?
2. Is my immediate behavior best for him or her?

- Contact your regional Center for Independent Living, a network of several hundred nonprofit agencies around the country that offer many free services. One of them includes matching your patient with the most appropriate in-home professional caregivers. Other free support services are benefits counseling, group support, and guidance on home modification projects, assistive technology, and the transition back home from a medical facility.[6]

- Build relationships. Help your patient get involved with the appropriate patient support association so that he or she can connect with other patients. The patient support association may help you to connect with other family caregivers. Make friends with others caring for a family member with a similar illness, and help your patient establish friendships with other patients. You both may find utility in chat rooms, message boards, listservs, and social media. Social media can help you connect with people around the world who are in your situation. However, never engage in any alternative treatments you learn about in these venues, even if promoted by a physician, without first consulting with your patient's doctors.

- Use this situation as an opportunity to become a positive agent of change. Being a family caregiver can provide you with a new sense of meaning and purpose. Use your anger, frustration, grief, and other unpleasant emotions to motivate you to not only help your loved one but help yourself grow into a more assertive, goal-directed person.

- Get additional opinions. If a doctor tells you that nothing can be done or wants to order a particularly invasive or otherwise high-risk diagnostic or treatment procedure, always get a second opinion at a large tertiary care center.[7]

- Become a researcher. Learn all you can about your loved one's diagnosis. Study everything you can find that will help you understand the disease process and all the possible treatments, and learn who the top authorities are on that particular condition. Go to sites like the National Institutes for Health, MedlinePlus, the Centers for Disease Control, and the Joint Commission, and do searches on Google Scholar, PubMed, and other evidence-based sites. Most .edu and .gov sites are reliable sources of information. Get detailed information from medical professionals. This will enable you to make informed decisions and help your loved one get the best care from the medical team. And it will give you a sense of mastery rather than frustration.
- Prepare your questions in advance of each medical appointment in order to get the most from treatment providers.
- When you go to medical appointments, bring all your patient's records, bottles of medications, and a list and description of his or her new symptoms since the last visit. Alternatively, keep all that information in your mobile device on a note or document so it will be readily and easily available.
- Be the social director. In chapter 19 on relationship building, I cited considerable research documenting that people with a large and high-quality social support network tend to recover faster when sick or disabled. It's up to you to schedule visits from friends for both of you.
- Empower the patient. Look for ways to create opportunities for him or her to make decisions. You can even do this with children as long as the options are all safe ones. Research has shown that simply having a sense of control over some of the choices that need to be made will improve health outcomes.[8]

Always be on the lookout for choices your patient

can make for him- or herself. Nursing home studies have proven that when patients are given choices, their health and state of mind improve. In some of these studies, half the patients were given more choices than they had before and half were deprived of choice.[9] The data showed that when choices were taken away from the patients who had been given them, they did worse than those who had no choices in the first place.

If your loved one isn't well enough to make choices, the next best thing is to fully explain what is being done and why. This is a way of helping your loved one maintain a sense of control. Make sure all home healthcare workers do this as well; anyone who won't comply needs to be replaced. Never let anyone treat your loved one like a piece of meat. For example, when the worker turns the patient over in bed, the patient should first be told that this is about to happen. When moving the patient for whatever reason, or changing anything, the healthcare worker should always first describe the process involved. If it is something that is performed repeatedly, simply naming the now familiar process will suffice.

- Get used to reaching out to family, friends, and your support community for help. For more on this, see Essential Caregiver Practice #2.

Essential Caregiver Practice #1: Practice Conscious Choice

As a caregiver, you may find yourself thinking in terms of all the things you *have to* do as if you have no choice. But if you read chapters 10 through 12 on Valued-Action Practice, you know that this is not conducive to mastery and wellbeing. By tuning in to your personal values, and by examining your power of choice, you can change the attribution you assign to each chore you undertake on your loved one's behalf. As you begin to realize that you do in fact choose to perform all the activities you do, you will be able to regain control. Whenever you find yourself thinking *I have to* or *I should,* ask yourself:

What am I choosing in this moment? If the task at hand is, for example, driving your loved one to the third medical appointment of the week, you may be *choosing* to do so because you value your loved one's health and want him or her to have the very best treatment available—if you examine it closely you will realize that you *want* to perform this task and that's why you have chosen to do so.

Making Choices as a Mindfulness-Based Mastery Practice

When you are in the role of family caregiver for someone who is very ill, you can easily fall into states of exhaustion, frustration, and helplessness. You may also feel resentful of the new one-sided relationship—*this is common.* An antidote for these feelings is to make a practice of framing all your activities throughout the day as choices, prefacing every action with *I'm choosing.*

For example:

- I'm choosing to turn her over in bed so she doesn't develop decubitus ulcers.
- I'm choosing to change his bed linens.
- I'm choosing to cook this special meal for her.
- I'm choosing to bathe him.
- I'm choosing to replace a particular home healthcare worker.

Patients can also benefit from learning this practice. For example:

- I'm choosing to allow this person to turn me over now.
- I'm choosing to request gentler handling.

Virtually every action can be prefaced with *I'm choosing to.* You will be surprised at how much difference this makes in restoring your sense of control over your life.

Essential Caregiver Practice #2:
Practice Loving Self-Care

Be aware that your role as caregiver will have profound effects on your physical and emotional state. In many ways, your experience parallels that of your beloved patient. You are likely to experience feelings of grief, despair, anxiety, and depression because you are coping with loss: often loss of income, loss of the ability to engage in all the activities that provide a sense of meaning and purpose—loss of the life you knew.

Caring for a family member who has a chronic and debilitating medical condition is extremely challenging and exhausting and can even be deadly. Make sure you are not so single-minded in your caregiving that you ignore your own self-care. You may feel reluctant to take time away from your caregiving activities, but at a time when your stress levels are stretched to the limit, don't make the common mistake of failing to take care of yourself. The stress of caring for a loved one who is very sick or disabled commonly results in anxiety-produced hypertension. Monitor your blood pressure and seek immediate medical attention as soon as you notice or have been told that it is too high.

Time Out

Although focusing all your attention on the caregiving task at hand can lead to living with greater mastery and wellbeing, there are times (if, for instance, you haven't been out of the house in a few days) when it's important to have someone else step in to help. This is also true of managing home healthcare workers, which can seem like a full-time job itself. Unless you make the time to get out in nature or involve yourself in your favorite activities, you will burn out, and that's not helpful for anyone.

Essential Caregiver Practice #3: See Life as a Mindfulness-Based Mastery Practice

What lies behind us and what lies before us are small matters to what lies within us.
—Ralph Waldo Emerson

You may think you don't have time to practice mindfulness-based mastery while going through this demanding period of your life, but this fundamental practice of acknowledging and accepting your thoughts and feelings will actually give you more energy, while suppressing your thoughts and feelings drains energy. Simply asking yourself the following question throughout the day—*What am I practicing and choosing and is it in harmony with my values and goals?*—can be an exceptionally effective mindfulness practice that requires no extra time; you can continue making the bed or feeding the dog while considering it. Asking and answering this question will serve to focus you on actions you can take to move back to center and live according to what matters most to you.

When we are faced with adversity, especially in situations such as serious illness, these practices can provide the skills to effectively meet the challenges we face and help us live with a sense of mastery and wellbeing, regardless of the seriousness of external circumstances.

It may seem counterintuitive, but focusing all our attention on the caregiving task at hand serves to make the task more rewarding and less exhausting. We may choose from innumerable distractions on our iPods, tablets, and mobile devices while performing undesirable tasks, but ironically, in doing this we create more rather than less anxiety and fatigue. The fewer things we focus on at any one time, the more satisfying and simpler the task.

As you go about your job as caregiver, always remember that a mindfulness practice is *any* action that is performed with full attention on the task.

Essential Caregiver Practice #4: Let Others Help

Be realistic: you alone can't do everything involved in caring for someone who is very ill or disabled. Many people believe that depending on others to do things for them means they are weak or helpless, but you can ask others to perform various tasks without adopting such beliefs. The fact is that when you reach out for help—and do the job of coordinating and managing it—you are very much in charge of the situation.

If you find yourself constantly exhausted, short-tempered, impatient, and burned out, it is time to hire professional in-home caregivers or find a way to get volunteer help. You can ask around and get names of individuals who do that work, contract with a home healthcare agency, get help from your regional Center for Independent Living, or use a combination of agency workers, individuals, and volunteers. Whichever you choose, if your loved one needs round-the-clock help, it will be your job to make sure there is someone to cover every shift. This is challenging in itself because you must observe each worker who comes into your home and replace those who are not doing a satisfactory job. This, unfortunately, is very common. Don't be afraid to ask a friend or family member to share this responsibility with you.[10]

Do Not Fear Being a Burden

The fear of becoming a burden is common for both chronically ill people and the family members who care for them. Patients are afraid to burden their family caregivers, who in turn are afraid to burden family, friends, and their support community. Yet living with mastery means recognizing your inability to do it all—and asking for help. This can be very difficult for some of us, and here is where it becomes useful to think about your personal life values, particularly the values of social support, relationship building, authentic self-expression, and mastery. Keeping those values in the front of your mind can help you take the valued action of picking up the phone and asking for help.

> Recruiting assistance from others is part of taking charge of your life.

It's also important to recognize that the very idea of being a "burden" is your own mental construct. The experience of giving you the help you need is entirely up to the person giving it, and it may actually be one of great joy and satisfaction. In fact, helping others is a behavior that builds self-esteem, and asking for help can become a mastery practice that builds a very healthy level of self-esteem.

When you need help and request it, you have an opportunity to practice mindfulness-based mastery: mindfully paying attention to the thoughts and feelings you experience when asking for help and consciously changing the stories you tell yourself about doing so. For example, an old story you may have told yourself is that you are helpless, useless, a burden. A healthy new story could involve acknowledging how powerful you've become by being able to ask for whatever you want from people, and recognizing the courage you exercise through such acts. Another healthy story is that you are giving your helpers a chance to feel better about themselves.

In addition to all these benefits, each time you ask for help, you have the opportunity to build relationships. This happens not just in the asking but also in the thanking, which can become a mastery practice and an art form in itself. Learning how to thank others for the help they so graciously give provides opportunities for meaningful connection.

Find a Caregiver Support Group
Just as healthy people cannot have any idea what it's like to live with chronic health challenges every day, people who have never been in the role of family caregiver to a spouse, child, or parent who is seriously ill cannot offer real un-

derstanding. It can be very healing and supportive to find others who know from personal experience what you're going through.

Essential Caregiver Practice #5: Disengage from Troubling Thoughts

When we are no longer able to change a situation—just think of an incurable disease such as inoperable cancer— we are challenged to change ourselves.
—Viktor Frankl

The emotional distress and resulting physiological stress on you as the family member caring for the sick or disabled person will take a toll on your health and wellbeing, but there are ways to reduce these effects. Even if you are very good at reaching out for help from family, friends, community, or a home healthcare agency, you may still have very troubling thoughts. These thoughts are common and are to be expected after a certain period of time spent coping with a protracted illness. For example, there will be times when you as well as your patient will feel very discouraged and think you can't go on. It's normal to have such thoughts, but they do not reflect reality—you *can* persevere and achieve mastery—and it can be extremely helpful and even life changing to learn how to avoid getting entangled in such thoughts. Don't become their passive victims; take action by labeling *I can't take this anymore!* as nothing but an insubstantial mental construct—a brain secretion!

A particularly troubling thought family caregivers quite often experience is that of wishing that the sick person would die, and this is associated with very painful feelings of shame and guilt for having such thoughts. It's important to acknowledge them and not try to suppress them, because that will only magnify the pain.

Joining a caregiver support group will give you the opportunity to realize that all these thoughts are normal—you are not a "bad person" for having them. And you can learn to disengage from them.

Essential Caregiver Practice #6: Renew Your Sense of Meaning and Purpose

You can't stop the waves, but you can learn to surf.
—Jon Kabat-Zinn

When bad things happen, as we've discussed, it is important to find meaning and purpose in the situation.[11] Many researchers have found that people who actively search for the benefits of having a serious disease develop a healthier state of mind; the same is true of seeking the benefits of focusing your time and energy on caring for your loved one. It's important for both of you to have hope and something to live for.

Helping your ill loved one is intrinsically meaningful—you are making a positive difference in this person's life, and that's important. Do not lose sight of this. Another purpose for your efforts is your own personal growth, which often takes place amid challenges.

We need energy to enhance our physiological functioning, and we can create more energy by placing our focus on those things we love, things that give meaning to our lives and make us feel alive. One of the most energizing things we can do is place our attention on and devote time to those people and things that give our lives joy, meaning, and purpose.[12] It is helpful to find even the smallest of things each day that help us feel joyful and are conducive to a healing mind state. Even neutral emotional states such as calm, peace, and tranquility are very health inducing. Spend more time with those people and activities that increase joy and deep fulfillment and less with those that leave you feeling depleted.

This advice is every bit as important for you, the caregiver, as it is for the patient; it is an aspect of your own loving self-care. You can support your loved one in making such meaningful choices, but don't forget to make them for yourself as well.

Essential Caregiver Practice #7: Take Valued Action Together

One way to improve the odds of your patient's recovery is for him or her to take advantage of every opportunity to act in accordance with personal values. Obviously, when patients are sick enough to require home healthcare, they are going to depend to a certain extent on others doing things for them. But as I described in some detail earlier in the section on your roles as caregiver, it is important to find ways for your loved one to make choices. Hospitalized patients in the ICU are too sick to make choices, but at home, you and your patient can collaborate in decision making. This will empower both of you and can bring you closer together. You both need to continue to engage in whatever normal activities you are capable of doing. Making decisions with you can even provide your loved one with the empowerment and mastery to manage pain; he or she will likely need less pain medication and will enjoy a healthier outlook.

Essential Caregiver Practice #8: Share Hope and Optimism Together

It's only natural to spend time thinking about what has gone wrong, or about what you don't like. But this is not conducive to anyone's health and wellbeing. Instead, focus on what you want, and learn to live with hope and optimism.

There is a big difference between optimism and positive thinking, which can actually be harmful. Positive thinking is not necessarily based on facts or anything you can control. For example, a person with cancer who engages in positive thinking might think, *I'm going to beat this cancer.* Optimistic thinking, on the other hand, might take this form: *Because of all I'm doing for my health, I know I'm improving my odds of beating the cancer.* Note the difference concerning "who's in charge." In positive thinking, there is no sense of control or mastery—the good result will magically happen. Optimistic thinking puts you in charge of creating the best outcome possible.

In every stage of life, optimists are healthier than pessimists. The challenge is in going from pessimism to optimism, and the clearest path is through cultivating mindfulness-based mastery. But all activities that give you and your loved one hope—whether it's enjoying upbeat movies, music, or lectures; practicing mental imagery; or getting visits from optimistic friends—are important, because hope and optimism consistently improve outcomes. Virtually everyone you and your loved one come into contact with will affect your state of mind, so be very careful to keep pessimistic, depressed people out of your home.

Also, although empathy is good, sympathy is not. People who are insensitive to what you are going through and who persist in telling you everything will be fine are not good to have around. You want to associate with people who empathize with you *and* who exude authentic hope and optimism.

It is conducive to health to focus on what we want rather than on what we don't want, so it's important to imagine our desired health outcome. For example, when one is in pain, it's more effective to imagine feeling good than to imagine the pain going away. One way to do this is to imagine a specific time and place when you felt great. Follow that up with thinking about and imagining a favored activity. Energy flows where our attention goes. Our imagination is the most powerful catalyst to getting well and staying well.[13]

It is important to:
- Imagine the disease as weak and yourself as strong.[14]
- Imagine the treatment as helpful. As you take a medicine or receive an infusion, imagine it working; you might see this in the form of a cartoon.[15]
- Imagine the body healing itself. Call up cartoon images of all the healing mechanisms of the body doing their jobs.[16]
- Imagine the desired outcome. Most of us are better at calling up catastrophic images, but when we use our

imagination to visualize what we want rather than what we dread, our physiological functioning improves, sometimes noticeably.[17]

- Imagine it in your own way. For many people, the cartoon images I have suggested work well. For others, drawing or painting can be helpful.

Life is what you make it; external circumstances are less important than how you react to them.

Accept the Diagnosis but Not the Prognosis

Mastery and wellbeing involve learning to experience bad news and difficult situations as challenges rather than as defeats. When he was diagnosed with advanced osteosarcoma and given only a few months to live, Ian Gawler fully accepted the diagnosis but refused to accept the prognosis. He decided that he would see if he could be the first person ever to recover from that particular disease—this was in 1974 and he is alive and well today.[18]

Essential Caregiver Practice #9: Practice Gratitude

Even while your loved one is sick, good things happen every day. You can both enhance your health by consciously focusing on these things. Conversations with your loved one should emphasize the good. Bad things that need attention and require decision making should be addressed as soon as possible, but you need to focus solely on what you have the power to influence. As I mentioned in chapter 13 on gratitude, the single most important skill-building practice to increase happiness is to learn to frequently express gratitude.[19] People who are consistently grateful are happier, more hopeful, and more energetic than other people, and gratitude is an antidote to unpleasant emotions. Because experiencing and expressing gratitude feel good, they improve physiological functioning and can often play a role in getting back to a normal life.[20]

Essential Caregiver Practice #10: Stop-Breathe-Feel

A very quick, easy practice from chapter 21 that requires no more than a minute of your time can be transformational when you are acting as the family caregiver.

Stop-Breathe-Feel is a quick way to tune in and step back from constant mind chatter. It helps you process uncomfortable emotions and clear your head.

1. Stop.
2. Consciously tune in to your breathing.
3. Feel whatever you are experiencing in the moment.[21]

Your Better Caregiving Future

As I have pointed out before, the goal of mastery is not to try to control people and situations (which is like trying to herd cats—a practical impossibility) but rather to simply be able to make conscious choices so you can regain a sense of control and live a happier, more satisfying life. To a certain extent, mindfulness will allow you to eliminate the "bad days," because mindfulness practices will help you build the ability to see the very thought that you or your loved one is having a bad day for what it is—an insubstantial mental construct.

Mastery is essential for wellbeing, but achieving mastery requires a strong and lifelong commitment. In her book, *The Butcher's Daughter: The Story of an Army Nurse with ALS*, Sandra Lesher Stuban describes how she managed to live with mastery and wellbeing despite requiring a respirator and feeding tube and being completely dependent on others to do everything for her. She refers to the Four A's: *Accept, Adapt, Attitude, and aggressively pursue Ambitions*.[22] Such fighting spirit is important for you as the caregiver as well as for your patient. Each time a new challenge presents itself, it's important to accept the change, grieve, and then adapt to it while simultaneously viewing it as a challenge, doing everything in your power to make things better.

In difficult times, it is especially important to consciously meet every new challenge with your full attention on the task at hand. Virtually everything goes better when your focus is on the here and now rather than on the past or the future, and this is an important reason why the mindfulness-based mastery practices I have presented in this chapter are so important to your wellbeing. Through these practices, you can build a better future for yourself as a caregiver—one moment at a time, in the present—as you become the master of your caregiving life.

Appendix

Some Science Behind the Mind's Influence on the Body

Introduction

I n this appendix, I'd like to expand on the topic of placebos, the endogenous pharmacy, and what is known about the way human behavior catalyzes physiological changes.

All cognition and behavior are associated with changes in brain structure and function, which can influence systemic physiological effects. Even the smallest changes in cognition and behavior affect neurotransmitter release at synapses. With repetition, these altered patterns of release lead to remodeling of neuronal connections, which in turn promote additional changes in cognition and behavior. Many of these changes are transient, but repetitive practice of any unhealthy behavior reinforces it along with its corresponding neurological and other physiological changes. If you want to achieve healthy durable changes, you will need to repeatedly practice a behavior that will reinforce them. In neuroscience this is known as *long-term potentiation*.

Neuropsychology researchers study the effects of specific thoughts and feelings on brain function using positron emission tomography (PET) and functional magnetic resonance imaging (fMRI). PET involves using a radioactive tracer to track the activity of neurotransmitters in the brain. The fMRI scanner allows researchers to observe and follow subtle shifts in oxygenation and perfusion in different areas of the brain. Electroencephalography (EEG) is another tool that allows researchers to pinpoint electrical activity in the brain by triangulating from electrodes attached to the scalp. EEG biofeedback, also known as neurofeedback, is often used to train people how to consciously create and reinforce healthy new neural circuits.

Every thought, emotion, and sensation affects the release of neurotransmitters at the synapse, which allow one cell to send signals to another across the synapse. All these messenger molecules are in constant dialogue with all our thoughts and emotions.[1] Neurotransmitters allow one cell to send signals to another across a synapse. When the sending cell releases a neurotransmitter, the molecules rapidly diffuse to the receiving neuron, where they interact with channels that regulate the flow of electrically charged atoms (ions) across the cell membrane. Depending on the change in electrical charge induced, the effect may be to excite or inhibit activity in the receiving cell. By altering ion flow, neurotransmitters mediate the passage of signals between the two neurons.[2]

With hyperstimulation over a period of time, cell membranes lose receptors, thereby becoming less sensitive, while cells that are understimulated tend to increase their receptors, thereby increasing their susceptibility to stimulation. Chronic use of either prescription or recreational drugs can also permanently alter cell function.[3]

Neurotransmitter substances (the same as neuropeptides) mediate between our thoughts, feelings, emotions, and sensations. They are the biochemical vehicles that bridge the synaptic cleft between an axon and a dendrite, or between two axons.

Just to give you an idea of the broad range of neuropeptides, they include norepinephrine (NE); acetylcholine (ACh); dopamine (DA); serotonin; the amino acids GABA, glutamate, aspartate, and glycine; as well as two peptides—endorphins and substance P. Examples of amino acid neurotransmitters are glutamate, GABA, and glycine. Examples of monoamine neurotransmitters are DA, NE, epinephrine (Epi), histamine, and serotonin. An example of an ester neurotransmitter is ACh. Nitric oxide (NO) is an example of a neurotransmitter gas.

In some cases, such as with NE, they can excite or inhibit depending on the context. For example, the receptor type to which the NE binds determines whether this neurotransmitter substance is excitatory or inhibitory.

When NE is secreted in the adrenal medulla, it acts as a hormone in the autonomic nervous system (ANS). Hormones differ from neurotransmitters in that they can travel great distances in the blood to stimulate or inhibit the growth or function in a specific organ or tissue. Chemicals that function as neurotransmitters in the brain are also found systemically and may help the brain communicate with immune, digestive, and cardiovascular structures.

I'll use serotonin in an example of the up-down and down-up processes. Low blood levels of serotonin lead to depression and negative schemas, whereas high blood levels of serotonin lead to positive affect and positive schemas. Interestingly, when we feel in control of our lives, serotonin levels rise. Conversely, when we feel overwhelmed by life circumstances, they drop.[4] In other words, our behavior influences our biochemistry.

Serotonin and cortisol are often inversely proportional. This is why many people suffer with both anxiety and depression. Just as high cortisol results in anxiety, low serotonin results in depression. High cortisol can be causal or secondary to anxiety and the physiological stress of disease or trauma.[5]

Contrary to popular notions, depression is not solely associated with low levels of serotonin, but also low levels of NE and DA, as well as hypocampal shrinkage. Despite the obvious biochemical imbalances, contrary to what the pharmaceutical industry would like us to believe, antidepressants are often not the best treatment. For example, entrainment

or neurofeedback training to 10 hertz has been shown to correct these biochemical imbalances without any medication.[6]
Mindfulness practice can do the same.[7] In fact, there are many
nonpharmacological ways of correcting these biochemical imbalances by actually reprogramming the brain.[8] Many people
living with major depressive disorder are able to live a full
life thanks to antidepressants, but for the vast majority of the
people taking antidepressants, behavioral therapy is superior
because of the absence of side effects and the cultivation of life
mastery skills that can reprogram the brain.[9]

The Basic Biochemistry of a Stressful Thought
The hypothalamic pituitary adrenal (HPA) axis[10]

1.   A stressful thought appears in the frontal cortex.
2.   The frontal cortex triggers the hypothalamus to secrete
     a peptide known as corticotropin-releasing factor (CRF)
     within seconds.
3.   The CRF then acts on membrane receptors in the anterior
     pituitary.
4.   Then, within about fifteen seconds, the anterior pitu-
     itary releases adrenocorticotropic hormone (ACTH) into
     the bloodstream, with the adrenal glands as the target
     organs.
5.   Blood flow rapidly delivers the ACTH to the adrenal
     glands, creating increased sympathetic activity.
6.   This increased sympathetic activity in the ANS then
     signals the adrenal medulla to secrete Epi into the blood-
     stream.
7.   Then, within a couple of minutes, the ACTH causes the
     adrenal cortex to secrete several hormones including
     cortisol into the bloodstream.
8.   The release of cortisol into the bloodstream triggers the
     pituitary to increase or decrease ACTH, depending on
     the cortisol level. This particular feedback loop gets inter-
     rupted during extreme emotional distress, resulting in
     continued release of cortisol into the bloodstream.

One of the reasons that knowledge of the HPA axis is important is that it helps explain medical as well as psychological problems. For example, the HPA axis has been found to become altered downward as a result of chronic emotional distress in childhood.

In addition to the HPA axis above, what follows below is the action of a second major stress-response system—the hypothalamic-adrenal medullary system. This system works as follows:

1. The hypothalamus activates the ANS.
2. ANS activation, including the action of NE, results in sympathetic arousal.
3. Sympathetic arousal results in release of the various stress-related hormones such as catecholamines, Epi, and NE.

The following basic information, provided by psychoneuroimmunology (PNI) researcher Dr. Margaret Kemeny, helps explain the connectivity of various physiological processes mentioned previously.[11]

Corticotropin-releasing hormone (CRH) causes production of ACTH, which then causes production of cortisol. One cause of unhealthy increased cortisol is depression. Increases in cortisol lead to apoptosis (programmed cell death) and decreased circulating leukocytes (WBCs). The reduced WBCs then migrate to the bone marrow, where they are sequestered, preventing them from doing their jobs. In addition, cortisol inhibits cytokine release. Cytokines are chemical messengers that are vital to fighting disease. They are released by WBCs, so the diminution of circulating WBCs acts to further reduce cytokine production.

WBCs have receptors for neurotransmitters and cytokines, allowing these substances to communicate with them, thereby altering WBC activity. A healthy WBC proliferative response is suppressed by sympathetic arousal. T and B cells are naturally suppressed in sympathetic arousal because they are functionally too slow to be effective in a fight-or-flight situation. This is a good thing when defending against a predator. However, when animals are finished fighting or fleeing, their immune function returns to normal. Humans, unfortunately, often live in a chronic state of sympathetic arousal, which contributes to a weakened immune system and increased disease—especially chronic illnesses.

Macrophages release interleukin 1 (IL-1) and T-cells release IL-2. Proinflammatory cytokines are directly related to depression in a reversible reaction, which manifests as follows: Proinflammatory cytokines can trigger depression, and depression can trigger higher levels of proinflammatory cytokines.

Depression is immunosuppressive, and people living with major depressive disorder get sick more frequently and severely, suffering from life-threatening diseases such as cancer more often than people who are free of any mood disorders. In addition, depressed people may possibly have more inflammation, as evidenced by increased leukocytes, especially monocytes and neutrophils, along with increased indicators of T-cell activation and increased levels of positive acute phase proteins such as C-reactive protein (CRP). Also, there is increased secretion of proinflammatory cytokines such as IL-6, IL-8, and other indirect indicators.[12]

Sympathetic arousal can create a three-hundred-fold increase in the production of Epi. Epi increases natural killer (NK) cells. NK cells and their activity diminish with a high allostatic load but increase with normal daily stressors, from which the ANS returns to homeostasis. Normal daily stressors from which we rapidly recover actually improve immune function.

Four Types of Allostatic Load

Allostasis refers to the deleterious effects of stressors and the adaptation to them. One type of allostatic load is the result of being repeatedly exposed to multiple novel stressors. A second type is the result of a lack of adaptation to those novel stressors. A third type is associated with a prolonged response that is due to delayed shutdown of the stress hormone response system. A fourth is due to an abnormal response, such as inadequate secretion of glucocorticoid, which in turn leads to elevated levels of inflammatory cytokines. Those cytokines are normally kept in check by the glucocorticoids.

Here is a bit more on the pathogenic nature of chronic emotional distress. It relates to the psychophysiology of allostatic load. Allostatic load can also be seen as the physiological cost of chronic exposure to fluctuating or elevated neural or neuroendocrine responses resulting from repeated or chronic emotional distress. This is important because increased allostatic load leads to immunosuppression, which can be permanent.

Allostatic load represents the physiological cost of chronic emotional distress, which, in addition to interfering with immune function, also has profound physiological effects on neurotransmitters and hormones. The heart is innervated by both the sympathetic and parasympathetic branches of the ANS. Parasympathetic fibers innervate the heart via the vagus nerve and release the neurotransmitter ACh on sinoatrial (SA) node cells. SA nodal cells serve as our biological pacemaker, generating the normal sinus rhythm that is easily identified on an EKG reading. ACh has an effect on the depolarization of SA nodal cells, slowing their firing rate. The increased parasympathetic stimulation has a negative chronotropic effect, slowing the heart rate (HR).

Increased HR is the result of the release of increased NE from the sympathetic fibers that innervate the heart. Emotional distress increases sympathetic activity and decreases parasympathetic activity, often resulting in tachycardia.

Sympathetic activation also results in NE being released on the ventricular cells, which leads to more forceful contractions. This increased sympathetic activation leads to increased HR, increased contractility, and increased vasoconstriction in all the major arteries. As I mentioned before, this is a good thing and healthy when we need to physically escape actual danger every once in a great while. However, emotional distress on a regular basis causes these same effects, and that chronicity is pathogenic to the entire cardiovascular system and beyond.

Emotional distress results in an alpha-adrenergic-mediated vasoconstriction in the entire GI tract, the kidneys, and the liver. Any negative impact on renal function can interfere with the ability to regulate blood pressure (BP) through fluid balancing. The release of angiotensin results in fluid retention and vasoconstriction, further contributing to hypertension. It is known that the renal arteries are not very responsive to alpha-adrenergic-mediated vasoconstriction.

During sympathetic arousal, skeletal and heart muscle receive increased oxygenation and perfusion while the GI tract receives less. This could be one of the reasons GI symptoms are so common in those with anxiety disorders.

Increased emotional distress results in the release of catecholamines, which is damaging to the intimal endothelium of the coronary arteries. That, in turn, leads to release of free fatty acids, which results in increased platelet aggregation and lipid deposition at the site of the endothelial damage. Subsequent increases in cortisol contribute to still further damage. (Catecholamines include DA, Epi, and NE.)

I have noticed that after a physically stressful event, such as a treadmill EKG stress test, blood pressure normalizes within minutes, but that after an emotionally stressful event, it can take many hours to normalize blood pressure. This is because the stress ends when we leave the treadmill, but in the case of emotional distress, the stress continues as long as we are emotionally distressed. Allostatic load increases in proportion to the length of time we experience emotional distress, and high allostatic load translates into catabolic processes.

A catabolic state results in:
- Cessation of protein, fat, and carbohydrate synthesis
- Increased breakdown of protein, fat, and carbohydrate
- Elevated blood levels of glucose, free fatty acids, and LDL cholesterol

- Decreased bone remodeling
- Decreased repair and replacement of cells that require high turnover
- Decreased production and circulation of WBCs, and general immune function impairment

The following are also part of sympathetic tone but are not part of catabolism:
- Increased salt and water retention
- Increased systolic and diastolic blood pressure (BP)
- Increased HR and stroke volume (SV)
- Increased serum uric acid levels
- Increased platelet adhesion and increased platelet aggregation
- Increased blood viscosity
- Constriction of peripheral resistance and capacitance vessels
- Arterial wall damage
- Impaired left ventricular (LV) function
- Lethal dysrhythmias
- Coronary vasospasm induced by hyperventilation.
- Increased BP leading to heart failure, atherosclerosis, heart attacks, kidney damage, ischemic strokes, and hemorrhagic strokes

Living in a catabolic state can present differently in different individuals. For example, generalized anxiety disorder (GAD) (unlike other anxiety disorders) does not typically manifest in sympathetic activation in the presence of worry, challenges, or threats. Instead, there is a reduction in heart rate variability (HRV—the interval between heartbeats) along with deficient parasympathetic tone. A high HRV is healthy, and a lack of variation in the beat-to-beat intervals is often a sign of congestive heart failure (CHF) as well as chronic debilitating emotional distress. (For more on HRV, see appendix B.) Frequent detection of threat with no place to run and no one to fight means that sympathetic activation is not adaptive, so it is suppressed. Nevertheless, people living with GAD live in a catabolic state.

Emotional distress and physiological stress have been measured through lab values, fMRI, biofeedback, and other methods.

Epigenetics

Epigenetics refers to the study of gene function changes that occur without changes to the DNA sequence.[13] *Genotype* refers to an individual's exact genetic makeup. *Phenotype* refers to the actual expression of genes present.

The significance of epigenetics is that phenotypal changes determine whether or not a gene will get expressed. The Human Genome Project revealed the sequence of all our protein-expressing genes, while epigenetics research is just beginning to reveal how the genes and other mechanisms of genetic activity are actually regulated. Epigenetics researchers explore the biological ramifications of how genes are altered by our internal and external environment.

Genetics and, to a larger extent, epigenetics, are very powerful determinants of health or illness. Examples of epigenetic factors are environmental toxins in the air, food, and water. Another epigenetic factor is chronic emotional distress, referred to as allostatic load, which is positively correlated with increased disease (see above). Alterations in gene expression can be caused by many types of physiological stress, such as trauma, disease, genetic mutations, expression of various genes, environmental stressors, and countless additional known and unknown factors.

Regardless of the etiology of the physiological stress, the specific diseases that manifest are most likely determined by genetic predispositions to those diseases, the type and amount of the environmental exposure to a toxin, any number of viruses, fungi, and bacteria, and unidentified factors. For example, when someone has a family history of cancer, neurological disease, cardiovascular disease, autoimmune disease, or some other class of diseases, the family genetics, combined with internal and external stressors most likely predispose that person to the specific disease to which she or he is also genetically predisposed.

Epigenetic factors can affect future generations. The spermatozoa or ova of a fetus can get altered by stress in the pregnant mother, which can then affect the future children of that fetus.[14]

Epigenetics deals with *methylation,* which is the process by which methyl groups are added to certain nucleotides in genomic DNA. That process has profound effects on gene expression. What happens is that once DNA has become methylated, it may not be able to go through the transcription process, which is where DNA is transcribed into RNA. Alterations in DNA methylation have been found in many types of tumors.

In addition to methylation, epigenetics also relates to histone markers, which refer to large proteins that surround and stabilize the long, linear, and highly flexible DNA molecule, forming the DNA/protein complex known as chromatin. Histones can affect gene expression by sequestering or exposing segments of DNA. This allows histone modification, like methylation, to function as an important epigenetic mechanism.[15]

Epigenetics researchers have demonstrated that the health of the physiological environment in which our genes reside determines whether certain genes turn on or off as well as determine the timing of genetic activation.

Every emotional change leads to a cascade of neurohormones and neurotransmitter substances, and can effect changes in shape, voltage, and biochemistry of cell membrane receptors.[16] It is possible that these psychophysiological processes may be able to effect healthy or unhealthy epigenetics processes.

The significance of physiological stress resulting in alterations in cell membrane function is that necessary substances may not be able to enter or exit cells at the appropriate times.

Our emotion-laden thoughts influence whether certain molecules will succeed in binding to the receptors for that molecule and whether or not the molecule will gain entrance to the cells where they are needed.[17]

Emotional distress activates the limbic-hypothalamic system to convert neural signals into neuropeptide messenger molecules that have direct effects on the endocrine and immune systems. Certain hormones are then synthesized, which then have an effect on which genes get expressed.[18]

Environmental Toxins
Environmental toxins to which we are all exposed every day enter cell membranes and then alter the shape of receptors on the surface of the cell membranes. Once a receptor has been altered, the exchange of molecules in and out of the cell also becomes altered. Some toxins, such as organophosphates and phthalates (plasticizers), bind to estrogen or testosterone receptors, resulting in increased breast and prostate cancer rates.[19] In addition to the toxins' alteration of cell membrane structure and function, arsenic may alter DNA methylation, which means it has an epigenetic mechanism. Cyanide inhibits cytochrome c oxidase, preventing the production of adenosine triphosphate (ATP). Organophosphates act as cholinesterase inhibitors and neuroendocrine disrupters.[20]

Stress and Immunosuppression
Psychoneuroimmunology researcher Janice Kiecolt-Glaser at Ohio State University Medical School has been studying medical students throughout her long career. One month prior to an intense period of academic exams, she tested medical students for their levels of messenger RNA expression of the proto-oncogenes c-myc and c-myb in their peripheral leukocytes. The blood draws and assays were repeated at the height of the academic exam period. The messenger RNA expression of these proto-oncogenes was elevated during the stressful academic exam period. It was already well known that emotional stress is immunosuppressive. This study demonstrated

that the immunosuppression as evidenced by the increased messenger RNA expression of proto-oncogenes resulted in actual genetic alterations of the type that lead to the turning on of oncogenes. In other words, the students' emotional distress created alterations in cell membrane function, which in turn resulted in transduction of signals to the DNA in the nucleus, and that in turn created alterations in the messenger RNA. We normally have molecular DNA repair mechanisms in place to prevent these genetic mutations from developing into actual tumors. However, chronic emotional distress interferes with the biochemical machinery of these repair mechanisms.[21]

Your Endogenous Pharmacy

The term *endogenous pharmacy* is used to describe drugs that are made by the body for the body. They are biological drugs synthesized by the endocrine, immune, GI, nervous, cardiovascular, renal, hepatic, and other systems. They are without side effects. If one is in perfect health, they are dispensed in exactly the right formula, dose, and schedule and are designed for the unique genetics of the individual. All of this occurs without any conscious awareness of the process.

A significant segment of the population lives with more than one health challenge. The pharmaceutical industry makes thousands of drugs, almost all of which have adverse effects. Because of a wide variation in human genotypes, every commercially made medicine has different effects on different people. Even within the same genotypes, commercial drugs commonly interact with each other, further complicating the effects. Although there are a few notable exceptions such as antibiotics, most commercially made drugs are designed to treat symptoms rather than to cure disease.

As we have seen, psychoneuroimmunology researchers have demonstrated that our thoughts, beliefs, images, and attitudes directly affect our emotions, and our emotions directly affect neurotransmitter substances such as the catecholamines—NE, Epi, and DA. For example, the biochemistry of the experience of hope is correlated with a decrease in corticosteroids. Joy is correlated with a decrease in the vasopressor catecholamines and therefore an improvement in oxygenation and perfusion in areas of injury.[22]

Endogenously produced drugs all have very specific effects. For example, DA activity relates to "wanting" and moving toward pleasure. Opioid activity relates to "liking" and has more to do with mindfulness—being in the moment.

One might wonder if the drugs the body naturally produces have fairly mild effects compared to those developed for a specific effect in the lab, but this is not the case. Endorphins are *three times more powerful than the exogenous analogs— the commercial drug morphine and its derivatives.* Endogenously produced serotonin is a more powerful anxiolytic and antidepressant than anything the pharmaceutical industry produces. Our endogenously produced pharmacopeia can produce profound results. The endogenous drug oxytocin causes us to bond with others, and the endogenous drug dopamine creates a feeling of well-being.[23]

The Endogenous Pharmacy and a Sense of Control

Patient-controlled analgesia (PCA) units commonly result in less pain and less anxiety among surgical post-op patients. One of the reasons for this is most likely that the sense of control mollifies the anxiety and fear of being overcome with pain. In fact, empowering the patient by offering PCA also results in less overall use of narcotics. PCA units are locked out at a certain level so that no patient can overdose, but ironically, patients with PCA units use less narcotic than those patients who must wait for the nurse to administer more analgesic. In the same study in which this was shown, it was also discovered that positive intraoperative suggestions while the patient was under general anesthesia resulted in lower post-operative needs for analgesia, lower rates of nausea and vomiting, and faster overall recovery.[24]

The Role of Beliefs and Expectancies

Our beliefs and expectancies are so powerful that the simple act of reading a drug package insert listing all its possible side effects can dramatically increase the odds of experiencing those side effects. The expectancies we hold about any drug we take are quite often more powerful than the pharmacological effects of the drug, as we shall see further on in a discussion of the placebo effect.

Just as various altered states of consciousness can be triggered with either prescription or recreational drugs, they can be triggered by various emotional states, because emotional states all influence, and are influenced by, the endogenous pharmacy. When we hold the belief *This day is going well,* that belief is likely to improve our experience of the day. The reverse can lead to a downward spiral.

The power of expectancy is so strong that in thousands of placebo studies, researchers have discovered very serious side effects from the placebos. For example, people have actually become addicted to placebos, believing them to be narcotics, and experienced all the side effects.

There have been cases where the subjects developed elevated liver enzymes and actually needed medical treatment to treat the damage done by their beliefs that they were taking a hepatotoxic drug.[25]

Imagination Triggers Digestive Enzymes

If you had never tasted a lemon, there would be no physiological correlates of thinking about eating a lemon. But if you have, just imagining doing so causes salivation, just as if the lemon were real. Positive expectancies do not have to be conscious; the mind remembers the actual experience of the lemon from the past and reacts as if the experience were happening in the moment. This is one of the ways in which the mind can be intentionally used to catalyze synthesis of various important substances.

The Power of Suggestion

The power of suggestion was at work in a British study of two hundred outpatients with a variety of complaints that did not require hospitalization. Half were given a diagnosis and told that they would be all better in a few days. The other half was told that it was a mystery why they were sick and that there was no way to determine when they would recover. Two weeks later, 64 percent of the patients in the first group reported full recovery; only 39 percent in the second group did so.[26]

One possible explanation for this is that the first group went home feeling reassured, and that reassurance served as a boost to their immune systems. The group who were told their illness was a mystery and recovery time uncertain presumably went home and worried, possibly assuming that they had some terrible disease that could kill them and ruminating about what the doctor told them; their subsequent emotional distress most likely had deleterious effects on their immune systems, interfering with their abilities to recover. There are, of course, some people who, when told there is a mystery, tend to think the best, or who may be well aware that doctors make mistakes all the time. These people may simply dismiss what they have been told, go home, and forget about it. Still others tend to get angry and become determined to prove the doctor wrong, and go home to fully recover.

Asthmatics Are Helped by Aerosolized Saline Solution

In an asthma study by Laver and Luparello in which forty asthma patients inhaled aerosolized saline believing it to be an allergen to which they were allergic, nineteen developed bronchoconstriction. In another asthma study, 29 asthma patients inhaled saline solution believing it to be an allergen and fifteen bronchoconstricted. Aerosolized saline normally does not create any effect at all. In experiments with asthmatic patients, it has consistently been found that the patient's belief that an inert inhalant (aerosolized saline) is an irritant triggers bronchoconstriction. In these same experiments, when the asthmatic patient's belief is that an irritant is an inert inhalant, the patient does not bronchoconstrict. When led to believe that aerosolized saline they were being given was in fact Albuterol (a sympathomimetic bronchodilator), the bronchoconstriction resolved.[27]

Messages Have Pharmacological Effects
In an independent replication of the studies by Luparello, asthmatic patients were part of a small study in which the same pharmacological treatment was administered to the same cohort of patients at two different times. A different message was delivered to the patients each time. Believing that what they had just inhaled caused bronchoconstriction, all of the patients experienced actual bronchoconstriction despite the fact that what they had been given was nothing more than aerosolized distilled water. Later, they were given the identical substance but were told that they were being given a powerful bronchodilator; all of them experienced immediate relief.[28]

In one study, a group of asthmatics were exposed to nebulized saline (a completely innocuous substance). When they were told they were inhaling allergens to which they were allergic, they all developed trouble breathing. Some developed full-blown asthma attacks. All the attacks were relieved completely as they were given the same saline solution to inhale when it was presented therapeutically.[29]

The Placebo Effect

> *The history of medicine is actually the history of the placebo effect.*
> —William Osler, MD

Nowhere are expectancies and beliefs more in evidence than in the phenomenon known as the placebo effect, in which people receiving what they believe to be an effective drug actually receive a benign substitute, yet still experience the drug's effect. I will illustrate this by drawing from a variety of studies.

Prescription Medication Placebo Effects
and Drug Packaging

Studies have determined very specific factors that contribute
to the efficacy of placebos. Price and Fields found placebo injections to be more effective than placebos by mouth. They
also discovered that placebos administered by a respected authority figure are more effective than placebos from a nurse.[30]

The drug companies also know that the size, shape, and
color of a tablet or capsule influence its popularity as well as
its efficacy. A study involving medical students revealed that
capsules are more effective than tablets, despite having identical ingredients. Two half-strength capsules have been found
to be more effective than one full-strength capsule. White
tablets are the most effective analgesics, but rheumatoid arthritis patients get more pain relief from red tablets or capsules. Aside from the effects of the active ingredient, orange
and yellow tablets have been found to be the most effective
antidepressants. Few doctors are willing to acknowledge that
the size, shape, and color of the capsule or tablet influences efficacy. For obvious reasons, no drug company would publicly
acknowledge it either.[31]

Dr. Allington and His Colored Water

In 1934 physician Herman Allington designed a study in
which sulpharsphenamine was administered to 105 patients.
Distilled water, which was colored to look like the drug, was
administered to 120 other patients. All the patients received
the drug or the water for the treatment of warts. This experiment was placebo-controlled, randomized, and double blind.
Complete remission occurred in 52 percent of the drug arm
and in 48 percent of those receiving colored water.[32] Again,
the power of positive expectancy is what cured all of the 48
percent who received the colored water. Of the 52 percent
who achieved complete remission, based on the placebo arm
results, the real drug may actually only have a 4 percent cure
rate rather than 52 percent. The remaining 48 percent were
cured by unidentified, endogenously produced drugs.

In a study involving arthritic patients, the results from a placebo were equivalent to the results from an active drug. Those who received no symptom relief from the drug were later given the placebo and got relief from the neutral substance.[33]

Pain, Morphine, and Placebo

A group of hospitalized patients suffering with severe, intractable pain were told they would be given morphine. A few were given the morphine, but most were given a placebo. Most of the placebo patients got relief from their pain.[34]

In one classic lab experiment, a blood pressure cuff is inflated to cause pain to the subjects. Biofeedback monitoring confirms sympathetic arousal. The blood pressure cuff is then deflated. Then the subjects are injected with a very small amount of morphine and the experiment is repeated. This time, there is no pain and no sympathetic arousal. After repeating this process a few times, the subjects are then injected with saline while believing that it is morphine. As you might expect by now, there is no pain and no sympathetic arousal. It appears that the belief that morphine is being injected is enough to catalyze a release of endorphins, a naturally produced molecule, which binds to the same opioid neuroreceptors, thereby blocking the pain signals.[35]

In another classic lab experiment, the same painful stimulus is delivered using the blood pressure cuff and the subjects quickly learn to expect pain before the next stimulus is delivered. Morphine is given just as in the previous experiment, blocking the pain. Then, Naloxone, a powerful drug that blocks the opioid receptors, is injected instead of morphine or saline. This means endorphins cannot have an effect because their receptors are occupied by Naloxone. This time, even though the subjects believe they are being injected with morphine, they experience pain and sympathetic arousal that can be measured by biofeedback equipment.[36] Substance P and cholecystokinin (CCK) are biological analogues of Naloxone. Belief and expectation that there will be pain relief can prevent CCK synthesis and enhance endorphin synthesis.

Studies like this make it clear that nothing is purely psychological or purely physiological. Cognition and emotion are continually altered by our physiology, and vice versa. The interplay between the two is extremely complex, and it would be quite difficult to distill out exactly which physiological process led to exactly which line of thinking and feeling. Of course, the reverse would be equally true.

In a study of postoperative wound pain, a placebo was found to be almost as effective as morphine. The researchers discovered that the effectiveness of the placebo is positively correlated with the degree of pain the patients experience. In a similar test of placebos to treat severe arthritis pain, the difference between the drug and the placebo was almost nonexistent. Later, some of the patients who had not had relief from the placebo tablet were given a placebo injection. Sixty-four percent of that group got relief.[37]

Placebo Beta Blockers

Beta-blockers are a very commonly used class of drugs for the treatment of a variety of cardiovascular diseases. In one study of these drugs, a large cohort of heart patients was divided into two groups. One group was treated with beta-blockers, and the second group was treated with a placebo. The most noncompliant patients—that is, the patients who often failed to take their medication each day—had a mortality rate of more than two and one-half times the rate of the compliant patients. One of the most interesting results of this study was that *the mortality rate for compliant versus noncompliant patients was identical in both groups.* In other words, it was the positive expectancy of all those who took their medications that improved their health, rather than the active ingredients of the drug itself.[38]

Parkinson's Disease and Placebo Dopamine

In another study, PET scanning was performed to assess dopaminergic activity in the affected parts of the brains of six Parkinson's patients, both before and after they were injected with either a placebo or a drug that stimulates dopamine synthesis. When the patients believed that they were receiving the real drug but were given the placebo, their brains *synthesized as much dopamine as when given the active drug* and their muscles showed the improvements that would normally be expected with the drug.[39]

When placebos outperform a real drug, it becomes clear that the most powerful drugs are the endogenous ones triggered by our beliefs and expectations.

The Wart-Killing Machine

Bruno Bloch was a Swiss physician who is most remembered for the spectacular success of a machine he invented and used in the 1920s to cure warts. Patients traveled great distances to be treated by Dr. Bloch, and most of them were cured of their warts. Interestingly, there was absolutely no scientific basis for the efficacy of the machine. It had a motor that produced varied sounds and some fancy electronics (for the time) that produced flashing lights. He explained to patients that the machine beamed lethal anti-wart rays at their hapless targets.

How could several hundred patients be completely cured of warts after being treated by a contraption that had absolutely no scientific or medical value? The cure was, in fact, synthesized in the patients' own endogenous pharmacies and by their deep faith in the doctor and the machine. This is no different from the dozens of cases of so-called terminal cancer patients who have made unexpected full recoveries after being treated by modern chemotherapeutic agents that had been proven to be completely ineffective.

Side Effects of Placebos Mimic Those of Real Drugs

Medical students in a pharmacology class listened to a lecture comparing the pharmacologic effects of stimulants with sedatives, including all the side effects of each class of drugs. Then the class was divided in half. Half the class then took a stimulant and the other half took a sedative. The students were then instructed to monitor their vitals and record them along with their symptoms. The professor actually had given half the class inert placebos that looked in every way like real sedatives, and the other half of the class received inert placebos that looked in every way like real stimulants. Despite the fact that everyone in both groups received nothing but a placebo, more than 60 percent of the students in each group, believing they had ingested the real thing, began to experience the precise physiological effects they expected, including side effects such as blurred vision, dizziness, cardiac dysrhythmia, and abdominal pain.[40]

In a full-page Prozac ad by Eli Lilly, I noticed a chart proudly revealing that in clinical trials, in many instances, the drug did not have significantly more side effects than the placebo. For example, 21 percent of the Prozac patients developed headache after going on the drug. I thought that was a high number until I noticed that 20 percent of the placebo-treated patients also developed headache after being given what they believed was Prozac. Five percent of the patients given Prozac developed a flu symptom, yet 4 percent on the placebo developed that symptom—again, not very different. Twelve percent of those given Prozac developed diarrhea, yet 8 percent on the placebo also developed diarrhea. Obviously, the drug did not cause diarrhea in the 8 percent because they didn't take it. Ten percent on Prozac developed dry mouth versus 7 percent on placebo. The placebo, a completely inert substance, could not have caused dry mouth in those patients. Eight percent of those on Prozac and 5 percent of those on placebo developed dyspepsia. Other symptoms included nervousness (13 percent versus 9); dizziness (10 percent versus 7); pharyngitis (5 percent versus 4); and rash (4 percent versus 3). That's quite a list, but the subjects in both groups experienced still more side effects: asthenia, fever, vasodilatation, palpitation, nausea, anorexia, flatulence, vomiting, insomnia, somnolence, tremor, decreased libido, sweating, pruritis, and abnormal vision.

Drug studies are double-blinded, meaning neither the people administering the drug or placebo nor the patients receiving either knew what was being given to them. The reason all drug studies are randomized, double-blind, and placebo-controlled is because the power of our beliefs is such that it is a powerful confounding variable for which researchers must control.

Meta-analyses of Placebo Studies

More evidence of the power of expectancy is evidenced by the results of a meta-analysis of a number of placebo studies. Here are just some of the physiological effects of various placebos given in studies: nausea, vomiting, diarrhea, dry mouth, heaviness, headache, concentration difficulties, drowsiness, fatigue, inability to stay awake, insomnia, weakness, heart palpitations, rashes, epigastric pain, urticaria, anaphylactic-like reactions, decreased libido, increased libido, abdominal bloating, dizziness, lumbar pain, tachycardia, euphoria, feeling drugged, incontinence, anxiety, dysmenorrhea, anorexia, acne, blurred vision, and many other symptoms, illnesses, and conditions. Not one of the patients experiencing any of these problems received any substance that could cause any effect at all.

A meta-analysis of fifteen placebo studies involving 1,082 patients revealed that 35 percent of placebo-treated patients with a wide variety of diagnoses consistently evidenced satisfactory relief whenever placebos were substituted for the regular medicine. The fifteen studies included patients with a range of medical problems including severe postoperative wound pain, headaches, various forms of degenerative arthritis, RBCs and WBCs out of reference range, hypertension, allergies, and many other diagnoses.[41]

Placebos and Cholesterol

A cohort of atherosclerotic, hypercholesterolemic heart patients was divided into two groups. The controls received a placebo and the treatment groups were given lipid-lowering drugs. At the five-year follow-up, the patients in both groups had similar mortality rates. However, the mortality of the most compliant patients was half the mortality rate of the less compliant patients; this was as true for those who had been taking placebos for the five years as it was for those on the actual lipid-lowering drugs. It was the positive expectancy of all those who took their medications that improved their health, rather than the active ingredients of the drug itself.[42]

The deep trust that the compliant patients had in their doctors may have contributed to the successful results in the placebo groups that were equal to the results in the treatment groups. In a sense, the actual treatment was not the medication given to the patients, but rather the trusting relationship between doctors and patients. This would also explain why some doctors consistently get better results than other doctors, despite prescribing the identical drugs.

Placebos and Gastric Activity

In 1964, a study was performed to specifically explore the power of belief. Subjects swallowed the identical placebo on three separate occasions. A magnetic tracer was in the capsule, allowing the experimenters to observe physiologic changes. The first time the subjects received the inert capsule, they were told that the drug they were being given would stimulate gastric activity. The second time they were told that the drug now being given would make them feel like their stomachs were full. The third time they swallowed the capsule they were told that it was a placebo. As hypothesized by the researchers, the physiological sensations experienced by the subjects mimicked the descriptions given to them as to what to expect.[43]

Beyond Placebo: Dr. Wolf
and Morning Sickness Sufferers

In 1950, physician Stewart Wolf performed an experiment with a group of women suffering with particularly severe morning sickness. Modern ethical regulations would forbid the study he performed on his patients in 1950, yet it helped the patients. The women were all told they would be receiving a new and powerful antiemetic, yet the drug he intentionally gave them, as an experiment in the power of suggestion, was syrup of ipecac. The patients' trust in the physician and in the power of this supposed new drug was powerful enough to not only counteract the emetogenic effects of the ipecac, but their nausea and vomiting actually abated.[44]

Further Experiments by Dr. Wolf

Wolf performed a number of case studies at that time. In one, a patient with Parkinson's disease was given a placebo but was told he was receiving a drug. His PD symptoms disappeared. As soon as the effects from the placebo wore off, Wolf put the same substance into the patient's milk without his knowledge. This time the substance had no effect.

In another study, 133 of Wolf's depressed patients were treated with a placebo. Twenty-five percent responded so well that they were kept on the placebo. When a group of patients were given a placebo instead of the usual antihistamine, 77.4 percent of them experienced drowsiness, which is a normal side effect of antihistamines.[45] (In the early 1950s, just prior to the introduction of tricyclics, antihistamines such as chlorpromazine and imipramine were used to treat depression.)

Physician Expectancies Dramatically Alter Treatment Outcomes

When a physician prescribes a drug or other treatment, the degree to which he or she believes in the treatment has a profound effect on its outcome. In three separate double-blind studies, vitamin E was given to treat angina pectoris. Two of the studies were conducted by physicians who believed vitamin E would be a useless treatment for angina. The patients of those two doctors did not experience any relief. The doctor in the third study enthusiastically believed the vitamin E would be effective. *The patients of that doctor experienced significant relief, despite the fact that vitamin E has been proven to be a useless treatment for angina.*[46]

Drugs Are Most Effective When First Introduced

> *You should treat as many patients as possible with new*
> *drugs while they still have the power to heal.*
> —Armand Trousseau (French physician, 1833)

As with most new drugs, the chemotherapeutic agent known as cis-platinum was first introduced by a pharmaceutical company with great fanfare. Enthusiastic oncologists reported success rates as high as 75 percent. Over time, though, the drug became far less effective. Physicians have hypothesized that "the atmosphere of positive expectation created by confident, gung-ho doctors who believed they had a magic bullet mobilized the patients' own healing response. When the agent was later administered by bored technicians minus the miracle drug fanfare, its effects may have been diminished."[47]

When meprobamate was first introduced in the 1950s as a tranquilizer, some doctors found it to be very effective while others found that their patients failed to get any effect. To explore these inconsistencies, researchers ran a double-blind study involving one physician who wholeheartedly believed in the drug's efficacy, and another physician who did not believe in it. Neither the two physicians nor any of the patients knew which pills were the real drugs and which were the placebos. In fact, neither the physicians nor the patients even knew they were in a study. The patients of the physician who believed in the meprobamate benefited from the real drug more than they did from the placebo. Interestingly, the patients of the physician who did not believe in the meprobamate got no effect from the meprobamate or from the placebo.[48] *This study was particularly interesting because neither the drug nor the placebo had any effect on the patients whose doctor did not expect any effect.*

Harvard cardiologist Herbert Benson has always taught his interns and residents that when a new medication is prescribed by an enthusiastic doctor who clearly has faith in the drug, the effects of the drug are considerably more impressive than when that same drug is prescribed a few years later by doctors who question the efficacy of the drug.

A new anxiolytic was tested against a placebo in 1955 by physicians who were very excited about the newly released drug. Side effects included nausea, dizziness, heart palpitations, and abdominal pain. The placebo groups experienced the identical levels of side effects as in those receiving the real drug. One of the patients in the placebo arm of the study developed a severe skin rash that resolved immediately upon discontinuation of her taking the placebo. Another patient not only developed sudden onset abdominal pain, but also developed ascites within ten minutes of taking the placebo.[49]

Drug Companies: Marketing for Maximum Effect

Pharmaceutical companies pour billions into marketing, an important aspect of which is promoting the name of the company itself. This is because they know that their products will not only sell better and be prescribed more as a result of name recognition, but that the efficacy of the drug is greater if people recognize it and have trust in it. They also know that if the prescribing doctor believes in the drug, the patients will do better on it than they would if the doctor had any doubts about its efficacy or safety.

Appendix

B

Conscious Breathing, Heart Rate Variability, Respiratory Sinus Arrhythmia, and Health

The role of breathing in health deserves special emphasis, so here I include some of the essential information about the physiology of respiration.

Research psychologists Joanna Arch and Michelle Craske at UCLA demonstrated that fifteen minutes of conscious attention to breathing allowed subjects to tune in to their emotional state and be present with it, even in the midst of aversive stimuli.[1] Neuroscience researcher Britta Hölzel and her team found that the reason for this is that conscious breathing practices serve to activate the anterior cingulate cortex, which regulates numerous autonomic as well as cognitive and emotional functions.[2] Neuroscience researcher John Allman and his team write that this part of the brain has been associated with resolution of conflict and adaptive responses to changing conditions.[3] This new research validates the attention that has been given to breathing methods in yoga, martial arts, and meditation practices for thousands of years.

Gas Exchange and Acid-Base Balance

Proper diaphragmatic breathing regulates acid-base balance as well as heart rate (HR) and rhythm. It also improves oxygenation and perfusion of tissues and organs, including the brain. In diaphragmatic breathing, gas exchange takes place in the lower, middle, and upper lobes of the lungs. In shallow chest breathing (hypoventilation), too much CO_2 is retained in the lower lobes, reducing blood pH and contributing to respiratory acidosis. If breathing becomes too shallow, the pH can get low enough to send us into metabolic compensation—a feedback process by which the kidneys secrete bicarb in order to raise blood pH. When we become very frightened, we may hyperventilate and blow off too much CO_2. This results in respiratory alkalosis.

Too much oxygen and too little oxygen are both toxic. Although metabolic compensation can correct respiratory acidosis and help maintain an acid-base balance, mindfulness practice and the cultivation of healthy breathing can often obviate the need for metabolic compensation, which could be especially important for anyone with renal problems.

Heart Rate Variability and Respiratory Sinus Arrhythmia

As I wrote in appendix A, HRV is the pattern of variation between beats of the heart. The greater the HRV, the better our health.[4] The HRV is also referred to as the standard deviation of beat-to-beat intervals, commonly referred to as the SDNN. It is measured by a computer program utilizing electrocardiography (EKG) or photoplethysmography (PPG) in a mathematical formula. When I was trained in physiology, I was taught that a wide HRV was unhealthy; new psychophysiology research has clearly disproved that old information. Contrary to what most of us (even physicians) were taught in physiology classes years ago, it is now known that increased variability in all biological rhythms optimizes physiological functioning. Biological rhythms evidence the greatest variability early in life and the least variability late in life. This is one reason why we are less able to regulate all the vast changes in our internal and external environments as we age.

Cardiologist J. Thomas Bigger at Columbia-Presbyterian Medical Center found that reduced HRV is a strong predictor of mortality following myocardial infarctions.[5] Karolinska Institute researcher Myriam Horsten and her team found that reduced HRV is often conceptualized as a lack of ability to respond by physiological variability and complexity, making the person physiologically rigid and, therefore, more vulnerable.[6] This translates into an underactive parasympathetic nervous system. Poor parasympathetic tone is a signal finding among people with reduced HRV; their autonomic nervous system is strikingly unbalanced in favor of sympathetic responses, and this is reflected in rigid (not variable) cardiac function. Medical researcher Hisako Tsuji and the Framingham Heart Study found that this rigidity is a clear-cut contributor to ventricular arrhythmias.[7] It is now common knowledge that parasympathetic tone and reasonably good HRV are essential for the maintenance of the electrical stability of the heart, which directly correlates with the prevention of lethal dysrhythmias. Even physically fit individuals who are depressed, anxious, or commonly feel hostile probably have low HRV. Researchers J. W. Hughes and C. M. Stoney at Ohio State Medical School found that preventricular contractions (PVCs) are a common symptom of people with reduced HRV.[8]

HRV at respiratory frequencies is called respiratory sinus arrhythmia (RSA). It is controlled by the vagus nerve. RSA is associated with a high frequency of HRV. RSA relates to the natural heart-rate fluctuations that are influenced by respiration, the baroreceptors, and limbic activity. In RSA breathing, exhalation, which is parasympathetic, is consciously self-regulated to be roughly twice as long as inhalation, which is sympathetic. One can intentionally reverse this at times to create specific physiological responses, such as to wake up when tired or when concentration is dull. Neurologist Richard Mendius, MD, once told a group of us that a treatment for daytime sleepiness is to focus on the in-breath in order to increase sympathetic drive. For example, sympathetic drive can intentionally be increased by making the inhalation longer than the exhalation. I often do this to increase alertness when I am getting sleepy at inopportune times. Although

drinking coffee has been strongly associated with health, re-
liance upon any drug is orthogonal to living with conscious
intention, mindfulness, and mastery. In addition, drinking
coffee in the evening in order to perk up can interfere with
sleep, whereas breathing as a form of self-regulation is easily reversible simply by switching from longer inhalations to
longer exhalations.

It has been known for a long time that RSA breathing
quiets sympathetic drive, normalizes HR as well as heart
rhythms, and is a very significant determinant of health. It is
also known to improve brain function.[9] The association with
improved brain function could simply be due to increased
oxygenation and perfusion, but most likely it is also related
to the balancing of numerous biological rhythms catalyzed by
the practice.

Utilizing biofeedback instrumentation, it is easy to learn
to maximize RSA and find the ideal breathing rate, which is
unique to each individual; this is referred to as resonant frequency.

Resonant frequency breathing is a type of RSA breathing,
but it is done at approximately six breaths per minute with
some minor variations depending on a person's size. The resonant frequency of each of us refers to the natural rhythm of
fluctuations in other biological functions such as HR, blood
pressure (BP), cerebral perfusion, and other measures. At resonant frequency, the synchronization is the rhythm of each
function resonating with all of the other functions, thereby
mutually reinforcing each other.

Although resonant frequency breathing is a practice that
brings forth the harmonization of biological rhythms for
health, researchers have found that twenty minutes a day is
optimum, and that breathing that way all day would actually
reduce HRV.[10] Resonant frequency breathing has been used
to control both HR and rhythm. It also serves to quiet sympathetic drive, regulate BP, and correct acid-base imbalances.

Also, RSA can enhance mindfulness practice because it
makes it possible to consciously correlate every subtle change

in breathing rate and rhythm with changes in cognition and emotion.[11] In addition, because the act of breathing involves communication with all the neuropeptides, it is one of the ways we can enhance psychophysiological functioning.[12]

Changes in rate and depth of respiration produce changes in the quantity and types of peptides (short amino acid chains) that are released from the brain stem. Conversely, peptide changes in the brain stem alter respiration. By consciously altering respiratory rate, we can effect changes in the rate at which peptides diffuse through the cerebral spinal fluid (CSF), in many cases contributing to a restoration of homeostasis.

Good vagal tone (related to the health of the parasympathetic nervous system) is associated with a state of happiness. The vagus nerve influences HR, HRV, immune responses, digestion, and absorption. RSA leads to increased vagal tone. Higher resting vagal tone is associated with improved immune function, health, and happiness.[13]

Bangkok researcher Sukanya Phongsuphap studied HRV in meditators and found that forms of meditation utilizing conscious breathing practices improve HRV, parasympathetic activity, and gas exchange.[14] They studied thirty-five meditators and seventy matched controls, and found that meditation improved cardiovascular function. They analyzed the HRV measures from the R-R intervals (time between two R-waves on an EKG reading). They concluded that meditation may have different effects on health depending on the frequency of the resonant peak that each meditator can achieve, which may relate both to the individual's physiology and the individual's method of practice. The possible effects include resetting the baroreflex sensitivity, increasing sympathetic tone, and improving efficiency of gas exchange.

Hyperventilation, Breath-Holding, and Optimal Respiration

Shallow thoracic breathing results in respiratory rates as high as 20 to 25 BPM, and that can induce a catabolic state. Slower diaphragmatic breathing produces an anabolic state.

Hyperventilation is characterized by rapid, shallow breathing, punctuated by frequent sighs. Hyperventilation results in blowing off too much CO_2. This then increases blood alkalinity and is one of the causes of hypertension, anxiety, and lightheadedness. In a type of reversible reaction, hyperventilation tends to trigger anxiety just as anxiety can trigger hyperventilation.

Breath-holding is common to many of us when we are concentrating on a tedious task. Although I have not been able to find documentation for this, it seems to be common knowledge among my colleagues that breath-holding on a chronic basis is a likely contributor to cardiac dysrhythmias. Some colleagues have agreed with me that breath-holding can even contribute to structural damage to the mitral valve. Shallow thoracic breathing increases the HR and BP. One colleague told me that she believes the reason for her damaged mitral valve was that she had been holding her breath whenever she felt any anxiety.

It is quite possible that she had also had some genetic predisposition to mitral valve problems or that the etiology of the mitral damage was a virus or other pathogen. Possibly, the unhealthy chronic breath-holding, may have simply been the last straw.

Psychophysiology researchers Dr. Paul Lehrer and Dr. Richard Gevirtz point out that it is essential to maintain a balance between sympathetic and parasympathetic stimulation in order to regulate the subtle exchange of sodium and potassium ions in the sinoatrial (SA) node of the heart.[15] Any electrical dysfunction in the SA node usually translates into atrial fibrillation (AF) and PVCs, and can sometimes even trigger a lethal dysrhythmia such as ventricular fibrillation.

Dysfunctional breathing such as hyperventilation, shallow thoracic breathing, sighing, and breath-holding can play a role in the etiology of any of the following conditions:

- Respiratory symptoms: asthma, dyspnea (shortness of breath), excessive sighing and yawning, and cough

- Cardiovascular symptoms: hypertension, ischemic as well as arrhythmic heart attacks, palpitations, tachycardia, angina, and cold hands and feet
- Neurological symptoms: dizziness, faintness, migraines, and paresthesias
- GI symptoms: dysphagia (swallowing difficulties), dry throat, belching, flatulence, globus (lump in throat), and abdominal discomfort
- Muscular symptoms: cramps, tremors, twitches, pain, and fatigue
- General symptoms: anxiety, fatigue, weakness, lack of concentration, impaired memory, sleep disturbances, nightmares[16]

Although there is some disagreement regarding optimal rates and depths of respiration, in talking to colleagues I have found a general consensus that diaphragmatic breathing at a respiration rate of approximately twelve to fourteen breaths per minute, with longer expiration than inspiration, is very healthy and optimizes gas exchange and acid-base balance.

Based on what we now know from psychophysiological research about the healthiest breathing patterns and the fact that they require a little training followed by a lot of practice, it would be advantageous to almost all of us to make conscious attention to respiration a priority in our lives.

Furthermore, this conscious attention to improving our respiratory patterns can be used as a mindfulness or concentration practice. Conscious respiration practices build mastery and wellbeing. This is because in addition to the direct benefits of healthy breathing patterns, just the act of practicing various forms of self-care—in this case related to an intentional breathing practice—you will feel more in control of your life. Mastery is not about finding cures or treatments; it is about taking valued action, regardless of the outcome.

Notes

Chapter 2

1. Kiecolt-Glaser J, Stephens R, Liepetz P, and Glaser R. Distress and DNA repair in human lymphocytes. *J of Behavioral Medicine,* 1985; 8:311–20.

Chapter 3

1. Roemer L and Orsillo S. *Mindfulness- and Acceptance-Based Behavioral Therapies in Practice.* New York: Guilford, 2009.

2. Luoma J, Hayes S, and Walser R. *Learning ACT: An Acceptance and Commitment Therapy Skills-Training Manual for Therapists.* Oakland, CA: New Harbinger, 2007.

3. Carlin G. *Brain Droppings.* New York: Hyperion, 1997.

4. Blackledge J. Disrupting verbal processes: Cognitive defusion in acceptance and commitment therapy and other mindfulness-based psychotherapies. *The Psychological Record,* 2007;57(4):555–76.

Roemer L and Orsillo S. *Mindfulness- and Acceptance-Based Behavioral Therapies in Practice.* New York: Guilford, 2009.

5. Roemer L and Orsillo S. *Mindfulness- and Acceptance-Based Behavioral Therapies in Practice.* New York: Guilford, 2009.

Chapter 4

1. Hayes S and Strosahl K. *A Practical Guide to Acceptance and Commitment Therapy.* New York: Springer, 2004.

2. Hayes S, Strosahl K, and Wilson K. *Acceptance and Commitment Therapy: An Experiential Approach to Behavioral Change.* New York: Guilford, 1999.

3. Langer E. *Mindfulness.* New York: Addison-Wesley, 1989.

Langer E and Rodin J. The effects of choice and enhanced personal responsibility for the aged: A Field Experiment in an Institutional Setting. *Journal of Personality and Social Psychology,* 1976;34;191–98.

4. Crane R. *Mindfulness-Based Cognitive Therapy.* London: Routledge, 2010.

5. Segal Z, Williams J, and Teasdale J. *Mindfulness-Based Cognitive Therapy for Depression.* New York: Guilford, 2002.

6. Dahl J, Wilson K, and Luciano C. *Acceptance and Commitment Therapy for Chronic Pain.* Reno, NV: Context Press, 2005.

7. Langer E. *Counter Clockwise: Mindful Health and the Power of Possibility.* New York: Ballantine, 2009.

8. Wilson K and Murrell A. Values work in acceptance and commitment therapy: Setting a course for behavioral treatment. In Hayes S, Follette V, and Linehan M (ed.), *Mindfulness and Acceptance: Expanding the Cognitive-Behavioral Tradition.* New York: Guilford, 2004.

9. Barsky A and Ahem D. Cognitive behavior therapy for hypochondriasis: a randomized controlled trial. *JAMA,* 2004;291:1464–70.

10. Achterberg J. *Imagery in Healing: Shamanism and Modern Medicine.* Boston: Shambhala, 1985.

Achterberg J and Lawless G. Imagery for Health and Healing — one-year training sponsored by Institute for Health and Healing, California Pacific Medical Center, 1998. Phase I: The Psychophysiological Model; Phase II: Assessment and Treatment for Modern Day Settings; Phase III: Psychoneuroimmunology, Advanced Topics and Protocols; Phase IV: Transpersonal Medicine.

11. Rossman M. *Guided Imagery for Self-Healing.* Novato, CA: H. J. Kramer, 2000.

12. Hayes S. *Get Out of Your Mind and Into Your Life: The New Acceptance and Commitment Therapy.* Oakland, CA: New Harbinger, 2006.

13. Teasdale J, Segal Z, and Williams J. Mindfulness and problem formulation. *Clinical Psychology: Science and Practice,* 2003; 10:157–60.

Chapter 5

1. Hayes S. Acceptance and commitment therapy, relational frame theory, and the third wave of behavioral and cognitive therapies. *Behavior Therapy,* 2004;35:639–65.

2. Hayes S. Hello darkness: Discovering our values by confronting our fears. *Psychotherapy Networker,* 2007;31(5):46–52.

3. Tull M and Roemer L. Emotion regulation difficulties associated with the experience of uncued panic attacks: Evidence of experiential avoidance, emotional nonacceptance, and decreased emotional clarity. *Behavior Therapy,* 2007;38:378–91.

4. Twohig M, Hayes S, and Masuda A. Increasing willingness to experience obsessions: Acceptance and Commitment Therapy as a treatment for obsessive-compulsive disorder. *Behavior Therapy,* 2006;37(1), 3–13.

5. Roemer L and Orsillo S. *Mindfulness- and Acceptance-Based Behavioral Therapies in Practice.* New York: Guilford, 2009.

6. Bugental J. Week-long residential training and weekly case consultation group, 1995 through 1998.

LeShan L. *Cancer as a Turning Point.* New York: Dutton, 1989.

Simonton O and Henson R. *The Healing Journey.* New York: Author's Choice, 2002.

7. Twohig M, Hayes S, and Masuda A. Increasing willingness to experience obsessions: Acceptance and Commitment Therapy as a treatment for obsessive-compulsive disorder. *Behavior Therapy,* 2006;37(1), 3–13.

8. Blackledge J. Disrupting verbal processes: Cognitive defusion in acceptance and commitment therapy and other mindfulness-based psychotherapies. *The Psychological Record,* 2007;57(4):555–76.

Davidson R. *Anxiety, Depression, and Emotion.* New York: Oxford University Press, 2000.

Fleshner M and Laudenslager M. Psychoneuroimmunology: then and now. *Behavioral and Cognitive Neuroscience Reviews,* 2004;3:114–30.

Kiecolt-Glaser J and Glaser R. Psychoneuroimmuology: Can psychological interventions modulate immunity? *J. of Consulting and Clinical Psychology,* 1992;60:569–75.

9. McCracken L, Carson J, Eccleston C, and Keefe F. Acceptance and change in the context of chronic pain. *Pain,*2004;109:4–7.

10. Borkovec T, Alcaine O, and Behar E. Avoidance theory of worry and generalized anxiety disorder. In Heimberg R, Turk C, and Mennin D (ed.), *Generalized Anxiety Disorder: Advances in Research and Practice.* New York: Guilford, 2004.

Cochrane A, Barnes-Holmes D, Barnes-Holmes Y, Steward I, and Luciano C. Experiential avoidance and aversive visual images: Response delays and event related potentials on a simple matching task. *Behavior Research and Therapy,* 2007;45:1379–88.

Eifert G and Heffner M. The effects of acceptance versus control contexts on avoidance of panic-related symptoms. *J. of Behavior Therapy and Experimental Psychiatry.* 2003;34:293–312.

Feldner M, Zvolensky M, Eifert G, and Spira A. Emotional avoidance: An experimental test of individual differences and response suppression during biological challenge. *Behaviour Research and Therapy.* 2003; 41:403–11.

Karekla M, Forsyth J, and Kelly M. Emotional avoidance and panicogenic responding to a biological challenge procedure. *Behavior Therapy,* 2004;35(4):725–46.

Salters-Pedneault K, Tull M, and Roemer L. The role of avoidance of emotional material in anxiety disorders. *Applied and Preventive Psychology: Current Scientific Perspectives*, 2004;11:95–114.

11. Karekla M, Forsyth J, and Kelly M. Emotional avoidance and panicogenic responding to a biological challenge procedure. *Behavior Therapy*, 2004;35(4):725–46.

12. Marcks B and Woods D. A comparison of thought suppression to an acceptance-based technique in the management of personal intrusive thoughts: A controlled evaluation. *Behaviour Research and Therapy*, 2005;43:433–45.

13. Wegner D. Ironic processes of mental control. *Psychological Review*, 1994;101:34–52.

14. Cioffi D and Holloway J. Delayed costs of suppressed pain. *Journal of Personality and Social Psychology*, Vol. 64(2), Feb 1993, 274–82.

15. Wenzlaff R and Wegner D. Thought suppression. *Annual Review of Psychology*, 2000;51:59–91.

16. Wegner D, Ansfield M, and Pilloff D. The putt and the pendulum: Ironic effects of the mental control of action. *Psychological Science*, 1998;9:196–99.

17. Hayes S, Masuda A, Bissett R, Luoma J, and Guerrero L. DBT, FAP, and ACT: How empirically oriented are the new behavior therapy technologies? *Behavior Therapy*, 2004; 35:35–54.

18. Roemer L and Orsillo S. *Mindfulness- and Acceptance-Based Behavioral Therapies in Practice*. New York: Guilford, 2009.

19. Hayes S and Strosahl K. *A Practical Guide to Acceptance and Commitment Therapy*. New York: Springer, 2004.

20. Kingston J, Chadwick P, Meron D, and Skinner T. A pilot randomized controlled trial investigating the effect of mindfulness practice on pain tolerance, psychological well-being, and physiological activity. *J. of Psychosomatic Research*, 2007;62:297–300.

21. Levitt J, Brown T, Orsillo S, and Barlow D. The effects of acceptance versus suppression of emotion on subjective and psychophysiological response to carbon dioxide challenge in patients with panic disorder. *Behavior Therapy*, 2004; 35:747–66.

22. Pennebaker J, Mayne T, and Francis M. Linguistic predictors of adaptive bereavement. *J of Personality and Social Psychology*, 1997;72:863–71.

Pennebaker J, Kiecolt-Glaser J, and Glaser R. Disclosures of traumas and immune function: health implications for psychotherapy. *J. of Consult. Clinical Psychol*, 1988;56:239–45.

23. Dworkin B. *Learning and Physiological Regulation*. Chicago: University of Chicago Press, 1993.

24. Gross J and Levenson R. Emotional suppression: Physiology, self-report, and expressive behavior. *J. of Personality and Social Psychology*, 1993;64:970–86.

Gross J and Levenson R. Hiding feelings: The acute effects of inhibiting negative and positive emotion. *J. of Abnormal Psychology*, 1997;106:95–103.

25. Levitt J, Brown T, Orsillo S, and Barlow D. The effects of acceptance versus suppression of emotion on subjective and psychophysiological response to carbon dioxide challenge in patients with panic disorder. *Behavior Therapy*, 2004; 35:747–66.

26. Ibid.

27. Dahl J, Wilson K, and Luciano C. *Acceptance and Commitment Therapy for Chronic Pain*. Reno, NV: Context Press, 2005.

28. McCracken L, Carson J, Eccleston C, and Keefe F. Acceptance and change in the context of chronic pain. *Pain,*2004;109:4–7.

Dahl J, Wilson K, and Luciano C. *Acceptance and Commitment Therapy for Chronic Pain*. Reno, NV: Context Press, 2005.

Chapter 6

1. Gardner-Nix J. *The Mindfulness Solution to Pain*. Oakland: New Harbinger, 2009.

Kabat-Zinn J. *Full Catastrophe Living: Using the Wisdom of Your Body and Mind to Face Stress, Pain, and Illness*, 15th edition. New York: Bantam, 2005.

2. Lau M. New developments in psychosocial interventions for adults with unipolar depression. *Current Opinions in Psychiatry*, 2008 Jan;21(1):30–36.

3. Levy S, Herberman R, and Lippman M. Correlation of stress factors with sustained depression of natural killer cell activity and predicted prognosis in patients with breast cancer. *J of Clinical Oncology*, 1987;5(3):348–53.

Reich M. Depression and cancer: recent data on clinical issues, research challenges and treatment approaches. *Current Opinion in Oncology*, 2008;20(4):353–59.

4. Finucane A and Mercer S. An exploratory mixed methods study of the acceptability and effectiveness of Mindfulness-Based Cognitive Therapy for patients with active depression and anxiety in primary care. *Biomed Central Psychiatry.* 2006 April 7;6:14.

5. Kennedy S, Kiecolt-Glaser J, and Glaser R. Immunological consequences of acute and chronic stressors: Mediating role of interpersonal relationships. *British J of Medical Psychology*, 1988;61:77–85.

6. Gellert G, Maxwell R, and Siegel B. Survival of breast cancer patients receiving adjunctive psychosocial support therapy: A 10-year follow-up study. *Journal of Clinical Oncology*, 1993;11:1; 66–69.

Chapter 7

1. Kabat-Zinn J. Foreword to Didonna F (ed.), *Clinical Handbook of Mindfulness*. New York: Springer, 2009.

2. Ibid.

3. Shapiro S and Carlson L. *The Art and Science of Mindfulness: Integrating Mindfulness into Psychology and the Helping Professions.* Washington, DC: American Psychological Association, 2009.

4. Bishop S, Lau M, Shapiro S, Carlson L, Anderson N, Carmody J, Segal Z, Abbey S, Speca M, Velting D, and Devins G. Mindfulness: A proposed operational definition. *Clinical Psychology: Science and Practice,* 2004;11(3):230–41.

5. Marlatt G and Kristeller J. Mindfulness and meditation. In Miller W (ed.), *Integrating Spirituality into Treatment.* Washington, DC: American Psychological Association, 1999.

6. Greeson J and Brantley J. Mindfulness and Anxiety Disorders: Developing a Wise Relationship with the Inner Experience of Fear. In Didonna F (ed.), *Clinical Handbook of Mindfulness.* New York: Springer, 2009.

7. Dimidjian S and Linehan M. Defining an agenda for future research on the clinical application of mindfulness practice. *Clinical Psychology: Science and Practice,* 2003;10(2):166.

8. Lipton B and Bhaerman S. *Sponaneous Evolution.* Carlsbad, CA: Hay House, 2009.

9. Csikszentmihalyi M. *Flow: The psychology of optimal experience.* New York: HarperCollins, 1991.

10. Crane R. *Mindfulness-Based Cognitive Therapy.* London: Routledge, 2010.

11. Kabat-Zinn J. *Full Catastrophe Living: Using the Wisdom of Your Body and Mind to Face Stress, Pain, and Illness,* 15th edition. New York: Bantam, 2005.

12. Ibid.

Langer E. *Mindfulness.* New York: Addison-Wesley, 1989.

13. Kabat-Zinn J. *Full Catastrophe Living: Using the Wisdom of Your Body and Mind to Face Stress, Pain, and Illness,* 15th edition. New York: Bantam, 2005.

Chapter 8

1. Tull M, Rodman S, and Roemer L. An examination of the fear of bodily sensations and body hypervigilance as predictors of emotion regulation difficulties among individuals with a recent history of uncued panic attacks. *J. of Anxiety Disorders,* 2008;22(4):750–60.

2. Hayes S, Follette V, and Linehan M. *Mindfulness and Acceptance: Expanding the Cognitive Behavioral Tradition.* New York: Guilford Press, 2004.

Segal Z, Williams J, and Teasdale J. *Mindfulness-Based Cognitive Therapy for Depression.* New York: Guilford, 2002.

Simonton Cancer Center—Certification Training, 2006, 2007, 2008. Most of the tools taught to the cancer patients at the Simonton retreats have been created by O. Carl Simonton, MD, and are unpublished.

Williams M, Teasdale J, Segal Z, and Kabat-Zinn J. *The Mindful Way through Depression: Freeing Yourself from Chronic Unhappiness.* New York: Guilford, 2007.

McQuade J, Carmona P, and Segal Z. *Peaceful Mind: Using Mindfulness and Cognitive Behavioral Psychology to Overcome Depression.* Oakland, CA: New Harbinger, 2004.

3. Peterson C, Seligman M, and Valliant G. Pessimistic explanatory style as a risk factor for physical illness: a thirty-five-year longitudinal study. *J. of Personality and Social Psychology,* 1988;55:23–27.

Gallo L and Mathews K. Understanding the association between socioeconomic status and physical health: Do negative emotions play a role? *Psychological Bulletin,* 2003;129:10–51.

4. McGaugh J. *Memory and Emotion: The Making of Lasting Memories.* New York: Columbia University Press, 2006.

5. Grossman P, Niemann L, Schmidt S, and Walach H. Mindfulness-based stress reduction and health benefits: A meta-analysis. *J. of Psychosomatic Research.* 2004;57:35–43.

6. Speca M, Carlson L, Goody E, and Angen M. A randomized wait-list controlled trial: The effect of a mindfulness meditation-based stress reduction program on mood and symptoms of stress in cancer outpatients. *Psychosomatic Medicine,* 2000;62:613–22.

7. Carlson L, Ursuliak Z, Goodey E, Angen M, and Speca M. The effects of a mindfulness meditation–based stress reduction program on mood and symptoms of stress in cancer outpatients: 6-month follow-up. *Supportive Care In Cancer,* 2001;9:112–23.

8. Massion A, Teas J, Hebert J, Wertheimer M, and Kabat-Zinn J. Meditation, melatonin, and breast/prostate cancer: Hypothesis and preliminary data. *Medical Hypotheses,* 1995;44:39–46.

9. Van Wielingen L, Carlson L, and Campbell T. Mindfulness-based stress reduction (MBSR), blood pressure, and psychological functioning in women with cancer. *Psychosomatic Medicine,* 2007;69:A43.

10. Simonton Cancer Center—Certification Training, 2006, 2007, 2008. Most of the tools taught to the cancer patients at the Simonton retreats have been created by O. Carl Simonton, MD, and are unpublished.

11. Tart C. *States of Consciousness,* Lincoln, NE: Authors Guild BackInPrint.com Edition, 2000.

12. Davidson R and Lutz A. Buddha's Brain: Neuroplasticity and Meditation. *IEEE Signal Processing* (2008),25(1),171–74.

13. Schwartz G. Psychobiology of repression and health: A systems approach. In Singer J. (ed.), *Repression and Dissociation: Implications for Personality Theory, Psychopathology, and Health.* Chicago: University of Chicago Press, 1990.

14. Creswell J, Way B, Eisenberger N, and Lieberman M. Neural correlates of dispositional mindfulness during affect labeling. *Psychosomatic Medicine,* 2007;69(6):560–65.

15. Treadway M and Lazar S. The Neurobiology of Mindfulness. In Didonna F (ed.), *Clinical Handbook of Mindfulness.* New York: Springer, 2009.

16. Hankey A. Studies of advanced stages of meditation in the Tibetan Buddhist and vedic traditions. *J. of Complementary and Alternative Medicine,* 2006;3:513–21.

Travis F and Arenander A. Cross-sectional and longitudinal study of effects of transcendental meditation practice on inter-hemispheric frontal asymmetry and frontal coherence. *International J. of Neuroscience,* 2006;116:1519–38.

17. Davidson R, Kabat-Zinn J, Schumacher J, Rosenkrantz M, Muller D, Santorelli S, Urbanowaki F, Harrington A, Bonus K, and Sheridan J. Alterations in brain and immune function produced by mindfulness meditation. *Psychosomatic Medicine,* 2003;65:564–70.

18. Farb N, Segal Z, Mayberg H, Bean J, McKeon D, Fatima Z, and Anderson A. Attending to the present: mindfulness meditation reveals distinct neural modes of self-reference. *Social Cognitive and Affective Neuroscience,* 2007;2(4), 313–22.

19. Shapiro S and Carlson L. *The Art and Science of Mindfulness: Integrating Mindfulness Into Psychology and the Helping Professions.* Washington DC: American Psychological Association, 2009.

20. Davidson R, Kabat-Zinn J, Schumacher J, Rosenkrantz M, Muller D, Santorelli S, Urbanowaki F, Harrington A, Bonus K, and Sheridan J. Alterations in brain and immune function produced by mindfulness meditation. *Psychosomatic Medicine,* 2003;65:564–70.

21. Davidson R and Lutz A. Buddha's Brain: Neuroplasticity and Meditation. *IEEE Signal Processing* (2008),25(1),171–74.

22. Ibid.

23. Creswell J, Way B, Eisenberger N, and Lieberman M. Neural correlates of dispositional mindfulness during affect labeling. *Psychosomatic Medicine,* 2007;69(6):560–65.

24. Davidson R, Kabat-Zinn J, Schumacher J, Rosenkrantz M, Muller D, Santorelli S, Urbanowaki F, Harrington A, Bonus K, and Sheridan J. Alterations in brain and immune function produced by mindfulness meditation. *Psychosomatic Medicine,* 2003;65:564–70.

Davidson R and Lutz A. Buddha's Brain: Neuroplasticity and Meditation. *IEEE Signal Processing* (2008),25(1),171–74.

25. Lazar S, Kerr C, Wasserman R, Gray J, Greve D, and Treadway M. Meditation experience is associated with increased cortical thickness. *NeuroReport,* 2005;16(17):1893–97.

26. Pagnoni G and Cekic M. Age effects on gray matter volume and attentional performance in Zen meditation. *Neurobiology of Aging,* 2007;28:1623–27.

27. Davidson R, Kabat-Zinn J, Schumacher J, Rosenkrantz M, Muller D, Santorelli S, Urbanowaki F, Harrington A, Bonus K, and Sheridan J. Alterations in brain and immune function produced by mindfulness meditation. *Psychosomatic Medicine,* 2003;65:564–70.

28. Creswell J, Way B, Eisenberger N, and Lieberman M. Neural correlates of dispositional mindfulness during affect labeling. *Psychosomatic Medicine,* 2007;69(6):560–65.

29. Hölzel B, Ott U, Gard T, Hempel H, Weygandt M, Morgen K, and Vaitl D. Investigation of mindfulness meditation practitioners with voxel-based morphometry. *Social Cognitive and Affective Neuroscience,* 2008;3:55–61.

30. Lazar S, Kerr C, Wasserman R, Gray J, Greve D, and Treadway M. Meditation experience is associated with increased cortical thickness. *NeuroReport,* 2005;16(17):1893–97.

31. Davidson R, Kabat-Zinn J, Schumacher J, Rosenkrantz M, Muller D, Santorelli S, Urbanowaki F, Harrington A, Bonus K, and Sheridan J. Alterations in brain and immune function produced by mindfulness meditation. *Psychosomatic Medicine,* 2003;65:564–70.

Davidson R and Lutz A. Buddha's Brain: Neuroplasticity and Meditation. *IEEE Signal Processing* (2008),25(1),171–74.

32. Lazar S, Kerr C, Wasserman R, Gray J, Greve D, and Treadway M. Meditation experience is associated with increased cortical thickness. *NeuroReport,* 2005;16(17):1893–97.

33. Treadway M and Lazar S. The Neurobiology of Mindfulness. In Didonna F (ed.), *Clinical Handbook of Mindfulness.* New York: Springer, 2009.

34. Langer E. Matters of mind: mindfulness/mindlessness in perspective. *Consciousness and Cognition,* 1992;1:289–305.

35. Langer E, Rodin J, Beck P, Weinman C, and Spitzer L. Environmental determinants of memory improvement in late adulthood. *J. of Personality and Social Psychology,* 1979;37:2003–13.

Alexander C, Langer E, Newman R, Chandler H, and Davies J. Aging, mindfulness and meditation. *J. of Personality and Social Psychology,* 1989;57:950–64.

Langer E. Matters of mind: mindfulness/mindlessness in perspective. *Consciousness and Cognition,* 1992;1:289–305.

36. Langer E. Matters of mind: mindfulness/mindlessness in perspective. *Consciousness and Cognition,* 1992;1:289–305.

37. Cousins N. *Head First: The Biology of Hope.* New York: Dutton, 1989.

38. Achterberg J. *Imagery in Healing: Shamanism and Modern Medicine.* Boston: Shambhala, 1985.

Achterberg J and Lawless G. Imagery for Health and Healing— one-year training sponsored by Institute for Health and Healing, California Pacific Medical Center, 1998. Phase I: The Psychophysiological Model; Phase II: Assessment and Treatment for Modern Day Settings; Phase III: Psychoneuroimmunology, Advanced Topics and Protocols; Phase IV: Transpersonal Medicine.

Murphy M. *The Future of the Body: Explorations into the Further Evolution of Human Nature.* Los Angeles: Tarcher, 1992.

Simonton Cancer Center—Certification Training, 2006, 2007, 2008. Most of the tools taught to the cancer patients at the Simonton retreats have been created by O. Carl Simonton, MD, and are unpublished.

LeShan L. *Cancer as a Turning Point.* New York: Dutton, 1989.

Rossman M and Bresler D. Academy for Guided Imagery Certification Training, 2007. "Special Place" and "Inner Advisor" guided imagery in the current form are the creation of Martin Rossman, MD, and David Bresler, PhD, originally adapted from the work of Irving Oyle, MD.

39. Davidson R, Kabat-Zinn J, Schumacher J, Rosenkrantz M, Muller D, Santorelli S, Urbanowaki F, Harrington A, Bonus K, and Sheridan J. Alterations in brain and immune function produced by mindfulness meditation. *Psychosomatic Medicine,* 2003;65:564–70.

Walsh R and Shapiro S. The meeting of meditative disciplines and Western psychology: A mutually enriching dialogue. *American Psychologist,* 2006;61:227–39.

Booth R and Ashbridge K. A fresh look at the relationship between the psyche and immune system: teleological coherence and harmony of purpose. *Advances, The Journal of Mind-Body Health,* 1993;9(2):4–23.

Carlson L, Ursuliak Z, Goodey E, Angen M, and Speca M. The effects of a mindfulness meditation–based stress reduction program on mood and symptoms of stress in cancer outpatients: 6-month follow-up. *Supportive Care In Cancer,* 2001;9:112–23.

Carlson L, Speca M, Patel K, and Goodey E. Mindfulness-based stress reduction in relation to quality of life, mood, symptoms of stress, and immune parameters in breast and prostate cancer outpatients. *Psychosomatic Medicine,* 2003;65:571–81.

Carlson L, Speca M, Faris P, and Patel K. One year pre-post intervention follow-up of psychological, immune, endocrine and blood pressure outcomes of mindfulness-based stress reduction (MBSR) in breast and prostate cancer outpatients. *Brain Behav Immun,* 2007;21(8):1038–49.

Solberg E, Halvorsen R, Sundgot-Borgen J, Ingjer F, and Holen A. Meditation: A modulator of the immune response to physical stress? A brief report. *British J. of Sport and Medicine,* 1995;29:255–57.

40. Davidson R, Kabat-Zinn J, Schumacher J, Rosenkrantz M, Muller D, Santorelli S, Urbanowaki F, Harrington A, Bonus K, and Sheridan J. Alterations in brain and immune function produced by mindfulness meditation. *Psychosomatic Medicine,* 2003;65:564–70.

Davidson R and Lutz A. Buddha's Brain: Neuroplasticity and Meditation. *IEEE Signal Processing* (2008),25(1),171–74.

LeDoux J. *Synaptic Self: How Our Brains Become Who We Are.* New York: Penguin, 2003.

Lehrer P and Gevirtz R. Two-day workshop at Association for Applied Psychophysiology and Biofeedback (AAPB) Annual Conference, Monterey, CA, 2007.

Lutz A, Dunne J, and Davidson R. Meditation and the Neuroscience of Consciousness: An Introduction. In Zelazo P, Moscovitch M, and Thompson E (ed.), *Cambridge Handbook of Consciousness.* New York: Cambridge University Press, 2007.

41. Davidson R, Kabat-Zinn J, Schumacher J, Rosenkrantz M, Muller D, Santorelli S, Urbanowaki F, Harrington A, Bonus K, and Sheridan J. Alterations in brain and immune function produced by mindfulness meditation. *Psychosomatic Medicine,* 2003;65:564–70.

42. Ibid.

43. Paul-Labrador M, Polk D, Dwyer J, Velazquez I, Nidich S, Rainforth M, Schneider R, and Merz N.Effects of randomized controlled trial of transcendental meditation on components of the metabolic syndrome in subjects with coronary heart disease. *Archives of Internal Medicine,* 2006;166:1218–24.

44. Solberg E, Halvorsen R, Sundgot-Borgen J, Ingjer F, and Holen A. Meditation: A modulator of the immune response to physical stress? A brief report. *British J. of Sport and Medicine,* 1995;29:255–57.

45. Kabat-Zinn J. Bringing mindfulness to medicine. *Alternative Therapies in Health and Medicine,* 2005;11(3):56–64.

46. Davidson R, Kabat-Zinn J, Schumacher J, Rosenkrantz M, Muller D, Santorelli S, Urbanowaki F, Harrington A, Bonus K, and Sheridan J. Alterations in brain and immune function produced by mindfulness meditation. *Psychosomatic Medicine,* 2003;65:564–70.

Davidson R and Lutz A. Buddha's Brain: Neuroplasticity and Meditation. *IEEE Signal Processing* (2008),25(1),171–74.

47. Kabat-Zinn J. Bringing mindfulness to medicine. *Alternative Therapies in Health and Medicine,* 2005;11(3):56–64.

Kabat-Zinn J. *Full Catastrophe Living: Using the Wisdom of Your Body and Mind to Face Stress, Pain, and Illness,* 15th edition. New York: Bantam, 2005.

Kabat-Zinn J, Lipworth L, and Burney R. The clinical use of mindfulness meditation for the self-regulation of chronic pain. *J. of Behavioral Medicine,* 1985;8:163–90.

Kabat-Zinn J, Lipworth L, Burney R, and Sellers W. Four-year follow-up of a meditation-based program for the self-regulation of chronic pain: Treatment outcome and compliance. *Clinical J. of Pain,* 1987;2:159–73.

48. Morone N, Lynch C, Greco C, Tindle H, and Weiner D. "I feel like a new person." The effects of mindfulness meditation on older adults with chronic pain: A qualitative narrative analysis of diary entries. *J. of Pain,* 2008;9:841–48.

49. Grossman P, Tiefenthaler-Gilmer U, Raysz A, and Kesper U. Mindfulness training as an intervention for fibromyalgia: Evidence of post-intervention and 3-year follow-up benefits in well-being. *Psychotherapy and Psychosomatics.* 2007;76:226–33.

Sephton S, Salmon P, Weissbecker I, Ulmer C, Floyd A, and Hoover K. Mindfulness meditation alleviates depressive symptoms in women with fibromyalgia: Results of a randomized clinical trial. *Arthritis and Rheumatism,* 2007;57(1):77–85.

50. McCracken L and Eccleston C. A prospective study of acceptance of pain and patient functioning with chronic pain. *Pain,* 2005;118:164–69.

51. Gardner-Nix J. *The Mindfulness Solution to Pain.* Oakland: New Harbinger, 2009.

52. Roth B and Stanley T. Mindfulness-based stress reduction and healthcare utilization in the inner city: Preliminary findings. *Alternative Therapies,* 2002;8:60–66.

53. McCracken L and Vowles K. Psychological flexibility and traditional pain management strategies in relation to patient functioning with chronic pain: An examination of a revised instrument. *J. of Pain,* 2007;8:700–7.

54. Carlson L et al. Mindfulness-based stress reduction in relation to quality of life, mood, symptoms of stress, and immune parameters in breast and prostate cancer outpatients. *Psychosomatic Medicine,* 2003;65:571–81.

Carlson L, Speca M, Patel K, and Goodey E. Mindfulness-based stress reduction in relation to quality of life, mood, symptoms of stress and levels of cortisol, dehydroepiandrosterone sulfate (DHEAS) and melatonin in breast and prostate cancer outpatients. *Psychoneuroendocrinology,* 2004;29:448–74.

55. Carlson L, Speca M, Faris P, and Patel K. One year pre-post intervention follow-up of psychological, immune, endocrine and blood pressure outcomes of mindfulness-based stress reduction (MBSR) in breast and prostate cancer outpatients. *Brain Behav Immun,* 2007;21(8):1038–49.

56. Speca M, Carlson L, Goody E, and Angen M. A randomized wait-list controlled trial: The effect of a mindfulness meditation-based stress reduction program on mood and symptoms of stress in cancer outpatients. *Psychosomatic Medicine,* 2000;62:613–22.

57. Meares A. What can a patient expect from intensive meditation? *Australian Family Physician,* 1980;9,322–25.

Cunningham A. *Can the Mind Heal Cancer?: A Clinician Scientist Examines the Evidence.* Toronto: Healing Journey Program at Ontario Cancer Institute, 2005.

58. Meares A. *Strange Places, Simple Truths*. London: Fontana, 1973.

59. Gawler I. *You Can Conquer Cancer: Prevention and Management*. South Yarra, VIC, Australia: Michelle Anderson Publishing, 2001.

60. Gawler I. *You Can Conquer Cancer: Prevention and Management*. South Yarra, VIC, Australia: Michelle Anderson Publishing, 2001.

Meares A. What can a patient expect from intensive meditation? *Australian Family Physician*, 1980;9,322–25.

LeShan L. *Cancer as a Turning Point*. New York: Dutton, 1989.

LeShan L. A new question in studying psychosocial interventions and cancer. *Advances, The Journal of Mind-Body Health*, 1991; 7(1).

LeShan L. Cancer as a Turning Point Residential Workshop, October–November 2007. Much of what is taught to those attending these workshops is published in the book *Cancer as a Turning Point*. The exercises have all been created by Lawrence LeShan, PhD.

Simonton O, Matthews-Simonton S, and Creighton J. *Getting Well Again*. Los Angeles: Tarcher, 1978.

Simonton O and Matthews-Simonton S. Cancer and stress: counseling the cancer patient. *Medical Journal of Australia*, 1981;27:679–83.

Simonton O and Henson R. *The Healing Journey*. New York: Author's Choice, 2002.

Simonton Cancer Center—Certification Training, 2006, 2007, 2008. Most of the tools taught to the cancer patients at the Simonton retreats have been created by O. Carl Simonton, MD, and are unpublished.

Cunningham A and Edmonds C. Delivering a very brief psychoeducational program to cancer patients and family members in a large group format. *Psycho-oncology*, 1999;8:177–82.

Cunningham A, Phillips C, Lockwood G, Hedley D and Edmonds C. Association of involvement in psychological self help with longer survival in patients with metastatic cancer: An exploratory study. *Advances in Mind-Body Medicine*, 2000;16:276–94.

Cunningham A, Edmonds C, Phillips C, Soots K, Hedley D, and Lockwood G. A prospective, longitudinal study of the relationship of psychological work to duration of survival in patients with metastatic cancer. *Psycho-oncology*, 2000;9:323–39.

Cunningham A. How psychological therapy may prolong survival in cancer patients: new evidence and a simple theory. *Integrative Cancer Therapies* 2004;3(3):214–29.

Chapter 9

1. Tart C. *States of Consciousness,* Lincoln, NE: Authors Guild BackInPrint.com Edition, 2000.

2. Crane R. *Mindfulness-Based Cognitive Therapy.* London: Routledge, 2010.

3. Ibid.

4. Krishnamurti J. *Discussions With Krishnamurti in Europe.* Ojai, CA: Krishnamurti Writings Inc, 1966.

5. Tull M, Rodman S, and Roemer L. An examination of the fear of bodily sensations and body hypervigilance as predictors of emotion regulation difficulties among individuals with a recent history of uncued panic attacks. *J. of Anxiety Disorders,* 2008;22(4):750–60.

6. Cochrane A, Barnes-Holmes D, Barnes-Holmes Y, Steward I, and Luciano C. Experiential avoidance and aversive visual images: Response delays and event related potentials on a simple matching task. *Behavior Research and Therapy,* 2007;45:1379–88.

7. Spiegel D. Effects of psychotherapy on cancer survival. *Nature Reviews Cancer,* 2002;2(5):383–89.

8. Hayes S, Strosahl K, and Wilson K. *Acceptance and Commitment Therapy: An Experiential Approach to Behavioral Change.* New York: Guilford, 1999.

Chapter 13

1. Emmons R. *Thanks!: How the new science of gratitude can make you happier.* New York: Houghton Mifflin, 2007.

2. Emmons R and McCullough M. Counting blessings versus burdens: An experimental investigation of gratitude and subjective well-being in daily life. *J of Personality and Social Psychology,* 2003;84(2):377–89.

3. Lyubomirsky S. *The How of Happiness: A Scientific Approach to Getting the Life You Want.* New York: Penguin, 2007.

Lyubomirsky S, King L, and Diener E. The benefits of frequent positive affect: Does happiness lead to success? *Psychological Bulletin,* 2005;131:803–55.

Lyubomirsky S, Sheldon K, and Schkade D. Pursuing happiness: The architecture of sustainable change. *Review of General Psychology,* 2005;9:111–31.

Lyubomirsky S. Why are some people happier than others?: The role of cognitive and motivational processes in well-being. *American Psychologist,* 2001;56:239–49.

Sheldon K and Lyubomirsky S. Achieving sustainable gains in happiness: Change your actions, not your circumstances. *J of Happiness Studies*, 2006;7:55–86.

4. Lyubomirsky S. *The How of Happiness: A Scientific Approach to Getting the Life You Want.* New York: Penguin, 2007.

5. Ibid.

6. Ong A, Bergeman C, Bisconti T, and Wallace K. Psychological resilience, positive emotions, and successful adaptation to stress in later life. *J of Personality and Social Psychology*, 2006;91:730–49.

7. Emmons R and McCullough M. Counting blessings versus burdens: An experimental investigation of gratitude and subjective well-being in daily life. *J of Personality and Social Psychology*, 2003;84(2):377–89.

8. Atkinson M, Carrios-Choplin B, McCraty R, Rozman D, and Watkins A. The impact of a new emotional self-management program on stress, emotions, HRV, DHEA, and cortisol. *Integrative Physiological and Behavioral Science*, 1998;33(2):151–70.

9. Gordon J. *Manifesto for a New Medicine.* Reading, MA: Addison-Wesley, 1996.

Gordon J. *Unstuck.* New York: Penguin, 2008.

Gordon J. Training in Mind-Body Medicine by the Center for Mind-Body Medicine, San Diego, September 2009.

Chapter 14

1. Schwartz G. Psychobiology of repression and health: A systems approach. In Singer J. (ed.), *Repression and Dissociation: Implications for Personality Theory, Psychopathology, and Health.* Chicago: University of Chicago Press, 1990.

Chapter 15

1. LeShan L. *Cancer as a Turning Point.* New York: Dutton, 1989.

2. Hayes S, Strosahl K, and Wilson K. *Acceptance and Commitment Therapy: An Experiential Approach to Behavioral Change.* New York: Guilford, 1999.

3. Conrad A, Muller A, Doberenz S et al. Psychophysiological effects of breathing instructions for stress management. *Applied Psychophysiology and Biofeedback;* 2007,32(2):89–98.

4. Vaschillo E, Vaschillo B, and Lehrer P. Characteristics of Resonance in Heart Rate Variability Stimulated by Biofeedback. *Applied Psychophysiology and Biofeedback*, 2006;31;2,129–42.

5. Luoma J, Hayes S, and Walser R. *Learning ACT: An Acceptance and Commitment Therapy Skills-Training Manual for Therapists.* Oakland, CA: New Harbinger, 2007.

6. Hayes S and Strosahl K. *A Practical Guide to Acceptance and Commitment Therapy.* New York: Springer, 2004.

7. Luoma J, Hayes S, and Walser R. *Learning ACT: An Acceptance and Commitment Therapy Skills-Training Manual for Therapists.* Oakland, CA: New Harbinger, 2007.

8. Tull M, Rodman S, and Roemer L. An examination of the fear of bodily sensations and body hypervigilance as predictors of emotion regulation difficulties among individuals with a recent history of uncued panic attacks. *J. of Anxiety Disorders,* 2008;22(4):750–60.

Tull M, Barrett H, McMillan E, and Roemer L. A preliminary investigation of the relationship between emotion regulation difficulties and posttraumatic stress symptoms. *Behavior Therapy,* 2007;38:303–13.

Dahl J, Wilson K, and Luciano C. *Acceptance and Commitment Therapy for Chronic Pain.* Reno, NV: Context Press, 2005.

9. Segal Z, Williams J, and Teasdale J. *Mindfulness-Based Cognitive Therapy for Depression.* New York: Guilford, 2002.

10. Tarrier N. Commentary: Yes, cognitive behaviour therapy may well be all you need. *BMJ,* 2002;324:291–92.

11. Rosenbaum E. *Here for Now: Living Well with Cancer Through Mindfulness.* Hardwick, MA: Satya House Publications, 2007.

12. Burch V. *Living Well with Pain and Illness: The Mindful Way to Free Yourself From Suffering.* Boulder, CO: Sounds True, 2010.

13. Hayes S, Strosahl K, Wilson K, Bissett R, Pistorello J, and Toarmino D. Measuring experiential avoidance: A preliminary test of a working model. *The Psychological Record,* 2004;54:553–78.

Kingston J, Chadwick P, Meron D, and Skinner T. A pilot randomized controlled trial investigating the effect of mindfulness practice on pain tolerance, psychological well-being, and physiological activity. *J. of Psychosomatic Research,* 2007;62:297–300.

14. McCracken L, Carson J, Eccleston C, Keefe F. Acceptance and change in the context of chronic pain. *Pain,* 2004;109:4–7.

McCracken L, Vowles K, and Eccleston C. Acceptance of Chronic Pain: Component analysis and a revised assessment method. *Pain,* 2004;107:159–66.

15. Cunningham A. *The Healing Journey: Overcoming the Crisis of Cancer.* Toronto: Key Porter, 2000.

Simonton Cancer Center—Certification Training, 2006, 2007, 2008. Most of the tools taught to the cancer patients at the Simonton retreats have been created by O. Carl Simonton, MD, and are unpublished.

Spiegel D and Classen C. *Group Therapy for Cancer Patients: A Research-Based Handbook of Psychosocial Care.* New York: Basic Books, 2000.

Fawzy F. Malignant melanoma: Effects of an early structured psychiatric intervention, coping, and affective state on recurrence and survival 6 years later. *Archives of General Psychiatry,* 1993;50:681–89.

Antoni M, Baggett L, Ironson, G, et al. Cognitive-behavioral stress management intervention buffers distress responses and immunological changes following notification of HIV-1 seropositivity. *Journal of Consulting and Clinical Psychology,* 1991;59: 905–15.

16. Krause J. Spinal cord injury and its rehabilitation. *Current Opinion in Neurology and Neurosurgery,* 1992;5:669–72.

17. Twohig M, Hayes S, and Masuda A. Increasing willingness to experience obsessions: Acceptance and Commitment Therapy as a treatment for obsessive-compulsive disorder. *Behavior Therapy,* 2006;37(1), 3–13.

18. Hayes S, Strosahl K, Wilson K, Bissett R, Pistorello J, and Toarmino D. Measuring experiential avoidance: A preliminary test of a working model. *The Psychological Record,* 2004;54:553–78.

19. Abramowitz J, Tolin D, and Street G. Paradoxical effects of thought suppression: A meta-analysis of controlled studies. *Clinical Psychology Review,* 2001;21(5):683–703.

20. Hayes S, Strosahl K, and Wilson K. *Acceptance and Commitment Therapy: An Experiential Approach to Behavioral Change.* New York: Guilford, 1999.

Chapter 16

1. Solomon G. Emotions, Stress and Immunity. In Ornstein R and Swencionis C (ed.), *The Healing Brain: A Scientific Reader.* New York: Guilford, 1990.

2. LeShan L. *Cancer as a Turning Point.* New York: Dutton, 1989.

LeShan L. Cancer as a Turning Point Residential Workshop, October–November 2007. Much of what is taught to those attending these workshops is published in the book *Cancer as a Turning Point.* The exercises have all been created by Lawrence LeShan, PhD.

3. Solomon G. Emotions, Stress and Immunity. In Ornstein R and Swencionis C (ed.), *The Healing Brain: A Scientific Reader.* New York: Guilford, 1990.

Ironson G, Balbin E, et al. Dispositional optimism and the mechanisms by which it predicts slower disease progression in HIV: proactive behavior, avoidant coping, and depression. *International J. of Behavioral Medicine,* 2005;12(2):86–97.

O'Cleirigh C, Ironson G, and Smits J. Does Distress Tolerance Moderate the Impact of Major Life Events on Psychosocial Variables and Behaviors Important in the Management of HIV? *Behavior Therapy,* 2007;vol. 38;3:314–23.

4. Solomon G. Emotions, Stress and Immunity. In Ornstein R and Swencionis C (ed.), *The Healing Brain: A Scientific Reader.* New York: Guilford, 1990.

5. Derogatis L, Abeloff M, and Melisaratos N. Psychological coping mechanisms and survival time in metastatic breast cancer. *JAMA,* 1979:242(14):1504–08.

LeShan L. *Cancer as a Turning Point.* New York: Dutton, 1989.

Stavraky K, Donner A, Kincade J, and Stewart M. The effect of psychosocial factors on lung cancer mortality at one year. *J of Clinical Epidemiology,* 1988;41:75–82.

6. Fawzy F. Immune effects of a short-term psychosocial intervention for cancer patients. *Advances: J. of Mind-Body Health,* 1994;10:32–33.

7. Greer S and Morris T. Psychological attributes of women who develop breast cancer: A controlled study. *J of Psychosomatic Research,* 1975;19:147–53.

Greer S, Morris T, Pettingale K, and Haybittle J. Psychological response to breast cancer and 15-year outcome. *The Lancet* 1990; 6: 335 (8680): 49–50.

Temoshok L. Biopsychosocial studies on cutaneous malignant melanoma: Psychosocial factors associated with prognostic indicators, progression, psychophysiology and tumor-host response. *Social Science and Medicine,* 1985;20(8):833–40.

Levy S, Herberman R, and Lippman M. Correlation of stress factors with sustained depression of natural killer cell activity and predicted prognosis in patients with breast cancer. *J of Clinical Oncology,* 1987;5(3):348–53.

Levy S, Herberman R, Whiteside T, Sanzo K, Lee J, and Kirkwood J. Perceived social support and tumor estrogen/progesterone receptor status as predictors of natural killer cell activity in breast cancer patients. *Psychosomatic Medicine,* 1990;52:73–85.

Levy S, Herberman R, Lippman M, d'Angelo T, and Lee J. Immunological and psychosocial predictors of disease recurrence in patients with early-stage breast cancer. *J of Behavioral Medicine*, 1991;17:67–75.

8. Levy S, Herberman R, Lippman M, d'Angelo T, and Lee J. Immunological and psychosocial predictors of disease recurrence in patients with early-stage breast cancer. *J of Behavioral Medicine*, 1991;17:67–75.

9. Pettingale K, Greer S, and Tee D. Serum IgA and emotional expression in breast cancer patients. *J. of Psychosomatic Research*, 1977;21(5):395–99.

10. Greer S and Morris T. Psychological attributes of women who develop breast cancer: A controlled study. *J of Psychosomatic Research*, 1975;19:147–53.

11. Jamner L and Schwartz G. Self-deception predicts self-report and endurance of pain. *Psychosomatic Medicine*, 1986;48:211–23.

12. Temoshok L. Personality, coping style, emotion and cancer: Towards an integrative model. *Cancer Surveys*, 1987;6(3):545–67.

Temoshok L and Dreher H. *The Type C Connection: The Behavioral Links to Cancer and Your Health*. New York: Random House, 1992.

13. Greer S. Mind-body research in psychooncology. *J. Advances in Mind-Body Medicine*, 1999;15(4):236–44.

14. Jensen M. Psychobiological factors predicting the course of cancer. *J. of Personality*, 1987;55:317–42.

15 Turner-Cobbs J, Sephton S, and Spiegel D. Psychosocial effects of immune function and disease progression in cancer: Human studies. In Ader R, Felton D, and Cohen N (ed.), *Psychoneuroimmunology*, 3rd edition. San Diego: Academic Press, 2001.

16. Barefoot J, Dahlstrom W, and Williams R. Hostility, CHD incidence, and total mortality: a 25-year follow-up study of 255 physicians. *Psychosomatic Medicine*, 1983;45:59–63.

Barefoot J, Dodge K, and Peterson B. The Cook-Medley Hostility Scale: Item content and ability to predict survival. *Psychosomatic Medicine*, 1989;51:46–57.

17. Suarez E and Blumenthal J. Ambulatory blood pressure responses during daily life in high and low hostile patients with a recent myocardial infarction. *J of Cardiopulmonary Rehabilitation*, 1991;11:169–75.

Suls J and Wan C. The relationship between trait hostility and cardiovascular reactivity: a quantitative analysis. *Psychophysiology*, 1993;30:615–26.

18. Kop W. Chronic and acute psychological risk factors for clinical manifestations of coronary artery disease. *Psychosomatic Medicine*, 1999;61:476–87.

19. Fricchione G, Bilfinger T, Hartman A, Liu Y, and Stefano G. Neuroimmunologic implications in coronary artery disease. *Advances in Neuroimmunology*, 1996;6:131–42.

20. Suarez E, Shiller A, Kuhn C, Schanberg S, Williams R, and Zimmermann E. The relationship between hostility and beta adrenergic receptor physiology in healthy young males. *Psychosomatic Medicine*, 1997;59:481–87.

21. Gorman J and Sloan R. Heart rate variability in depressive and anxiety disorders. *Amer Heart J*, 2000;140:77–83.

Kop W and Cohen N. Psychological risk factors and immune system involvement in cardiovascular disease. In Ader R, Felton D, and Cohen N (ed.), *Psychoneuroimmuology*, 3rd edition, Vol. 2. New York: Academic Press, 2001.

22. Pennebaker J. Writing about emotional experiences as a therapeutic process. *Psychological Science*, 1997;8:162–66.

Pennebaker J and Graybeal A. Patterns of natural language use: Disclosure, personality, and social integration. *Current Directions in Psychological Science*, 2001;10:90–93.

23. Pennebaker J. Writing about emotional experiences as a therapeutic process. *Psychological Science*, 1997;8:162–66.

24. Thomas C, Duszynski K, and Shaffer J. Family attitudes reported in youth as potential predictors of cancer. *J of Psychosomatic Medicine*, 1979;41:287–482.

Shaffer J, Duszynski K, and Thomas C. Family attitudes in youth as a possible precursor of cancer among physicians: A search for explanatory mechanisms. *J of Behavioral Medicine*, 1982;5:143–63.

Shaffer J, Graves P, Swank R, and Pearson T. Clustering of personality traits in youth and the subsequent development of cancer among physicians. *J of Behavioral Medicine*, 1987;10:441–47.

Graves P, Thomas C, and Mead L. Familial and psychological predictors of cancer. *Cancer Detection Review*, 1991;15:59–64.

25. Price M, Tennant C, and Butow P. The role of psychosocial factors in the development of breast carcinoma: Part II: Life event stressors, social support, defense style, and emotional control and their interactions. *Cancer*, 2001;91(4):686–97.

Reich M. Depression and cancer: recent data on clinical issues, research challenges and treatment approaches. *Current Opinion in Oncology*, 2008;20(4):353–59.

Scherg H. Psychosocial factors and disease bias in breast cancer patients. *J of Psychosomatic Medicine*, 1987;49:302–12.

Siegel B. Mind over cancer: An exclusive interview with Yale surgeon Dr. Bernie Siegel. *Prevention*, 1988;March:59–64.

Temoshok L and Dreher H. *The Type C Connection: The Behavioral Links to Cancer and Your Health.* New York: Random House, 1992.

Walker L, Hays S, and Walker M. Psychosocial factors can predict the response to primary chemotherapy in patients with locally advanced breast cancer. *European J of Cancer,* 1999;35:1783–88.

Antoni M, Lutgendorf S, and Cole S. The influence of biobehavioral factors on tumor biology: Pathways and mechanisms. *Nature Reviews Cancer,* 2006;6(3):240–48.

Classen C, Kraemer H, Blasey C, Giese-Davis J, Koopman C, Palesh O, Atkinson A, Dimiceli S, Stonisch-Riggs G, Westendorp J, Morrow G, and Spiegel D. Supportive-expressive group therapy for primary breast cancer patients: a randomized prospective multicenter trial. *Psychooncology,* 2008;17(5):438–47.

Cunningham A. How psychological therapy may prolong survival in cancer patients: new evidence and a simple theory. *Integrative Cancer Therapies* 2004;3(3):214–29.

Derogatis L. Psychology in cancer medicine: a perspective and overview. *J. of Consulting and Clinical Psychology,* October 1986:632–38.

Derogatis L, Abeloff M, and Melisaratos N. Psychological coping mechanisms and survival time in metastatic breast cancer. *JAMA,* 1979:242(14):1504–08.

Dreher H. Beyond fighting spirit: What mind-states influence cancer survival? *Advances in Mind-Body Medicine,* Spring 2000; 16(2): 120–27.

Eysenck H. Personality, stress, and cancer: prediction and prophylaxis. *British J of Medical Psychology,* 1988;61:57–75.

Faller H, Bulzebruck H, Schilling S, Drings P, and Lang H. Do psychological factors modify survival of cancer patients? II: Results of an empirical study with bronchial carcinoma patients. *Psychotherapy Psychosomatic Medicine Psychology,* 1997;47:206–18.

Greer S and Morris T. Psychological attributes of women who develop breast cancer: A controlled study. *J of Psychosomatic Research,* 1975;19:147–53.

Grossarth-Maticek R. Interpersonal repression as a predictor of cancer. *Social Science Medicine,* 1982;16:493–98.

Kreitler S, Peleg D, and Ehrenfeld M. Stress, self-efficacy and quality of life in cancer patients. *Psychooncology,* 2007;16(4):329-41.

LeShan L. *Cancer as a Turning Point.* New York: Dutton, 1989.

Morris T, Greer S, Pettingale K, and Watson M. Patterns of expression of anger and their psychological correlates in women with breast cancer. *J of Psychosomatic Research,* 1981;25:111–17.

26. House J, Landis K, and Umberson D. Social relationships and health. *Science,* 1988;241:540–45.

Chapter 17

1. LeShan L. *Cancer as a Turning Point.* New York: Dutton, 1989. Simonton O and Henson R. *The Healing Journey.* New York: Author's Choice, 2002.

2. Katz R, Flasher L, Cacciapaglia H, and Nelson S. The psychosocial impact of cancer and lupus: A cross validation study that extends the generality of "benefit-finding" in patients with chronic disease. *J. of Behavioral Medicine,* 2001;24:561–71.

3. Manne S, Ostroff J, Winkel G, Goldstein L, Fox K, and Grana G. Posttraumatic growth after breast cancer: Patient, partner, and couple perspectives. *Psychosomatic Medicine,* 2004;66:442–54.

4. Solomon G, Fiatarone M, Benton D, Morley J, Bloom E, and Makinodan T. Psychoneuroimmunologic and endorphin function in the aged. *Annals of the New York Academy of Sciences,* 1988;521:43–58.

5. Solomon G. Emotions, Stress and Immunity. In Ornstein R and Swencionis C (ed.), *The Healing Brain: A Scientific Reader.* New York: Guilford, 1990.

6. Butler R. The inequality of longevity: Life expectancy gap widens between industrialized world and developing nations. *Geriatrics,* 1999;Dec.

7. LeShan L. *Cancer as a Turning Point.* New York: Dutton, 1989.

8. Simonton Cancer Center—Certification Training, 2006, 2007, 2008. Most of the tools taught to the cancer patients at the Simonton retreats have been created by O. Carl Simonton, MD, and are unpublished.

9. Davidson R. *Anxiety, Depression, and Emotion.* New York: Oxford University Press, 2000.

10. King L. The health benefits of writing about life goals. *Personality and Social Psychology Bulletin,* 2001;27:798–807.

11. Lyubomirsky S, King L, and Diener E. The benefits of frequent positive affect: Does happiness lead to success? *Psychological Bulletin,* 2005;131:803–55.

12. Sheldon K and Elliot A. Goal striving, need satisfaction, and longitudinal well-being: The self-concordance model. *J of Personality and Social Psychology,* 1999;76:546–57.

Elliot A and Sheldon K. Avoidance personal goals and the personality-illness relationship. *J. of Personality and Social Psychology,* 1998;75:1282–99.

13. Bower J, Kemeny M, Taylor S, and Fahey J. Cognitive processing, discovery of meaning, CD4 decline, and AIDS-related mortality among bereaved HIV-seropositive men. *J of Consulting and Clinical Psychology*, 1998;66:979–86.

14. Frankl V. *Man's Search for Meaning*. New York: Pocket Books, 1984.

15. LeShan L. *Cancer as a Turning Point*. New York: Dutton, 1989.

Chapter 18

1. Lyubomirsky S. *The How of Happiness: A Scientific Approach to Getting the Life You Want*. New York: Penguin, 2007.

2. Andrews H. Helping and health: The relationship between volunteer activity and health-related outcomes. *Advances*, 1990;7(1):25–34.

3 Brown S. A boon for caregivers. *Psychology Today*, Nov 1, 2003.

4. House J, Landis K, and Umberson D. Social relationships and health. *Science*, 1988;241:540–45.

5. Andrews H. Helping and health: The relationship between volunteer activity and health-related outcomes. *Advances*, 1990;7(1):25–34.

6. Vaillant G. *Aging Well*. New York: Little, Brown, 2003.

7. Schulz U, Pischke C, Weidner G, Daubenmier J, Elliot-Eller M, Scherwitz L, Bullinger M, and Ornish D. Social support group attendance is related to blood pressure, health behaviours, and quality of life in the Multicenter Lifestyle Demonstration Project. *Psychology Health Medicine*, 2008;13(4):423–27.

8. Seligman M. *Learned Optimism: How to Change Your Mind and Your Life*. New York: Random House, 2006.

9. Oliner S. *Do Unto Others: Extraordinary Acts of Ordinary People*. New York: Basic Books, 2004.

10. Ibid.

11. Brown S. A boon for caregivers. *Psychology Today*, Nov 1, 2003.

12. Lyubomirsky S. *The How of Happiness: A Scientific Approach to Getting the Life You Want*. New York: Penguin, 2007.

13. Gordon. Training in Mind-Body Medicine, San Diego, 2009.

Chapter 19

1. Sobel D. The cost-effectiveness of mind-body medicine interventions. *Progress in Brain Research*, 2000;122:393–412.

2. Berkman L and Syme L. Social networks, host resistance, and mortality: a nine-year follow-up study of Alameda County residents. *American Journal of Epidemiology* 1982;109:186–204.

3. Ibid.

4. House J, Landis K, and Umberson D. Social relationships and health. *Science,* 1988;241:540–45.

5. Uchino B, Cacioppo J, and Kiecolt-Glaser J. The relationship between social support and physiological processes: a review with emphasis on underlying mechanisms and implications for health. *Psychological Bulletin,* 1996;119(3):4480–531.

6. Kiecolt-Glaser J, Glaser R, Williger D, et al. Psychosocial enhancement of immunocompetence in a geriatric population. *Health Psychology,* 1985; 4(1): 25-41.

7. Arnetz B, Thorell T, Levi L, Kallner A, and Eneroth P. An experimental study of social isolation of elderly people: psychoendocrine and metabolic effects. *Psychosomatic Medicine,* 1983;45:395–406.

8. Ornstein R and Sobel D. *The Healing Brain: Breakthrough Medical Discoveries About How the Brain Manages Health.* New York: Simon and Schuster, 1987.

9. Kaplan G. Outcomes of the North Karetic, Sweden project. *Am J. of Epidemiology,* 1988;128(2):370–80.

10. Buettner D. *The Blue Zones: Lessons for Living Longer from the People Who've Lived the Longest.* Washington, DC: National Geographic, 2008.

11. Depner C and Ingersoll-Dayton B. Supportive relationships in later life. *Psychology and Aging,* 1988;3(4):348–57.

12. Orth-Gomer K, Rosengren A, and Wilhelmsen L. Lack of social support and incidence of coronary heart disease in middle-aged Swedish men. *Psychosomatic Medicine,* 1993;55(1):37–43.

13. Schulz U, Pischke C, Weidner G, Daubenmier J, Elliot-Eller M, Scherwitz L, Bullinger M, and Ornish D. Social support group attendance is related to blood pressure, health behaviours, and quality of life in the Multicenter Lifestyle Demonstration Project. *Psychology Health Medicine,* 2008;13(4):423–27.

14. Marmot M, Syme S, Kagan A, Kato H, Cohen J, and Belsky J. Epidemiologic studies of coronary heart disease and stroke in Japanese men living in Japan, Hawaii and California: prevalence of coronary and hypertensive heart disease and associated risk factor. *American J. of Epidemiology,* 1975;102(6):514–25.

15. Hanson B, Isacsson S, Janzon L, and Lindell S. Social network and social support influence on mortality in elderly men. *American J of Epidemiology.* 1989;130(1):110–11.

16. Orth-Gomer K and Unden A. Type A behavior, social support, and coronary risk: Interaction and significance for mortality in cardiac patients. *Psychosomatic Medicine,* 1990;52:59–72.

17. Kiecolt-Glaser J, Glaser R, Williger D, et al. Psychosocial modifiers of immunocompetence in medical students. *Psychosomatic Medicine,* 1984;46:7–14.

18. Kennedy S, Kiecolt-Glaser J, and Glaser R. Immunological consequences of acute and chronic stressors: Mediating role of interpersonal relationships. *British J of Medical Psychology,* 1988;61:77–85.

19. Glaser R, Kiecolt-Glaser J, and Malarkey W. The effect of stress on viral vaccine responses. Procedings of the Congress of the International Society for Neuroimmunomodulation. 1996;56:13–15.

20. Waxler-Morrison N, Hislop T, Meares B, and Kan L. Effects of social relationships on survival for women with breast cancer: a prospective study. *Society for Science in Medicine,* 1991;33:177–83.

Maunsell E, Brisson J, and Deschenes L. Social support and survival among women with breast cancer. *Cancer,* 1995;76:631–37.

Brown J, Butow P, Culjak G, Coates A, and Dunn S. Psychosocial predictors of outcome: Time to relapse and survival in patients with early stage melanoma. *British J of Cancer,* 2000;83:1448–53.

21. Lyubomirsky S, Sheldon K, and Schkade D. Pursuing happiness: The architecture of sustainable change. *Review of General Psychology,* 2005;9:111–31.

22. Maunsell E, Brisson J, and Deschenes L. Social support and survival among women with breast cancer. *Cancer,* 1995;76:631–37.

23. Wolf S, Grace K, Bruhn J, and Stout C. Roseto revisited. *Transactions of the American Clinical Climatological Assoc,* 1974.

24. Ibid.

25. Peterson C, Seligman M, and Valliant G. Pessimistic explanatory style as a risk factor for physical illness: a thirty-five-year longitudinal study. *J. of Personality and Social Psychology,* 1988;55:23–27.

Peterson C, Maier S, and Seligman M. *Learned Helplessness.* New York: Oxford University Press, 1993.

26. McClelland D. Some reflections on the two psychologies of love. *J of Personality,* 1986;54:334–53.

McClelland D and Kirshnit C. The effect of motivational arousal through films on salivary immunoglobulin A. *Psychology and Health,* 1988;2:31–52.

27. McKay J. Assessing aspects of object relations associated with immune function: Development of the Affiliative Trust-Mistrust coding system. *Psychological Assessment,* 1991;3(4):641–47.

McClelland D. Some reflections on the two psychologies of love. *J of Personality,* 1986;54:334–53.

McClelland D. Motivational factors in health and disease. *American Psychologist,* 1989;44(4):675–83.

28. Borysenko J. Healing motives: An interview with David C. McClelland. *Advances,* 1985;2(2):29–41.

29. Ibid.

30. Moore T. *Care of the Soul.* New York: HarperCollins, 1993.

31. Rook K. The negative side of social interaction: Impact on psychological well-being. *J of Personality and Social Psychology,* 1984;46:1097–1108.

32. Spiegel D. Effects of psychotherapy on cancer survival. *Nature Reviews Cancer,* 2002;2(5):383–89.

Fawzy F. Immune effects of a short-term psychosocial intervention for cancer patients. *Advances: J. of Mind-Body Health,* 1994;10:32–33.

Antoni M, Lutgendorf S, and Cole S. The influence of biobehavioral factors on tumor biology: Pathways and mechanisms. *Nature Reviews Cancer,* 2006;6(3):240–48.

Cunningham A. *Bringing Spirituality into Your Healing Journey.* Toronto: Key Porter, 2002.

Chapter 20

1. Keltner D and Bonanno G. A study of laughter and dissociation: Distinct correlates of laughter and smiling during bereavement. *J. Personality and Social Psychology,* 1997;73:687–702.

2. Keltner D and Bonanno G. A study of laughter and dissociation: Distinct correlates of laughter and smiling during bereavement. *J. Personality and Social Psychology,* 1997;73:687–702.

Berk L, Tan S, and Westengard J. Beta-endorphin and HGH increase are associated with both the anticipation and experience of mirthful laughter. Annual Meeting of Experimental Biology, San Francisco, 2006.

Chapter 21

1. Nielsen L and Kasczniak A. Awareness of subtle emotional feelings: a comparison of long-term meditators and nonmeditators. *Emotion,* 2006;6:392–405.

2. Lehrer P and Gevirtz R. Two-day workshop at Association for Applied Psychophysiology and Biofeedback (AAPB) Annual Conference, Monterey, CA, 2007.

3. Wolever R and Best J. Mindfulness-based approaches to eating disorders. In Didonna (ed.), *Clinical Handbook of Mindfulness.* New York: Springer, 2009.

4. Rosenberg I. An Exercise to Train Heart and Breath without Equipment. *Newsletter of the California Society of Biofeedback,* 1988;4(1).

5. Vaschillo E, Vaschillo B, and Lehrer P. Characteristics of Resonance in Heart Rate Variability Stimulated by Biofeedback. *Applied Psychophysiology and Biofeedback,* 2006;31;2,129–42.

Chapter 22

1. Damasio A. *Descartes' Error: Emotion, Reason, and the Human Brain.* New York: Putnam, 1994.

2. Futterman A. Immunological variability associated with experimentally induced positive and negative affective states. *Psychosomatic Medicine,* 1994;22:231–68.

3. Achterberg J and Lawless G. Imagery for Health and Healing—one-year training sponsored by Institute for Health and Healing, California Pacific Medical Center, 1998. Phase I: The Psychophysiological Model; Phase II: Assessment and Treatment for Modern Day Settings; Phase III: Psychoneuroimmunology, Advanced Topics and Protocols; Phase IV: Transpersonal Medicine.

4. Murphy M. *The Future of the Body: Explorations into the Further Evolution of Human Nature.* Los Angeles: Tarcher, 1992.

5. Kunzendorf R and Sheikh A (ed.), *The Psychophysiology of Mental Imagery: Theory, Research, and Application.* Amityville, NY: Baywood Publishing, 1990.

Achterberg J. *Imagery in Healing: Shamanism and Modern Medicine.* Boston: Shambhala, 1985.

Achterberg J and Lawless G. Imagery for Health and Healing—one-year training sponsored by Institute for Health and Healing, California Pacific Medical Center, 1998. Phase I: The Psychophysiological Model; Phase II: Assessment and Treatment for Modern Day Settings; Phase III: Psychoneuroimmunology, Advanced Topics and Protocols; Phase IV: Transpersonal Medicine.

Borysenko J. *Minding the Body: Mending the Mind.* Reading, MA: Addison-Wesley, 1987.

Murphy M. *The Future of the Body: Explorations into the Further Evolution of Human Nature.* Los Angeles: Tarcher, 1992.

6. LeShan L. *Cancer as a Turning Point.* New York: Dutton, 1989.

Block K. Psychooncology and total survivorship. *Advances in Mind-Body Medicine,* 1999;15(4):244–81.

Hirshberg C and Barasch M. *Remarkable Recovery: What Extraordinary Healings Tell Us About Getting Well and Staying Well.* New York: Riverhead, 1995.

O'Regan B and Hirshberg C. *Spontaneous Remission: An Annotated Bibliography.* Sausalito, CA: Institute of Noetic Sciences, 1993.

7. Simonton Cancer Center—Certification Training, 2006, 2007, 2008. Most of the tools taught to the cancer patients at the Simonton retreats have been created by O. Carl Simonton, MD, and are unpublished.

8. Gawler I. *You Can Conquer Cancer: Prevention and Management.* South Yarra, VIC, Australia: Michelle Anderson Publishing, 2001.

9. LeShan L. *Cancer as a Turning Point.* New York: Dutton, 1989.

10. Simonton Cancer Center—Certification Training, 2006, 2007, 2008. Most of the tools taught to the cancer patients at the Simonton retreats have been created by O. Carl Simonton, MD, and are unpublished.

LeShan L. *Cancer as a Turning Point.* New York: Dutton, 1989.

11. Achterberg J and Lawless G. Imagery for Health and Healing—one-year training sponsored by Institute for Health and Healing, California Pacific Medical Center, 1998. Phase I: The Psychophysiological Model; Phase II: Assessment and Treatment for Modern Day Settings; Phase III: Psychoneuroimmunology, Advanced Topics and Protocols; Phase IV: Transpersonal Medicine.

LeShan L. *Cancer as a Turning Point.* New York: Dutton, 1989.

Simonton Cancer Center—Certification Training, 2006, 2007, 2008. Most of the tools taught to the cancer patients at the Simonton retreats have been created by O. Carl Simonton, MD, and are unpublished.

12. Murphy M. *The Future of the Body: Explorations into the Further Evolution of Human Nature.* Los Angeles: Tarcher, 1992.

Chapter 23

1. Ironson G, Balbin E, et al. Dispositional optimism and the mechanisms by which it predicts slower disease progression in HIV: proactive behavior, avoidant coping, and depression. *International J. of Behavioral Medicine,* 2005;12(2):86–97.

2. Murdock R. *Patient Number One: A True Story of How One CEO Took on Cancer and Big Business in the Fight of His Life.* New York: Crown, 2000.

3. Wachter R. *Understanding Patient Safety.* New York: McGraw-Hill, 2012.

4. Ruggieri P. *Confessions of a Surgeon: The Good, the Bad, and the Complicated.* New York: Berkley, 2012.

5. Hallisy J. *The Empowered Patient.* Empowered Patient Coalition Press, 2008.

6. Groopman J. *Your Medical Mind: How to Decide What Is Right for You.* New York: Penguin, 2012.

7. Ibid.

8. Schneider S. *The Patient from Hell.* New York: Da Capo, 2005.

9. Ibid.

10. Ibid.

11. Ibid.

12. Hallisy J. *The Empowered Patient.* Empowered Patient Coalition Press, 2008.

13. Murdock R. *Patient Number One: A True Story of How One CEO Took on Cancer and Big Business in the Fight of His Life.* New York: Crown, 2000.

14. Williams J. *The Patient Advocate's Handbook.* Panglossian Press, 2007.

15. Hallisy J. *The Empowered Patient.* Empowered Patient Coalition Press, 2008.

Chapter 24

1. Frankl V. *Man's Search for Meaning.* New York: Pocket Books, 1984.

2. Cousins N. *Head First: The Biology of Hope.* New York: Dutton, 1989.

3. Chou R, Huffman L. Nonpharmacologic therapies for acute and chronic low back pain: a review of the evidence for an American Pain Society/American College of Physicians clinical practice guideline. *Ann Intern Med* 2007; 147(7):492–504.

4. Krause J. Spinal cord injury and its rehabilitation. *Current Opinion in Neurology and Neurosurgery,* 1992;5:669–72.

5. Brown S. A boon for caregivers. *Psychology Today,* Nov 1, 2003.

6. Olian S. Caring for a Loved One at Home, Interview published on my website 9/12/12.

7. Ubel P. *Critical Decisions.* New York: Harper Collins, 2012.

8. Bolletino R and LeShan L. Cancer. In Watkins A. (ed.), *Mind-Body Medicine*. New York: Churchill Livingstone, 1997.

9. Langer E and Rodin J. The effects of choice and enhanced personal responsibility for the aged: A Field Experiment in an Institutional Setting. *Journal of Personality and Social Psychology*, 1976;34;191–98.

10. Olian S. Caring for a Loved One at Home, Interview published on my website 9/12/12.

11. Brown S. A boon for caregivers. *Psychology Today*, Nov 1, 2003.

12. Simonton Cancer Center—Certification Training, 2006, 2007, 2008. Most of the tools taught to the cancer patients at the Simonton retreats have been created by O. Carl Simonton, MD, and are unpublished.

13. Simonton Cancer Center—Certification Training, 2006, 2007, 2008. Most of the tools taught to the cancer patients at the Simonton retreats have been created by O. Carl Simonton, MD, and are unpublished.

LeShan L. *Cancer as a Turning Point*. New York: Dutton, 1989.

14. Simonton Cancer Center—Certification Training, 2006, 2007, 2008. Most of the tools taught to the cancer patients at the Simonton retreats have been created by O. Carl Simonton, MD, and are unpublished.

15. Ibid.

16. Achterberg J. *Imagery in Healing: Shamanism and Modern Medicine*. Boston: Shambhala, 1985.

17. Simonton Cancer Center—Certification Training, 2006, 2007, 2008. Most of the tools taught to the cancer patients at the Simonton retreats have been created by O. Carl Simonton, MD, and are unpublished.

18. Gawler I. *You Can Conquer Cancer: Prevention and Management*. South Yarra, VIC, Australia: Michelle Anderson Publishing, 2001.

19. Lyubomirsky S, King L, and Diener E. The benefits of frequent positive affect: Does happiness lead to success? *Psychological Bulletin*, 2005;131:803–55.

Lyubomirsky S, Sheldon K, and Schkade D. Pursuing happiness: The architecture of sustainable change. *Review of General Psychology*, 2005;9:111–31.

20. Emmons R and McCullough M. Counting blessings versus burdens: An experimental investigation of gratitude and subjective well-being in daily life. *J of Personality and Social Psychology,* 2003;84(2):377–89.

21. Wolever R and Best J. Mindfulness-based approaches to eating disorders. In Didonna F (ed.), *Clinical Handbook of Mindfulness.* New York: Springer, 2009.

22. Stuban S. *The Butcher's Daughter: The Story of an Army Nurse with ALS.* Virtualbookworm.com, 2009.

Appendix A

1. Pert C. *Molecules of Emotion: Why You Feel the Way You Feel.* New York: Simon and Schuster, 1997.

2. Meecham W. Consultation with physician and visionary Will Meecham in early January 2013.

3. Benefiel D. Personal conversation, May 2011. (Dr. David Benefiel is a retired anesthesiologist whose nickname is "The Whiz" because of his encyclopedic knowledge of biochemistry.)

4. King B. *How the Brain Forms New Habits: Why Willpower Is Not Enough.* Symposium sponsored by Institute for Brain Potential, held in Berkeley, CA, January 2012.

5. Benefiel D. Personal conversation, May 2011. (Dr. David Benefiel is a retired anesthesiologist whose nickname is "The Whiz" because of his encyclopedic knowledge of biochemistry.)

6. Siever D. *The role of audio-visual entrainment in seniors' issues.* Annual AAPB Meeting, 2006.

7. Davidson R. *Anxiety, Depression, and Emotion.* New York: Oxford University Press, 2000.

Finucane A and Mercer S. An exploratory mixed methods study of the acceptability and effectiveness of Mindfulness-Based Cognitive Therapy for patients with active depression and anxiety in primary care. *Biomed Central Psychiatry.* 2006 April 7;6:14.

Segal Z, Williams J, and Teasdale J. *Mindfulness-Based Cognitive Therapy for Depression.* New York: Guilford, 2002.

8. Gordon J. *Unstuck.* New York: Penguin, 2008.

9. Gordon J. *Manifesto for a New Medicine.* Reading, MA: Addison-Wesley, 1996.

Gordon J. *Unstuck.* New York: Penguin, 2008.

10. Cacioppo J and Tassinary L (ed.), *Principles of Psychophysiology: Physical, Social, and Inferential Elements.* New York: Cambridge University Press, 1999.

11. Kemeny M. *Psychobiology of Mental Control: Focus on the Immune System, Pain, and Emotions.* Workshop taught by Margaret Kemeny, PhD, San Rafael, CA, April 2000.

12. Kiecolt-Glaser J, McGuire L, Robles T, and Glaser R. Psychoneuroimmunology and psychosomatic medicine: Back to the future. *Psychosomatic Medicine,* 2002;64(1):15–18.

13. Lucier G. The next revolution in life science? *Quest,* 2008;5(1):4.

14. Benefiel D. Personal conversation, May 2011. (Dr. David Benefiel is a retired anesthesiologist whose nickname is "The Whiz" because of his encyclopedic knowledge of biochemistry.)

15. Meecham W. Consultation with physician and visionary Will Meecham in early January 2013.

16. Pert C. *Molecules of Emotion: Why You Feel the Way You Feel.* New York: Simon and Schuster, 1997.

Achterberg J and Lawless G. Imagery for Health and Healing — one-year training sponsored by Institute for Health and Healing, California Pacific Medical Center, 1998. Phase I: The Psychophysiological Model; Phase II: Assessment and Treatment for Modern Day Settings; Phase III: Psychoneuroimmunology, Advanced Topics and Protocols; Phase IV: Transpersonal Medicine.

17. Pert C. *Molecules of Emotion: Why You Feel the Way You Feel.* New York: Simon and Schuster, 1997.

18. Rossi E. *Psychobiology of Mind-Body Healing.* New York: Norton, 1993.

19. Pert C. *Molecules of Emotion: Why You Feel the Way You Feel.* New York: Simon and Schuster, 1997.

20. Benefiel D. Personal conversation, May 2011. (Dr. David Benefiel is a retired anesthesiologist whose nickname is "The Whiz" because of his encyclopedic knowledge of biochemistry.)

21. Kiecolt-Glaser J, Stephens R, Liepetz P, and Glaser R. Distress and DNA repair in human lymphocytes. *J of Behavioral Medicine,* 1985; 8:311–20.

22. Achterberg J. *Intentional Healing: Consciousness and Connection for Health and Well-Being.* Boulder, CO: Sounds True CD set, 2008.

23. Pert C. *Molecules of Emotion: Why You Feel the Way You Feel.* New York: Simon and Schuster, 1997.

24. McLintock T, Aitken H, Downie C, and Kenny G. Postoperative analgesic requirements in patients exposed to intraoperative suggestions. *British Medical J.* 1990;301:788–90.

25. Harrington A (ed.). *The Placebo Effect: An Interdisciplinary Exploration.* Cambridge, MA: Harvard University Press, 1997.

26. Evans F. Expectancy, therapeutic instructions and the placebo response. In White L, Tursky B, and Schwartz G (ed.), *Placebo: Theory, Research, and Mechanisms.* New York: Guilford, 1985.

27. Luparello T, Leist N, Lourie C, and Sweet P. The interaction of psychologic stimuli and pharmacologic agents on airway reactivity in asthmatic subjects. *Psychosomatic Medicine,* 1970;32:509–13.

28. Butler C and Steptoe A. Placebo responses: An experimental study of psychophysiological processes in asthmatic volunteers. *British J. of Clinical Psychology,* 1986;25:173–83.

29. Sobel D. Rethinking medicine: improving health outcomes with cost-effective psychosocial interventions. *Psychosomatic Medicine,* 1995;57,234–44.

30. Price D and Fields H. The Contribution of Desire and Expectation to Placebo Analgesia: Implications for New Research Strategies. In Harrington A (ed.). *The Placebo Effect: An Interdisciplinary Exploration.* Cambridge, MA: Harvard University Press, 1997.

31. Blackwell B, Bloomfield S, and Buncher C. Demonstration to medical students of placebo responses and non-drug factors. *The Lancet,* 1972;1:1279–82.

32. Luparello T, Leist N, Lourie C, and Sweet P. The interaction of psychologic stimuli and pharmacologic agents on airway reactivity in asthmatic subjects. *Psychosomatic Medicine,* 1970;32:509–13.

33. Achterberg J and Lawless G. Imagery for Health and Healing — one-year training sponsored by Institute for Health and Healing, California Pacific Medical Center, 1998. Phase I: The Psychophysiological Model; Phase II: Assessment and Treatment for Modern Day Settings; Phase III: Psychoneuroimmunology, Advanced Topics and Protocols; Phase IV: Transpersonal Medicine.

34. Evans F. Expectancy, therapeutic instructions and the placebo response. In White L, Tursky B, and Schwartz G (ed.), *Placebo: Theory, Research, and Mechanisms.* New York: Guilford, 1985.

35. Amanzio M, Pollo A, Maggi G, and Benedetti F. Response variability to analgesics: A role for non-specific activation of endogenous opioids. *Pain,* 2001;90:205–15.

36. Ibid.

37. Beecher H. The powerful placebo. *JAMA,* 1955;159:1602–6.

38. Horwitz R, Viscoli C, Berkman L, Donaldson R, Horwitz S, Murray C, Ransohoff D, and Sindelar J. Treatment adherence and risk of death after myocardial infarction. *The Lancet,* 1990;336:542–45.

39. Fuente-Sernandez R, Ruth T, Sossi V, Schulzer M, Calne D, and Stossl A. Expectation and dopamine release: Mechanisms of the placebo effect in Parkinson's Disease. *Science*, 2001;293:1164–66.

40. Ornstein R and Sobel D. *The Healing Brain: Breakthrough Medical Discoveries About How the Brain Manages Health*. New York: Simon and Schuster, 1987.

41. Beecher H. The powerful placebo. *JAMA*, 1955;159:1602–6.

42. Coronary Drug Project Research Group. Influence of adherence to treatment and response of cholesterol on mortality in the Coronary Drug Project. *New England J. of Medicine*, 1980;303:1038–41.

43. Sternbach, R. The effects of instructional sets on autonomic responsivity. *Psychophysiology*, 1964;1(1):67–72.

44. Harrington A (ed.). *The Placebo Effect: An Interdisciplinary Exploration*. Cambridge, MA: Harvard University Press, 1997.

45. Wolf S and Pinsky R. Effects of placebo administration and occurence of toxic reactions. *JAMA*, 1974;155:339.

46. Davis M. Don't let placebos fool you. *Postgraduate Medicine*, 1990;88(4):22.

47. Barasch M. *The Healing Path*. New York: Penguin, 1995.

48. Davis. Don't let placebos fool you. *Postgraduate Medicine*, 1990;88(4):22.

48. Beecher H. The powerful placebo. *JAMA*, 1955;159:1602–6.

Appendix B

1. Arch J and Craske M. Mechanisms of mindfulness: Emotion regulation following a focused breathing induction. *Behaviour Research and Therapy*, 2006;44:1849–58.

2. Hölzel B, Ott U, Hempel H, Hackl A, Wolf K, Stark R, and Vaitl D. Differential engagement of anterior cingulate and adjacent medial frontal cortex in adept meditators and non-meditators. *Neuroscience Letters*, 2007;421(1):16–21.

3. Allman J, Hakeem A, Erwin J, Nimchinsky E, and Hof P. The anterior cingulate cortex: The evolution of an interface between emotion and cognition. *Annals of The New York Academy of Science*, 2001;935:107–17.

4. Lehrer P and Gevirtz R. Two-day workshop at Association for Applied Psychophysiology and Biofeedback (AAPB) Annual Conference, Monterey, CA, 2007.

5. Bigger J, Fleiss J, Steinman R, Rolnitzky L, Kleiger R, and Rottman J. Frequency domain measures of heart period variability and mortality after myocardial infarction. *Circulation,* 1992;85:164–71.

6. Horsten M, Ericson M, and Perski A. Psychosocial factors and heart rate variability in women. *Psychosomatic Medicine.* 1999;61:49–57.

7. Tsuji H, Venditti F, and Manders E. Reduced heart rate variability and mortality risk in an elderly cohort: The Framingham Heart Study. *Circulation,* 1994;90(2):878–83.

8. Hughes J and Stoney C. Depressed mood is related to high-frequency heart rate variability during stressors. *Psychosomatic Medicine,* 2000;62:796–803.

9. Lehrer P and Gevirtz R. Two-day workshop at Association for Applied Psychophysiology and Biofeedback (AAPB) Annual Conference, Monterey, CA, 2007.

10. Ibid.

11. Peper E. Applied Psychophysiology and Biofeedback Annual Conference, 2008.

12. Atkinson M, Carrios-Choplin B, McCraty R, Rozman D, and Watkins A. The impact of a new emotional self-management program on stress, emotions, HRV, DHEA, and cortisol. *Integrative Physiological and Behavioral Science,* 1998;33(2):151–70.

13. Preston J. Integrating Psychotherapy, Neuroscience, and Eastern Healing Traditions. Professional conference, San Rafael, CA, March 7, 2009.

14. Phongsuphap S, Pongsupap Y, Chandanmattha P, and Lursinsap C. Changes in heart rate variability during concentration meditation. *J. of Cardiology,* 2008;130(3):481–84.

15. Lehrer P and Gevirtz R. Two-day workshop at Association for Applied Psychophysiology and Biofeedback (AAPB) Annual Conference, Monterey, CA, 2007.

16. Cacioppo J and Tassinary L (ed.), *Principles of Psychophysiology: Physical, Social, and Inferential Elements.* New York: Cambridge University Press, 1999.

Dworkin B. *Learning and Physiological Regulation.* Chicago: University of Chicago Press, 1993.

Hugdahl K. *Psychophysiology: The Mind-Body Perspective.* Cambridge, MA: Harvard University Press, 1998.

Bibliography

Abramowitz J, Tolin D, and Street G. Paradoxical effects of thought suppression: A meta-analysis of controlled studies. *Clinical Psychology Review,* 2001;21(5):683–703.

Achterberg J. *Intentional Healing: Consciousness and Connection for Health and Well-Being.* Boulder, CO: Sounds True CD set, 2008.

———. *Imagery in Healing: Shamanism and Modern Medicine.* Boston: Shambhala, 1985.

Achterberg J and Lawless G. Imagery for Health and Healing — one-year training sponsored by Institute for Health and Healing, California Pacific Medical Center, 1998. Phase I: The Psychophysiological Model; Phase II: Assessment and Treatment for Modern Day Settings; Phase III: Psychoneuroimmunology, Advanced Topics and Protocols; Phase IV: Transpersonal Medicine.

Alexander C, Langer E, Newman R, Chandler H, and Davies J. Aging, mindfulness and meditation. *J. of Personality and Social Psychology,* 1989;57:950–64.

Allman J, Hakeem A, Erwin J, Nimchinsky E, and Hof P. The anterior cingulate cortex: The evolution of an interface between emotion and cognition. *Annals of The New York Academy of Science,* 2001;935:107–17.

Amanzio M, Pollo A, Maggi G, and Benedetti F. Response variability to analgesics: A role for non-specific activation of endogenous opioids. *Pain,* 2001;90:205–15.

Andrews H. Helping and health: The relationship between volunteer activity and health-related outcomes. *Advances,* 1990;7(1):25–34.

Antoni M, Baggett L, Ironson, G, et al. Cognitive-behavioral stress management intervention buffers distress responses and immunological changes following notification of HIV-1 seropositivity. *Journal of Consulting and Clinical Psychology,* 1991;59:905–15.

Antoni M, Lutgendorf S, and Cole S. The influence of biobehavioral factors on tumor biology: Pathways and mechanisms. *Nature Reviews Cancer,* 2006;6(3):240–48.

Arch J and Craske M. Mechanisms of mindfulness: Emotion regulation following a focused breathing induction. *Behaviour Research and Therapy,* 2006;44:1849–58.

Arnetz B, Thorell T, Levi L, Kallner A, and Eneroth P. An experimental study of social isolation of elderly people: psychoendocrine and metabolic effects. *Psychosomatic Medicine,* 1983;45:395–406.

Atkinson M, Carrios-Choplin B, McCraty R, Rozman D, and Watkins A. The impact of a new emotional self-management program on stress, emotions, HRV, DHEA, and cortisol. *Integrative Physiological and Behavioral Science,* 1998;33(2):151–70.

Barasch M. *The Healing Path.* New York: Penguin, 1995.

Barefoot J, Dahlstrom W, and Williams R. Hostility, CHD incidence, and total mortality: a 25-year follow-up study of 255 physicians. *Psychosomatic Medicine,* 1983;45:59–63.

Barefoot J, Dodge K, and Peterson B. The Cook-Medley Hostility Scale: Item content and ability to predict survival. *Psychosomatic Medicine,* 1989.51:46–57.

Barsky A and Ahem D. Cognitive behavior therapy for hypochondriasis: a randomized controlled trial. *JAMA,* 2004;291:1464–70.

Beecher H. The powerful placebo. *JAMA,* 1955;159:1602–6.

Benefiel D. Personal conversation, May 2011. (Dr. David Benefiel is a retired anesthesiologist whose nickname is "The Whiz" because of his encyclopedic knowledge of biochemistry.)

Berk L, Tan S, and Westengard J. Beta-endorphin and HGH increase are associated with both the anticipation and experience of mirthful laughter. Annual Meeting of Experimental Biology, San Francisco, 2006.

Berkman L and Syme L. Social networks, host resistance, and mortality: a nine-year follow-up study of Alameda County residents. *American Journal of Epidemiology,* 1982;109:186–204.

Bigger J, Fleiss J, Steinman R, Rolnitzky L, Kleiger R, and Rottman J. Frequency domain measures of heart period variability and mortality after myocardial infarction. *Circulation,* 1992;85:164–71.

Bishop S, Lau M, Shapiro S, Carlson L, Anderson N, Carmody J, Segal Z, Abbey S, Speca M, Velting D, and Devins G. Mindfulness: A proposed operational definition. *Clinical Psychology: Science and Practice,* 2004;11(3):230–41.

Blackledge J. Disrupting verbal processes: Cognitive defusion in acceptance and commitment therapy and other mindfulness-based psychotherapies. *The Psychological Record,* 2007;57(4):555–76.

Blackwell B, Bloomfield S, and Buncher C. Demonstration to medical students of placebo responses and non-drug factors. *The Lancet,* 1972;1:1279–82.

Block K. Psychooncology and total survivorship. *Advances in Mind-Body Medicine,* 1999;15(4):244–81.

Bolletino R and LeShan L. Cancer. In Watkins A. (ed.), *Mind-Body Medicine.* New York: Churchill Livingstone, 1997.

Booth R and Ashbridge K. A fresh look at the relationship between the psyche and immune system: teleological coherence and harmony of purpose. *Advances, The Journal of Mind-Body Health,* 1993; 9(2):4–23.

Borkovec T, Alcaine O, and Behar E. Avoidance theory of worry and generalized anxiety disorder. In Heimberg R, Turk C, and Mennin D (ed.), *Generalized Anxiety Disorder: Advances in Research and Practice.* New York: Guilford, 2004.

Borysenko J. Healing motives: An interview with David C. Mc-Clelland. *Advances,* 1985;2(2):29–41.

———. *Minding the Body: Mending the Mind.* Reading, MA: Addison-Wesley, 1987.

Bower J, Kemeny M, Taylor S, and Fahey J. Cognitive processing, discovery of meaning, CD4 decline, and AIDS-related mortality among bereaved HIV-seropositive men. *J of Consulting and Clinical Psychology,* 1998;66:979–86.

Brawley O and Goldberg P. *How We Do Harm: A Doctor Breaks Ranks About Being Sick in America.* New York: St. Martin's, 2011.

Brown J, Butow P, Culjak G, Coates A, and Dunn S. Psychosocial predictors of outcome: Time to relapse and survival in patients with early stage melanoma. *British J of Cancer,* 2000;83:1448–53.

Brown S. A boon for caregivers. *Psychology Today,* Nov 1, 2003.

Buettner D. *The Blue Zones: Lessons for Living Longer from the People Who've Lived the Longest.* Washington, DC: National Geographic, 2008.

Bugental J. Week-long residential training and weekly case consultation group, 1995 through 1998.

Burch V. *Living Well with Pain and Illness: The Mindful Way to Free Yourself From Suffering.* Boulder, CO: Sounds True, 2010.

Butler C and Steptoe A. Placebo responses: An experimental study of psychophysiological processes in asthmatic volunteers. *British J. of Clinical Psychology,* 1986;25:173–83.

Butler R. The inequality of longevity: Life expectancy gap widens between industrialized world and developing nations. *Geriatrics,* 1999;Dec.

Cacioppo J and Tassinary L (ed.), *Principles of Psychophysiology: Physical, Social, and Inferential Elements.* New York: Cambridge University Press, 1999.

Carlin G. *Brain Droppings.* New York: Hyperion, 1997.

Carlson L, Speca M, Faris P, and Patel K. One year pre-post intervention follow-up of psychological, immune, endocrine and blood pressure outcomes of mindfulness-based stress reduction (MBSR) in breast and prostate cancer outpatients. *Brain Behav Immun,* 2007;21(8):1038–49.

Carlson L, Speca M, Patel K, and Goodey E. Mindfulness-based stress reduction in relation to quality of life, mood, symptoms of stress, and immune parameters in breast and prostate cancer outpatients. *Psychosomatic Medicine,* 2003;65:571–81.

————. Mindfulness-based stress reduction in relation to quality of life, mood, symptoms of stress and levels of cortisol, dehydroepiandrosterone sulfate (DHEAS) and melatonin in breast and prostate cancer outpatients. *Psychoneuroendocrinology,* 2004;29:448–74.

Carlson L, Ursuliak Z, Goodey E, Angen M, and Speca M. The effects of a mindfulness meditation–based stress reduction program on mood and symptoms of stress in cancer outpatients: 6-month follow-up. *Supportive Care In Cancer,* 2001;9:112–23.

Cioffi D and Holloway J. Delayed costs of suppressed pain. *Journal of Personality and Social Psychology,* Vol. 64(2), Feb 1993, 274–82.

Classen C, Kraemer H, Blasey C, Giese-Davis J, Koopman C, Palesh O, Atkinson A, Dimiceli S, Stonisch-Riggs G, Westendorp J, Morrow GR, and Spiegel D. Supportive-expressive group therapy for primary breast cancer patients: a randomized prospective multicenter trial. *Psychooncology,* 2008;17(5):438–47.

Cochrane A, Barnes-Holmes D, Barnes-Holmes Y, Steward I, and Luciano C. Experiential avoidance and aversive visual images: Response delays and event related potentials on a simple matching task. *Behavior Research and Therapy,* 2007;45:1379–88.

Cohen E. *The Empowered Patient.* New York: Ballantine, 2010.

Conrad A, Muller A, Doberenz S et al. Psychophysiological effects of breathing instructions for stress management. *Applied Psychophysiology and Biofeedback,* 2007;32(2):89–98.

Coronary Drug Project Research Group. Influence of adherence to treatment and response of cholesterol on mortality in the Coronary Drug Project. *New England J. of Medicine,* 1980;303:1038–41.

Cousins N. *Head First: The Biology of Hope.* New York: Dutton, 1989.

Crane R. *Mindfulness-Based Cognitive Therapy.* London: Routledge, 2010.

Creswell J, Way B, Eisenberger N, and Lieberman M. Neural correlates of dispositional mindfulness during affect labeling. *Psychosomatic Medicine,* 2007;69(6):560–65.

Csikszentmihalyi M. *Flow: The psychology of optimal experience.* New York: HarperCollins, 1991.

Cunningham A. *Bringing Spirituality into Your Healing Journey.* Toronto: Key Porter, 2002.

———. *Can the Mind Heal Cancer?: A Clinician Scientist Examines the Evidence.* Toronto: Healing Journey Program at Ontario Cancer Institute, 2005.

———. *The Healing Journey: Overcoming the Crisis of Cancer.* Toronto: Key Porter, 2000.

———. How psychological therapy may prolong survival in cancer patients: new evidence and a simple theory. *Integrative Cancer Therapies,* 2004;3(3):214–29.

Cunningham A and Edmonds C. Delivering a very brief psychoeducational program to cancer patients and family members in a large group format. *Psycho-oncology,* 1999;8:177–82.

Cunningham A, Edmonds C, Phillips C, Soots K, Hedley D, and Lockwood G. A prospective, longitudinal study of the relationship of psychological work to duration of survival in patients with metastatic cancer. *Psycho-oncology,* 2000;9:323–39.

Cunningham A, Phillips C, Lockwood G, Hedley D, and Edmonds C. Association of involvement in psychological self help with longer survival in patients with metastatic cancer: An exploratory study. *Advances in Mind-Body Medicine,* 2000;16:276–94.

Dahl J, Wilson K, and Luciano C. *Acceptance and Commitment Therapy for Chronic Pain.* Reno, NV: Context Press, 2005.

Damasio A. *Descartes' Error: Emotion, Reason, and the Human Brain.* New York: Putnam, 1994.

Davidson R. *Anxiety, Depression, and Emotion.* New York: Oxford University Press, 2000.

Davidson, R, Kabat-Zinn, J, Schumacher J, Rosenkrantz M, Muller D, Santorelli S, Urbanowaki F, Harrington A, Bonus K, and Sheridan J. Alterations in brain and immune function produced by mindfulness meditation. *Psychosomatic Medicine,* 2003;65:564–70.

Davidson R and Lutz A. Buddha's Brain: Neuroplasticity and Meditation. *IEEE Signal Processing* (2008);25(1),171–74.

Davis M. Don't let placebos fool you. *Postgraduate Medicine,* 1990;88(4):22.

Depner C and Ingersoll-Dayton B. Supportive relationships in later life. *Psychology and Aging,* 1988;3(4):348–57.

Derogatis L. Psychology in cancer medicine: a perspective and overview. *J. of Consulting and Clinical Psychology,* October 1986:632–38.

Derogatis L, Abeloff M, and Melisaratos N. Psychological coping mechanisms and survival time in metastatic breast cancer. *JAMA,* 1979:242(14):1504–08.

Dimidjian S and Linehan M. Defining an agenda for future research on the clinical application of mindfulness practice. *Clinical Psychology: Science and Practice,* 2003;10(2):166.

Dreher H. Beyond fighting spirit: What mind-states influence cancer survival? *Advances in Mind-Body Medicine,* Spring 2000; 16(2):120–27.

Dworkin B. *Learning and Physiological Regulation.* Chicago: University of Chicago Press, 1993.

Eifert G and Heffner M. The effects of acceptance versus control contexts on avoidance of panic-related symptoms. *J. of Behavior Therapy and Experimental Psychiatry,* 2003;34:293–312.

Elliot A and Sheldon K. Avoidance personal goals and the personality-illness relationship. *J. of Personality and Social Psychology,* 1998;75:1282–99.

Emmons R. *Thanks!: How the new science of gratitude can make you happier.* New York: Houghton Mifflin, 2007.

Emmons R and McCullough M. Counting blessings versus burdens: An experimental investigation of gratitude and subjective well-being in daily life. *J of Personality and Social Psychology,* 2003;84(2):377–89.

Evans F. Expectancy, therapeutic instructions and the placebo response. In White L, Tursky B, and Schwartz G (ed.), *Placebo: Theory, Research, and Mechanisms.* New York: Guilford, 1985.

Eysenck H. Personality, stress, and cancer: prediction and prophylaxis. *British J of Medical Psychology,* 1988;61:57–75.

Faller H, Bulzebruck H, Schilling S, Drings P, and Lang H. Do psychological factors modify survival of cancer patients? II: Results of an empirical study with bronchial carcinoma patients. *Psychotherapy Psychosomatic Medicine Psychology,* 1997;47:206–18.

Farb N, Segal Z, Mayberg H, Bean J, McKeon D, Fatima Z, and Anderson A. Attending to the present: mindfulness meditation reveals distinct neural modes of self-reference. *Social Cognitive and Affective Neuroscience*, 2007;2(4), 313–22.

Fawzy F. Immune effects of a short-term psychosocial intervention for cancer patients. *Advances: J. of Mind-Body Health*, 1994; 10:32–33.

———. Malignant melanoma: Effects of an early structured psychiatric intervention, coping, and affective state on recurrence and survival 6 years later. *Archives of General Psychiatry*. 1993;50:681–89.

Feldner M, Zvolensky M, Eifert G, and Spira A. Emotional avoidance: An experimental test of individual differences and response suppression during biological challenge. *Behaviour Research and Therapy*. 2003; 41:403–11.

Finucane A and Mercer S. An exploratory mixed methods study of the acceptability and effectiveness of Mindfulness-Based Cognitive Therapy for patients with active depression and anxiety in primary care. *Biomed Central Psychiatry*, 2006;April 7;6:14.

Fleshner M and Laudenslager M. Psychoneuroimmunology: then and now. *Behavioral and Cognitive Neuroscience Reviews*, 2004;3:114–30.

Frankl V. *Man's Search for Meaning*. New York: Pocket Books, 1984.

Fricchione G, Bilfinger T, Hartman A, Liu Y, and Stefano G. Neuroimmunologic implications in coronary artery disease. *Advances in Neuroimmunology*. 1996;6:131–42.

Fuente-Sernandez R, Ruth T, Sossi V, Schulzer M, Calne D, and Stossl A. Expectation and dopamine release: Mechanisms of the placebo effect in Parkinson's Disease. *Science*, 2001;293:1164–66.

Futterman A. Immunological variability associated with experimentally induced positive and negative affective states. *Psychosomatic Medicine*, 1994;22:231–68.

Gallin P. *How to Survive Your Doctor's Care*. Washington, DC: LifeLine Press, 2003.

Gallo L and Mathews K. Understanding the association between socioeconomic status and physical health: Do negative emotions play a role? *Psychological Bulletin*, 2003;129:10–51.

Gardner-Nix J. *The Mindfulness Solution to Pain*. Oakland: New Harbinger, 2009.

Gawande A. *Better*. New York: Holt, 2007.

———. *The Checklist Manifesto*. New York: Holt, 2009.

———. *Complications.* New York: Holt, 2002.

Gawler I. *You Can Conquer Cancer: Prevention and Management.* South Yarra, VIC, Australia: Michelle Anderson Publishing, 2001.

Gellert G, Maxwell R, and Siegel B. Survival of breast cancer patients receiving adjunctive psychosocial support therapy: A 10-year follow-up study. *Journal of Clinical Oncology,* 1993;11:1;66–69.

Gibson R. and Singh J. *Wall of Silence: The Untold Story of the Medical Mistakes That Kill and Injure Millions of Americans.* Washington, DC: LifeLine Press, 2003.

Giller C. *Port in the Storm: How to Make a Medical Decision and Live to Tell About It.* Washington, DC: 004, Washington, DC: Life-Line Press, 2004.

Glaser R, Kiecolt-Glaser J, and Malarkey W. The effect of stress on viral vaccine responses. Procedings of the Congress of the International Society for Neuroimmunomodulation. 1996;56:13–15.

Gordon J. *Manifesto for a New Medicine.* Reading, MA: Addison-Wesley, 1996.

———. Training in Mind-Body Medicine by the Center for Mind-Body Medicine, San Diego, September 2009.

———. *Unstuck.* New York: Penguin, 2008.

Gorman J and Sloan R. Heart rate variability in depressive and anxiety disorders. *Amer Heart J,* 2000;140:77–83.

Graves P, Thomas C, and Mead L. Familial and psychological predictors of cancer. *Cancer Detection Review,* 1991;15:59–64.

Greer S. Mind-body research in psychooncology. *J. Advances in Mind-Body Medicine,* 1999;15(4):236–44.

Greer S and Morris T. Psychological attributes of women who develop breast cancer: A controlled study. *J of Psychosomatic Research,* 1975;19:147–53.

Greer S, Morris T, Pettingale K, and Haybittle J. Psychological response to breast cancer and 15-year outcome. *The Lancet* 1990; 6: 335 (8680): 49–50.

Greeson J and Brantley J. Mindfulness and Anxiety Disorders: Developing a Wise Relationship with the Inner Experience of Fear. In Didonna F (ed.), *Clinical Handbook of Mindfulness.* New York: Springer, 2009.

Groopman J. *How Doctors Think.* New York: Houghton Mifflin, 2008.

———. *Second Opinions.* New York: Viking Penguin, 2000.

———. *Your Medical Mind: How to Decide What Is Right for You.* New York: Penguin, 2012.

Gross J and Levenson R. Emotional suppression: Physiology, self-report, and expressive behavior. *J. of Personality and Social Psychology*, 1993;64:970–86.

———. Hiding feelings: The acute effects of inhibiting negative and positive emotion. *J. of Abnormal Psychology*, 1997;106:95–103.

Grossarth-Maticek R. Interpersonal repression as a predictor of cancer. *Social Science Medicine*, 1982;16:493–98.

Grossman P, Niemann L, Schmidt S, and Walach H. Mindfulness-based stress reduction and health benefits: A meta-analysis. *J. of Psychosomatic Research*. 2004;57:35–43.

Grossman P, Tiefenthaler-Gilmer U, Raysz A, and Kesper U. Mindfulness training as an intervention for fibromyalgia: Evidence of post-intervention and 3-year follow-up benefits in well-being. *Psychotherapy and Psychosomatics*. 2007;76:226–33.

Hallisy J. *The Empowered Patient*. Empowered Patient Coalition Press, 2008.

Hankey A. Studies of advanced stages of meditation in the Tibetan Buddhist and vedic traditions. *J. of Complementary and Alternative Medicine*, 2006;3:513–21.

Hanson B, Isacsson S, Janzon L, and Lindell S. Social network and social support influence on mortality in elderly men. *American J of Epidemiology*. 1989;130(1):110–11.

Harrington A (ed.). *The Placebo Effect: An Interdisciplinary Exploration*. Cambridge, MA: Harvard University Press, 1997.

Hayes S. Acceptance and commitment therapy, relational frame theory, and the third wave of behavioral and cognitive therapies. *Behavior Therapy*, 2004;35:639–65.

———. *Get Out of Your Mind and Into Your Life: The New Acceptance and Commitment Therapy*. Oakland, CA: New Harbinger, 2006.

———. Hello darkness: Discovering our values by confronting our fears. *Psychotherapy Networker*, 2007;31(5):46–52.

Hayes S, Follette V, and Linehan M. *Mindfulness and Acceptance: Expanding the Cognitive Behavioral Tradition*. New York: Guilford Press, 2004.

Hayes S, Masuda A, Bissett R, Luoma J, and Guerrero L. DBT, FAP, and ACT: How empirically oriented are the new behavior therapy technologies? *Behavior Therapy*, 2004; 35:35–54.

Hayes S and Strosahl K. *A Practical Guide to Acceptance and Commitment Therapy*. New York: Springer, 2004.

Hayes S, Strosahl K, and Wilson K. *Acceptance and Commitment Therapy: An Experiential Approach to Behavioral Change.* New York: Guilford, 1999.

Hayes S, Strosahl K, Wilson K, Bissett R, Pistorello J, and Toarmino D. Measuring experiential avoidance: A preliminary test of a working model. *The Psychological Record,* 2004;54:553–78.

Hirshberg C and Barasch M. *Remarkable Recovery: What Extraordinary Healings Tell Us About Getting Well and Staying Well.* New York: Riverhead, 1995.

Hölzel B, Ott U, Gard T, Hempel H, Weygandt M, Morgen K, and Vaitl D. Investigation of mindfulness meditation practitioners with voxel-based morphometry. *Social Cognitive and Affective Neuroscience,* 2008;3:55–61.

Hölzel B, Ott U, Hempel H, Hackl A, Wolf K, Stark R, and Vaitl D. Differential engagement of anterior cingulate and adjacent medial frontal cortex in adept meditators and non-meditators. *Neuroscience Letters,* 2007;421(1):16–21.

Horsten M, Ericson M, and Perski A. Psychosocial factors and heart rate variability in women. *Psychosomatic Medicine,* 1999;61:49–57.

Horwitz R, Viscoli C, Berkman L, Donaldson R, Horwitz S, Murray C, Ransohoff D, and Sindelar J. Treatment adherence and risk of death after myocardial infarction. *The Lancet,* 1990;336:542–45.

House J, Landis K, and Umberson D. Social relationships and health. *Science,* 1988;241:540–45.

Hugdahl K. *Psychophysiology: The Mind-Body Perspective.* Cambridge, MA: Harvard University Press, 1998.

Hughes J and Stoney C. Depressed mood is related to high-frequency heart rate variability during stressors. *Psychosomatic Medicine,* 2000;62:796–803.

Ironson G, Balbin E, et al. Dispositional optimism and the mechanisms by which it predicts slower disease progression in HIV: proactive behavior, avoidant coping, and depression. *International J. of Behavioral Medicine,* 2005;12(2):86–97.

Jamner L and Schwartz G. Self-deception predicts self-report and endurance of pain. *Psychosomatic Medicine,* 1986;48:211–23.

Jensen M. Psychobiological factors predicting the course of cancer. *J. of Personality,* 1987;55:317–42.

Kabat-Zinn J. Bringing mindfulness to medicine. *Alternative Therapies in Health and Medicine,* 2005;11(3):56–64.

———. Foreword to Didonna F (ed.), *Clinical Handbook of Mindfulness.* New York: Springer, 2009.

———. *Full Catastrophe Living: Using the Wisdom of Your Body and Mind to Face Stress, Pain, and Illness,* 15th edition. New York: Bantam, 2005.

Kabat-Zinn J, Lipworth L, and Burney R. The clinical use of mindfulness meditation for the self-regulation of chronic pain. *J. of Behavioral Medicine,* 1985;8:163–90.

Kabat-Zinn J, Lipworth L, Burney R, and Sellers W. Four-year follow-up of a meditation-based program for the self-regulation of chronic pain: Treatment outcome and compliance. *Clinical J. of Pain,* 1987;2:159–73.

Kaplan G. Outcomes of the North Karetic, Sweden project. *Am J. of Epidemiology,* 1988;128(2):370–80.

Karekla M, Forsyth J, and Kelly M. Emotional avoidance and panicogenic responding to a biological challenge procedure. *Behavior Therapy,* 2004;35(4):725–46.

Katz R, Flasher L, Cacciapaglia H, and Nelson S. The psychosocial impact of cancer and lupus: A cross validation study that extends the generality of "benefit-finding" in patients with chronic disease. *J. of Behavioral Medicine,* 2001;24:561–71.

Keene N. *Working with Your Doctor.* Sebastopol, CA: O'Reilly & Associates, 1998.

Keltner D and Bonanno G. A study of laughter and dissociation: Distinct correlates of laughter and smiling during bereavement. *J. Personality and Social Psychology,* 1997;73:687–702.

Kemeny M. *Psychobiology of Mental Control: Focus on the Immune System, Pain, and Emotions.* Workshop taught by Margaret Kemeny, PhD. San Rafael, CA, April 2000.

Kennedy S, Kiecolt-Glaser J, and Glaser R. Immunological consequences of acute and chronic stressors: Mediating role of interpersonal relationships. *British J of Medical Psychology,* 1988;61:77–85.

Kiecolt-Glaser J and Glaser R. Psychoneuroimmuology: Can psychological interventions modulate immunity? *J. of Consulting and Clinical Psychology,* 1992;60:569–75.

Kiecolt-Glaser J, Glaser R, Williger D, et al. Psychosocial modifiers of immunocompetence in medical students. *Psychosomatic Medicine,* 1984;46:7–14.

Kiecolt-Glaser J, McGuire L, Robles T, and Glaser R. Psychoneuroimmunology and psychosomatic medicine: Back to the future. *Psychosomatic Medicine,* 2002;64(1):15–18.

Kiecolt-Glaser J, Stephens R, Liepetz P, and Glaser R. Distress and DNA repair in human lymphocytes. *J of Behavioral Medicine,* 1985;8:311–20.

King B. *How the Brain Forms New Habits: Why Willpower Is Not Enough.* Symposium sponsored by Institute for Brain Potential, held in Berkeley, CA, January 2012.

King L. The health benefits of writing about life goals. *Personality and Social Psychology Bulletin,* 2001;27:798–807.

Kingston J, Chadwick P, Meron D, and Skinner T. A pilot randomized controlled trial investigating the effect of mindfulness practice on pain tolerance, psychological well-being, and physiological activity. *J. of Psychosomatic Research,* 2007;62:297–300.

Kop W. Chronic and acute psychological risk factors for clinical manifestations of coronary artery disease. *Psychosomatic Medicine,* 1999;61:476–87.

Kop W and Cohen N. Psychological risk factors and immune system involvement in cardiovascular disease. In Ader R, Felton D, and Cohen N (ed.), *Psychoneuroimmuology,* 3rd edition, Vol. 2. New York: Academic Press, 2001.

Krause J. Spinal cord injury and its rehabilitation. *Current Opinion in Neurology and Neurosurgery,* 1992;5:669–72.

Kreitler S, Peleg D, and Ehrenfeld M. Stress, self-efficacy and quality of life in cancer patients. *Psychooncology,* 2007;16(4):329-41.

Krishnamurti J. *Discussions With Krishnamurti in Europe.* Ojai, CA: Krishnamurti Writings Inc, 1966.

Kunzendorf R and Sheikh A (ed.), *The Psychophysiology of Mental Imagery: Theory, Research, and Application.* Amityville, NY: Baywood Publishing, 1990.

Langer E. *Counter Clockwise: Mindful Health and the Power of Possibility.* New York: Ballantine, 2009.

———. Matters of mind: mindfulness/mindlessness in perspective. *Consciousness and Cognition,* 1992;1:289–305.

———. *Mindfulness.* New York: Addison-Wesley, 1989.

Langer E and Rodin J. The effects of choice and enhanced personal responsibility for the aged: A field experiment in an institutional setting. *Journal of Personality and Social Psychology,* 1976;34;191–98.

Langer E, Rodin J, Beck P, Weinman C, and Spitzer L. Environmental determinants of memory improvement in late adulthood. *J. of Personality and Social Psychology,* 1979;37:2003–13.

Lau M. New developments in psychosocial interventions for adults with unipolar depression. *Current Opinions in Psychiatry,* 2008 Jan;21(1):30–36.

Lazar S, Kerr C, Wasserman R, Gray J, Greve D, and Treadway M. Meditation experience is associated with increased cortical thickness. *NeuroReport,* 2005;16(17):1893–97.

LeDoux J. *Synaptic Self: How Our Brains Become Who We Are.* New York: Penguin, 2003.

Lehrer P and Gevirtz R. Two-day workshop at Association for Applied Psychophysiology and Biofeedback (AAPB) Annual Conference, Monterey, CA, 2007.

LeShan L. A new question in studying psychosocial interventions and cancer. *Advances, The Journal of Mind-Body Health,* 1991;7(1).

———. *Cancer as a Turning Point.* New York: Dutton, 1989.

———. Cancer as a Turning Point Residential Workshop, October–November 2007. Much of what is taught to those attending these workshops is published in the book *Cancer as a Turning Point.* The exercises have all been created by Lawrence LeShan, PhD.

Levitt J, Brown T, Orsillo S, and Barlow D. The effects of acceptance versus suppression of emotion on subjective and psychophysiological response to carbon dioxide challenge in patients with panic disorder. *Behavior Therapy,* 2004; 35:747–66.

Levy S, Herberman R, and Lippman M. Correlation of stress factors with sustained depression of natural killer cell activity and predicted prognosis in patients with breast cancer. *J of Clinical Oncology,* 1987;5(3):348–53.

Levy S, Herberman R, Lippman M, d'Angelo T, and Lee J. Immunological and psychosocial predictors of disease recurrence in patients with early-stage breast cancer. *J of Behavioral Medicine,* 1991;17:67–75.

Levy S, Herberman R, Whiteside T, Sanzo K, Lee J, and Kirkwood J. Perceived social support and tumor estrogen/progesterone receptor status as predictors of natural killer cell activity in breast cancer patients. *Psychosomatic Medicine,* 1990;52:73–85.

Lipton B and Bhaerman S. *Sponaneous Evolution.* Carlsbad, CA: Hay House, 2009.

Lucier G. The next revolution in life science? *Quest,* 2008;5(1):4.

Luoma J, Hayes S, and Walser R. *Learning ACT: An Acceptance and Commitment Therapy Skills-Training Manual for Therapists.* Oakland, CA: New Harbinger, 2007.

Luparello T, Leist N, Lourie C, and Sweet P. The interaction of psychologic stimuli and pharmacologic agents on airway reactivity in asthmatic subjects. *Psychosomatic Medicine*, 1970;32: 509–13.

Lutz A, Dunne J, and Davidson R. Meditation and the Neuroscience of Consciousness: An Introduction. In Zelazo P, Moscovitch M, and Thompson E (ed.), *Cambridge Handbook of Consciousness*. New York: Cambridge University Press, 2007.

Lyubomirsky S. *The How of Happiness: A Scientific Approach to Getting the Life You Want*. New York: Penguin, 2007.

———. Why are some people happier than others?: The role of cognitive and motivational processes in well-being. *American Psychologist*, 2001;56:239–49.

Lyubomirsky S, King L, and Diener E. The benefits of frequent positive affect: Does happiness lead to success? *Psychological Bulletin*, 2005;131:803–55.

Lyubomirsky S, Sheldon K, and Schkade D. Pursuing happiness: The architecture of sustainable change. *Review of General Psychology*, 2005;9:111–31.

Manne S, Ostroff J, Winkel G, Goldstein L, Fox K, and Grana G. Posttraumatic growth after breast cancer: Patient, partner, and couple perspectives. *Psychosomatic Medicine*, 2004;66:442–54.

Marcks B and Woods D. A comparison of thought suppression to an acceptance-based technique in the management of personal intrusive thoughts: A controlled evaluation. *Behaviour Research and Therapy*, 2005;43:433–45.

Marlatt G and Kristeller J. Mindfulness and meditation. In Miller W (ed.), *Integrating Spirituality into Treatment*. Washington, DC: American Psychological Association, 1999.

Marmot M, Syme S, Kagan A, Kato H, Cohen J, and Belsky J. Epidemiologic studies of coronary heart disease and stroke in Japanese men living in Japan, Hawaii and California: prevalence of coronary and hypertensive heart disease and associated risk factor. *American J. of Epidemiology*, 1975;102(6):514–25.

Massion A, Teas J, Hebert J, Wertheimer M, and Kabat-Zinn J. Meditation, melatonin, and breast/prostate cancer: Hypothesis and preliminary data. *Medical Hypotheses*, 1995;44:39–46.

Maunsell E, Brisson J, and Deschenes L. Social support and survival among women with breast cancer. *Cancer*, 1995;76:631–37.

McClelland D. Motivational factors in health and disease. *American Psychologist*, 1989;44(4):675–83.

———. Some reflections on the two psychologies of love. *J of Personality*, 1986;54:334–53.

McClelland D and Kirshnit C. The effect of motivational arousal through films on salivary immunoglobulin A. *Psychology and Health*, 1988;2:31–52.

McCracken L, Carson J, Eccleston C, Keefe F. Acceptance and change in the context of chronic pain. *Pain*,2004;109:4–7.

McCracken L and Eccleston C. A prospective study of acceptance of pain and patient functioning with chronic pain. *Pain*, 2005;118:164–69.

McCracken L and Vowles K. Psychological flexibility and traditional pain management strategies in relation to patient functioning with chronic pain: An examination of a revised instrument. *J. of Pain*, 2007;8:700–7.

McCracken L, Vowles K, and Eccleston C. Acceptance of Chronic Pain: Component analysis and a revised assessment method. *Pain*, 2004;107:159–66.

McGaugh J. *Memory and Emotion: The Making of Lasting Memories.* New York: Columbia University Press, 2006.

McKay J. Assessing aspects of object relations associated with immune function: Development of the Affiliative Trust-Mistrust coding system. *Psychological Assessment*, 1991;3(4):641–47.

McLintock T, Aitken H, Downie C, and Kenny G. Postoperative analgesic requirements in patients exposed to intraoperative suggestions. *British Medical J*, 1990;301:788–90.

McQuade J, Carmona P, and Segal Z. *Peaceful Mind: Using Mindfulness and Cognitive Behavioral Psychology to Overcome Depression.* Oakland, CA: New Harbinger, 2004.

Meares A. *Strange Places, Simple Truths.* London: Fontana, 1973.

———. What can a patient expect from intensive meditation? *Australian Family Physician*, 1980;9,322–25.

Meecham W. Consultation with physician and visionary Will Meecham in early January 2013.

Moore T. *Care of the Soul.* New York: HarperCollins, 1993.

Morone N, Lynch C, Greco C, Tindle H, and Weiner D. "I feel like a new person." The effects of mindfulness meditation on older adults with chronic pain: A qualitative narrative analysis of diary entries. *J. of Pain*, 2008;9:841–48.

Morris T, Greer S, Pettingale K, and Watson M. Patterns of expression of anger and their psychological correlates in women with breast cancer. *J of Psychosomatic Research*, 1981;25:111–17.

Murdock R. *Patient Number One: A True Story of How One CEO Took on Cancer and Big Business in the Fight of His Life.* New York: Crown, 2000.

Murphy M. *The Future of the Body: Explorations into the Further Evolution of Human Nature.* Los Angeles: Tarcher, 1992.

Nielsen L and Kaszniak A. Awareness of subtle emotional feelings: a comparison of long-term meditators and nonmeditators. *Emotion,* 2006;6:392–405.

Null G. *Death by Medicine.* Mt. Jackson, VA: Praktikos Books, 2010.

O'Cleirigh C, Ironson G, and Smits J. Does Distress Tolerance Moderate the Impact of Major Life Events on Psychosocial Variables and Behaviors Important in the Management of HIV? *Behavior Therapy,* 2007;vol. 38;3:314–23.

Olian S. Caring for a Loved One at Home. Interview published on my website 9/12/12.

Oliner S. *Do Unto Others: Extraordinary Acts of Ordinary People.* New York: Basic Books, 2004.

Oliver C. *Cautious Care: A Guide for Patients.* Self-published, 2009.

Ong A, Bergeman C, Bisconti T, and Wallace K. Psychological resilience, positive emotions, and successful adaptation to stress in later life. *J of Personality and Social Psychology,* 2006;91:730–49.

O'Regan B and Hirshberg C. *Spontaneous Remission: An Annotated Bibliography.* Sausalito, CA: Institute of Noetic Sciences, 1993.

Ornstein R and Sobel D. *The Healing Brain: Breakthrough Medical Discoveries About How the Brain Manages Health.* New York: Simon and Schuster, 1987.

Orth-Gomer K, Rosengren A, and Wilhelmsen L. Lack of social support and incidence of coronary heart disease in middle-aged Swedish men. *Psychosomatic Medicine,* 1993;55 (1):37–43.

Orth-Gomer K and Unden A. Type A behavior, social support, and coronary risk: Interaction and significance for mortality in cardiac patients. *Psychosomatic Medicine,* 1990;52:59–72.

Oster N, Thomas L, and Joseff D. *Making Informed Medical Decisions.* Sebastopol, CA: O'Reilly & Associates, 2000.

Pagnoni G and Cekic M. Age effects on gray matter volume and attentional performance in Zen meditation. *Neurobiology of Aging,* 2007;28:1623–27.

Paul-Labrador M, Polk D, Dwyer J, Velazquez I, Nidich S, Rainforth M, Schneider R, and Merz N. Effects of randomized controlled trial of transcendental meditation on components of the metabolic syndrome in subjects with coronary heart disease. *Archives of Internal Medicine,* 2006;166:1218–24.

Pennebaker J. Writing about emotional experiences as a therapeutic process. *Psychological Science,* 1997;8:162–66.

Pennebaker J and Graybeal A. Patterns of natural language use: Disclosure, personality, and social integration. *Current Directions in Psychological Science,* 2001;10:90–93.

Pennebaker J, Kiecolt-Glaser J, and Glaser R. Disclosures of traumas and immune function: health implications for psychotherapy. *J. of Consult. Clinical Psychol,* 1988;56:239–45.

Pennebaker J, Mayne T, and Francis M. Linguistic predictors of adaptive bereavement. *J of Personality and Social Psychology,* 1997;72:863–71.

Peper E. Applied Psychophysiology and Biofeedback Annual Conference, 2008.

Pert C. *Molecules of Emotion: Why You Feel the Way You Feel.* New York: Simon and Schuster, 1997.

Peterson C, Maier S, and Seligman M. *Learned Helplessness.* New York: Oxford University Press, 1993.

Peterson C, Seligman M, and Valliant G. Pessimistic explanatory style as a risk factor for physical illness: a thirty-five-year longitudinal study. *J. of Personality and Social Psychology,* 1988;55: 23–27.

Pettingale K, Greer S, and Tee D. Serum IgA and emotional expression in breast cancer patients. *J. of Psychosomatic Research,* 1977;21 (5):395–99.

Pettus M. *The Savvy Patient.* Hendon, VA: Capital Books, 2004.

Phongsuphap S, Pongsupap Y, Chandanmattha P, and Lursinsap C. Changes in heart rate variability during concentration meditation. *J. of Cardiology,* 2008;130(3):481–84.

Preston J. Integrating Psychotherapy, Neuroscience, and Eastern Healing Traditions. Professional conference, San Rafael, CA, March 7, 2009.

Price D and Fields H. The Contribution of Desire and Expectation to Placebo Analgesia: Implications for New Research Strategies. In Harrington A (ed.), *The Placebo Effect: An Interdisciplinary Exploration.* Cambridge, MA: Harvard University Press, 1997.

Price M, Tennant C, and Butow P. The role of psychosocial factors in the development of breast carcinoma: Part II: Life event stressors, social support, defense style, and emotional control and their interactions. *Cancer,* 2001;91(4):686–97.

Pronovost P and Vohr E. *Safe Patients, Smart Hospitals.* New York: Plume, 2011.

Reich M. Depression and cancer: recent data on clinical issues, research challenges and treatment approaches. *Current Opinion in Oncology*, 2008;20(4):353–59.

Roemer L and Orsillo S. *Mindfulness- and Acceptance-Based Behavioral Therapies in Practice*. New York: Guilford, 2009.

Rook K. The negative side of social interaction: Impact on psychological well-being. *J of Personality and Social Psychology*, 1984;46:1097–1108.

Rosenbaum E. *Here for Now: Living Well with Cancer Through Mindfulness*. Hardwick, MA: Satya House Publications, 2007.

Rosenberg I. An Exercise to Train Heart and Breath without Equipment. *Newsletter of the California Society of Biofeedback*, 1988;4(1).

Rossi E. *Psychobiology of Mind-Body Healing*. New York: Norton, 1993.

Rossman M. *Guided Imagery for Self-Healing*. Novato, CA: H. J. Kramer, 2000.

Rossman M and Bresler D. Academy for Guided Imagery Certification Training, 2007. "Special Place" and "Inner Advisor" guided imagery in the current form are the creation of Martin Rossman, MD, and David Bresler, PhD, originally adapted from the work of Irving Oyle, MD.

Roth B and Stanley T. Mindfulness-based stress reduction and healthcare utilization in the inner city: Preliminary findings. *Alternative Therapies*, 2002;8:60–66.

Ruggieri P. *Confessions of a Surgeon: The Good, the Bad, and the Complicated*. New York: Berkley, 2012.

Russell T. *I Need an Operation… Now What?* Montvale, NJ: Thomson Healthcare, 2008.

Salters-Pedneault K, Tull M, and Roemer L. The role of avoidance of emotional material in anxiety disorders. *Applied and Preventive Psychology: Current Scientific Perspectives*, 2004;11:95–114.

Scherg H. Psychosocial factors and disease bias in breast cancer patients. *J of Psychosomatic Medicine*, 1987;49:302–12.

Schneider S. *The Patient from Hell*. New York: Da Capo, 2005.

Schulz U, Pischke C, Weidner G, Daubenmier J, Elliot-Eller M, Scherwitz L, Bullinger M, and Ornish D. Social support group attendance is related to blood pressure, health behaviours, and quality of life in the Multicenter Lifestyle Demonstration Project. *Psychology Health Medicine*, 2008;13(4):423–27.

Schwartz G. Psychobiology of repression and health: A systems approach. In Singer J. (ed.), *Repression and Dissociation: Implications for Personality Theory, Psychopathology, and Health.* Chicago: University of Chicago Press, 1990.

Segal Z, Williams J, and Teasdale J. *Mindfulness-Based Cognitive Therapy for Depression.* New York: Guilford, 2002.

Seligman M. *Learned Optimism: How to Change Your Mind and Your Life.* New York: Random House, 2006.

Sephton S, Salmon P, Weissbecker I, Ulmer C, Floyd A, and Hoover K. Mindfulness meditation alleviates depressive symptoms in women with fibromyalgia: Results of a randomized clinical trial. *Arthritis and Rheumatism,* 2007;57(1):77–85.

Shaffer J, Duszynski K, and Thomas C. Family attitudes in youth as a possible precursor of cancer among physicians: A search for explanatory mechanisms. *J of Behavioral Medicine,* 1982;5:143–63.

Shaffer J, Graves P, Swank R, and Pearson T. Clustering of personality traits in youth and the subsequent development of cancer among physicians. *J of Behavioral Medicine,* 1987;10:441–47.

Shapiro S and Carlson L. *The Art and Science of Mindfulness: Integrating Mindfulness into Psychology and the Helping Professions.* Washington, DC: American Psychological Association, 2009.

Sheldon K and Elliot A. Goal striving, need satisfaction, and longitudinal well-being: The self-concordance model. *J of Personality and Social Psychology,* 1999;76:546–57.

Sheldon K and Lyubomirsky S. Achieving sustainable gains in happiness: Change your actions, not your circumstances. *J of Happiness Studies,* 2006;7:55–86.

Siegel B. Mind over cancer: An exclusive interview with Yale surgeon Dr. Bernie Siegel. *Prevention,* 1988;March:59–64.

Siever D. *The role of audio-visual entrainment in seniors' issues.* Annual AAPB Meeting, 2006.

Simonton O and Henson R. *The Healing Journey.* New York: Author's Choice, 2002.

Simonton O and Matthews-Simonton S. Cancer and stress: counseling the cancer patient. *Medical Journal of Australia,* 1981;27:679–83.

Simonton O, Matthews-Simonton S, and Creighton J. *Getting Well Again.* Los Angeles: Tarcher, 1978.

Simonton Cancer Center—Certification Training, 2006, 2007, 2008. Most of the tools taught to the cancer patients at the Simonton retreats have been created by O. Carl Simonton, MD, and are unpublished.

Sobel D. The cost-effectiveness of mind-body medicine interventions. *Progress in Brain Research,* 2000;122:393–412.

———. Rethinking medicine: improving health outcomes with cost-effective psychosocial interventions. *Psychosomatic Medicine,* 1995;57,234–44.

Solberg E, Halvorsen R, Sundgot-Borgen J, Ingjer F, and Holen A. Meditation: A modulator of the immune response to physical stress? A brief report. *British J. of Sport and Medicine,* 1995;29: 255–57.

Solomon G. Emotions, Stress and Immunity. In Ornstein R and Swencionis C (ed.), *The Healing Brain: A Scientific Reader.* New York: Guilford, 1990.

Solomon G, Fiatarone M, Benton D, Morley J, Bloom E, and Makinodan T. Psychoneuroimmunologic and endorphin function in the aged. *Annals of the New York Academy of Sciences,* 1988;521:43–58.

Speca M, Carlson L, Goody E, and Angen M. A randomized wait-list controlled trial: The effect of a mindfulness meditation-based stress reduction program on mood and symptoms of stress in cancer outpatients. *Psychosomatic Medicine,* 2000;62: 613–22.

Spiegel D. Effects of psychotherapy on cancer survival. *Nature Reviews Cancer,* 2002;2(5):383–89.

Spiegel D and Classen C. *Group Therapy for Cancer Patients: A Research-Based Handbook of Psychosocial Care.* New York: Basic Books, 2000.

Stavraky K, Donner A, Kincade J, and Stewart M. The effect of psychosocial factors on lung cancer mortality at one year. *J of Clinical Epidemiology,* 1988;41:75–82.

Sternbach R. The effects of instructional sets on autonomic responsivity. *Psychophysiology,* 1964;1(1):67–72.

Stuban S. *The Butcher's Daughter: The Story of an Army Nurse with ALS.* Virtualbookworm.com, 2009.

Suarez E and Blumenthal J. Ambulatory blood pressure responses during daily life in high and low hostile patients with a recent myocardial infarction. *J of Cardiopulmonary Rehabilitation,* 1991;11:169–75.

Suarez E, Shiller A, Kuhn C, Schanberg S, Williams R, and Zimmermann E. The relationship between hostility and beta adrenergic receptor physiology in healthy young males. *Psychosomatic Medicine,* 1997;59:481–87.

Suls J and Wan C. The relationship between trait hostility and cardiovascular reactivity: a quantitative analysis. *Psychophysiology,* 1993;30:615–26.

Tarrier N. Commentary: Yes, cognitive behaviour therapy may well be all you need. *BMJ*, 2002;324:291–92.

Tart C. *States of Consciousness*. Lincoln, NE: Authors Guild Back-InPrint.com Edition, 2000.

Teasdale J, Segal Z, and Williams J. Mindfulness and problem formulation. *Clinical Psychology: Science and Practice*, 2003; 10:157–60.

Temoshok L. Biopsychosocial studies on cutaneous malignant melanoma: Psychosocial factors associated with prognostic indicators, progression, psychophysiology and tumor-host response. *Social Science and Medicine*, 1985;20(8):833–40.

———. Personality, coping style, emotion and cancer: Towards an integrative model. *Cancer Surveys*, 1987;6(3):545–67.

Temoshok L and Dreher H. *The Type C Connection: The Behavioral Links to Cancer and Your Health*. New York: Random House. 1992.

Thomas C, Duszynski K, and Shaffer J. Family attitudes reported in youth as potential predictors of cancer. *J of Psychosomatic Medicine*, 1979;41:287–482.

Torrey T. *You Bet Your Life! The 10 Mistakes Every Patient Makes*. Baldwinsville, NY: Langdon Street Press, 2010.

Travis F and Arenander A. Cross-sectional and longitudinal study of effects of transcendental meditation practice on interhemispheric frontal asymmetry and frontal coherence. *International J. of Neuroscience*, 2006;116:1519–38.

Treadway M and Lazar S. The Neurobiology of Mindfulness. In Didonna F (ed.), *Clinical Handbook of Mindfulness*. New York: Springer, 2009.

Tsuji H, Venditti F, and Manders E. Reduced heart rate variability and mortality risk in an elderly cohort: The Framingham Heart Study. *Circulation*, 1994;90(2):878–83.

Tull M, Barrett H, McMillan E, and Roemer L. A preliminary investigation of the relationship between emotion regulation difficulties and posttraumatic stress symptoms. *Behavior Therapy*, 2007;38:303–13.

Tull M, Rodman S, and Roemer L. An examination of the fear of bodily sensations and body hypervigilance as predictors of emotion regulation difficulties among individuals with a recent history of uncued panic attacks. *J. of Anxiety Disorders*, 2008;22(4):750–60.

Tull M and Roemer L. Emotion regulation difficulties associated with the experience of uncued panic attacks: Evidence of experiential avoidance, emotional nonacceptance, and decreased emotional clarity. *Behavior Therapy*. 2007;38:378–91.

Turner-Cobbs J, Sephton S, and Spiegel D. Psychosocial effects of immune function and disease progression in cancer: Human studies. In Ader R, Felton D, and Cohen N (ed.), *Psychoneuroimmunology*, 3rd edition. San Diego: Academic Press, 2001.

Twohig M, Hayes S, and Masuda A. Increasing willingness to experience obsessions: Acceptance and Commitment Therapy as a treatment for obsessive-compulsive disorder. *Behavior Therapy,* 2006;37(1),3–13.

Ubel P. *Critical Decisions.* New York: Harper Collins, 2012.

Uchino B, Cacioppo J, and Kiecolt-Glaser J. The relationship between social support and physiological processes: a review with emphasis on underlying mechanisms and implications for health. *Psychological Bulletin,* 1996;119(3):4480–531.

Vaillant G. *Aging Well.* New York: Little, Brown, 2003.

Van Wielingen L, Carlson L, and Campbell T. Mindfulness-based stress reduction (MBSR), blood pressure, and psychological functioning in women with cancer. *Psychosomatic Medicine,* 2007;69:A43.

Vaschillo E, Vaschillo B, and Lehrer P. Characteristics of Resonance in Heart Rate Variability Stimulated by Biofeedback. *Applied Psychophysiology and Biofeedback,* 2006;31;2,129–42.

Wachter R. *Understanding Patient Safety.* New York: McGraw-Hill, 2012.

Wachter R and Shojania K. *Internal Bleeding.* New York: Rugged Land, 2004.

Walker L, Hays S, and Walker M. Psychosocial factors can predict the response to primary chemotherapy in patients with locally advanced breast cancer. *European J of Cancer,* 1999;35:1783–88.

Walsh R and Shapiro S. The meeting of meditative disciplines and Western psychology: A mutually enriching dialogue. *American Psychologist,* 2006;61:227–39.

Waxler-Morrison N, Hislop T, Meares B, and Kan L. Effects of social relationships on survival for women with breast cancer: a prospective study. *Society for Science in Medicine,* 1991;33:177–83.

Wegner D. Ironic processes of mental control. *Psychological Review,* 1994;101:34–52.

Wegner D, Ansfield M, and Pilloff D. The putt and the pendulum: Ironic effects of the mental control of action. *Psychological Science,* 1998;9:196–99.

Wenzlaff R and Wegner D. Thought suppression. *Annual Review of Psychology*, 2000;51:59–91.

Williams J. *The Patient Advocate's Handbook.* Panglossian Press, 2007.

Williams M, Teasdale J, Segal Z, and Kabat-Zinn J. *The Mindful Way through Depression: Freeing Yourself from Chronic Unhappiness.* New York: Guilford, 2007.

Wilson K and Murrell A. Values work in acceptance and commitment therapy: Setting a course for behavioral treatment. In Hayes S, Follette V, and Linehan M (ed.), *Mindfulness and Acceptance: Expanding the Cognitive-Behavioral Tradition.* New York: Guilford, 2004.

Wolever R and Best J. Mindfulness-based approaches to eating disorders. In Didonna F (ed.), *Clinical Handbook of Mindfulness.* New York: Springer, 2009.

Wolf S, Grace K, Bruhn J, and Stout C. Roseto revisited: further data on the incidence of myocardial infarction in Roseto and neighboring Pennsylvania communities. *Transactions of the American Clinical Climatological Assoc.,* 1974;85:100–8.

Wolf S and Pinsky R. Effects of placebo administration and occurence of toxic reactions. *JAMA,* 1954;155(4):339.

Index

Abamowitz, Jonathan, 177

ACC (anterior cingulate cortex), 83

acceptance, 48–49, 102. *see also* non-acceptance; self-acceptance
of disability, 94
of disease, 173–74
in mindfulness, 67
of pain, 94, 115, 174–75
and suffering, 175

Acceptance and Commitment Therapy (ACT), 40, 50, 57, 70, 80, 95

ACT. *see* Acceptance and Commitment Therapy

actors, 262

addictions, 41–42, 88

Addison's disease, 3

advance directives, 292–93

aggressiveness, 186

aging, 88–91, 221–24

AIDS, 182

alertness, 345–46

alexithymia, 184, 190

Allington, Herman, 332

Allman, John, 343

allostatic load, 12, 320–24

alpha/theta training, 81–82

altered state of consciousness (ASC), 25, 31

altruism, 205–8, 209–10. *see also* caregiving

Alzheimer's disease, 211

anabolic state, 347

analysis, 105, 113
and energy, 80
and suffering, 45

Andrews, Howard, 206–7, 208

anger, 172, 184, 186–88

anterior cingulate cortex (ACC), 83

antidepressants, 55, 213, 318

anxiety, 44, 58, 259
acceptance of, 175–76
and brain activity, 84
generalized anxiety disorder, 323–24
and immune system, 97
and PCA, 328

Arch, Joanna, 343

Arnetz, Bengt, 222

ASC (altered state of consciousness), 25, 31

assertiveness, 186, 193, 289

asthma, and placebos, 330–31

atrial fibrillation, 252

attachment to outcomes, 30

attachment to recovery, 94

attributions, 29–30

authenticity, 176, 181–82, 191–95

autogenic imagery, 152

autoimmune diseases, 3. *see also* immune system

aversions and fears, 172

avoidance, 20. *see also* experiential avoidance
of unpleasant states, 173

awareness, 68–69, 141–45

bare attention, 105–6

Barefoot, John, 186

beginner's mind, 71–72

behavior
    changes in, 261–62
    and symptoms, 275

belief. *see also* core beliefs
    and drug marketing, 341
    and language, 45
    and placebos, 329–31 *(see also* placebos)
    power of, 338

belonging, 209, 220, 230–31, 233–34

Benson, Herbert, 340

Berk, Lee, 238

Berkman, Lisa, 220

beta blockers, 334

Bhaerman, Steve, 69

Bigger, J. Thomas, 344

biomarkers, 275–76

bipolar disorder, 18

Bishop, Scott, 67

blame, 140

Blindsided (Cohen), 173

Bloch, Bruno, 335

Blumenthal, James, 187

body mechanics, 163, 164–65

body scan, 115

Bonanno, George, 238, 241

borderline personality disorder, 18

Bower, Julienne, 202

Brain Droppings (Carlin), 18

brain function
    biochemistry of stressful thoughts, 318–20
    and immune system, 92
    long-term potentiation and, 315

mindfulness practice and, 83–88
    neurotransmitters, 316–18

Brantley, Jeffrey, 67–68

breath-holding, 348

breathing, 174, 248–53, 312
    and alertness, 345–46
    breath-holding, 348
    and control, 167, 347
    as form of self-regulation, 346
    gas exchange and, 343–44
    and happiness, 347
    and health, 343–49
    hyperventilation, 348
    optimal rate, 349
    and peptides, 347
    research on, 343
    resonant frequency breathing, 346
    respiratory sinus arrhythmia (RSA), 345–47
    and self-esteem, 164

bringing awareness, 68–69

Brown, Stephanie, 208

Buddhism
    and effects of mindfulness practice, 84–85
    vipassana, 81, 88, 104–5, 225

Burch, Vidyamala, 174

burden, fear of being, 305–6

The Butcher's Daughter (Stuban), 312

Butler, Robert, 199

caffeine, 346

cancer
    causes of, 95–96
    and emotional suppression, 184
    gratitude and, 153
    mindfulness practice and, 95–99

purpose and, 199, 202
and self-expression,
187–88, 190
support and, 228–29

cardiac disease. *see* heart
disease

cardiovascular disease. *see*
heart disease

caregivers, professional, 299,
301

caregiving
asking for help, 305–6
benefits of, 210–11, 298 (*see
also* altruism)
conscious choice and,
301–2
effects of on health, 210–11
gratitude and, 311–12
grieving and, 295–96
hope and optimism and,
309–11
loss of identity and, 295
and loving self-care, 303,
308
mindfulness practice and,
304
personality changes and,
297
proactive caregiving,
298–301
reevaluation and, 296
sense of meaning and
purpose and, 308–9
spouses and, 297–98
Stop-Breathe-Feel, 312
troubling thoughts and,
307–8
values and, 309

caring, 212. *see also* service

Carlin, George, 18

Carlson, Linda, 66–67, 79, 96

catabolic state, 322–24, 347

catecholamine, 187

categorical and judgmental
thought, 33

celiac disease, 4

cell function, 316

cell phones, 274

Center for Independent Living, 299

chemotherapy, 96, 153

choice, 309
in caregiving, 301–2
confluence with practice,
141
declaring, 133–36
empowerment and,
300–301
examples of, 130–31
and gratitude, 155
guidelines for, 132–33
living by, 128–30
practices, 132–36
of self-care, 158–59

choice, conscious, 128, 301–2

choice, unconscious, 133

cholesterol, 337–38

chronic illness. *see* illness,
chronic

chronic pain, 93–95

cis-platinum, 340

clinical trials, 279, 292

Cobb, Julie, 186

coffee, 346

cognitive decline, effects of
mindfulness on, 88–91

cognitive fusion
antidotes to, 109
attachment to outcomes
and, 30
attributions and, 29–30
core beliefs and, 20–21, 28,
34–35
dangers of, 30–33
definition and overview,
25–26
FEAR and, 19–20
forms of, 27–30

language and, 33–34
mindfulness and, 26
new symptoms and, 57
questions for self-study,
   35–37
rumination, 28–29
suffering and, 16–17, 27
Cohen, Richard, 173
communication, respectful,
   288–89
community, joining, 233. *see
   also* belonging; support/
   support groups
compartmentalization, 246
concentration, 84, 90
conceptualized self, 17–18, 27
conflicts of interest, 281
connectedness, 205–8, 220. *see
   also* relationships; service;
   support/support groups;
   volunteer work
   and medical appoint-
      ments, 213–14
   practicing, 214–16
consciousness, shifting,
   265–67
control, 5, 61–62, 90–91,
   246–47
   and breathing, 347
   and outcomes, 300–301
   and PCA, 328
   and serotonin levels, 317
core beliefs, 20–21, 28, 34–35
cortisol, 79–80, 83, 96, 153,
   187, 317
Costa Rica, 211
Cousins, Norman, 241–42
cramping, 258
Crane, Rebecca, 28
Craske, Michelle, 343
Crohn's disease, 3
Csikszentmihalyi, Mihali, 70

curiosity, 67

Dalai Lama, 22, 84
Davidson, Richard, 83, 84, 86,
   87, 92, 201
DBT (Dialectical Behavior
   Therapy), 68
death
   approaching, 203
   dying mode, 203
   dying phase, 60–61
   of loved ones, 202
decision making, 39, 309, 311
dehydroepiandrosterone
   (DHEA), 153
dependence, *vs.* mastery, 259
Depner, Charlene, 223
depression
   and brain activity, 84
   and chronic illness, 55, 58
   and gratitude, 154
   and immune system, 320
   and meaning and purpose,
      213
   and placebos, 339
   and rumination, 28
   and self-care mastery, 271
   and serotonin levels, 317
   treatment for, 317–18
describing, in mindfulness,
   69, 70
DHEA (dehydroepiandros-
   terone), 153
diagnoses, idiopathic, 284
diagnosis, differential, 274–75
diagnosis, reaction to, 53
diagnostic tests, 275–76
Didonna, Fabrizio, 72
differential diagnosis, 274–75
Dimidjian, Sona, 68–69
discomfort. *see also* distress,
   emotional; suffering

avoiding, 173
experiential avoidance
and, 44
mindfulness practice and,
109–11
need for changes and,
255–67
pain, 93–95, 115–16
and unconscious choices,
133
disengaging, 106
dissociation, 46–47, 245–46,
247–48
dissociative identity disorder, 262–63, 266
distraction, 46–47, 245,
246–47
distress, emotional. *see also*
discomfort; stress, physiological; suffering
allostatic loads, 320–24
avoiding, 173
biochemistry of stressful
thoughts, 318–20
denying, 185
effects of, 11–14, 321–24
epigenetics and, 324–26
immunosuppression and,
326–27
memories and, 22–23
mindfulness practice and,
109–11
prodromes and, 81
self-expression and,
186–88
DNR (do not resuscitate), 293
doctors. *see* physicians
documentation, 289–93
dopamine, 87–88, 334–35
drug packaging, 332
drugs. *see* medication
drugs, endogenously pro-
duced, 327–28
drug studies, 336–37

durable power of attorney for
healthcare, 293
dying mode, 203
dying phase, 60–61
dysthymia, 28. *see also* depression

economics of screening tests,
276
ego, 18
Eisenhower, Dwight D., 3
Ekman, Paul, 21–22
elderly people. *see* aging
Elliot, Andrew, 201
emergency departments, 273
Emerson, Ralph Waldo, 169
Emmons, Robert, 149, 151
emotions. *see also* experiential
avoidance
function of, 39
recognizing, 188, 192–93,
244
suppressing, 184
suppression *vs.* repression,
185–86
emotions, negative, 181, 184,
186
empathy, 60, 234
The Empowered Patient (Hallisy), 285
emWave, 152, 252
endogenous pharmacy,
327–28
energy levels, 80–81
epigenetics, 324–26
equanimity, 86
evaluating/judging, 20–21,
105
in mindfulness, 71–72
exercise, 163, 257, 259

expectations, 329–31, 339–41.
    see also placebos
experience, present, 71, 73,
    313
experiential avoidance. see
    also acceptance
    as cause of suffering, 17
    definition and overview,
    39–40
    discomfort and, 44
    dissociation/distraction
    and, 46–47
    effects of, 39
    examples of, 41–45
    FEAR and, 20
    healthy, 46–47
    "healthy" techniques, 43
    intimacy and, 46
    mindfulness and, 40
    paradox and, 44–45, 47, 48
    physiology of, 47–49
    self-acceptance and,
    170–71
    writing exercise for, 49–50
explanatory style, 73–74, 75,
    78. see also self-talk
eye of hurricane, 243–44

fatigue, 93–95
Fawzy, Fawzy, 183
FEAR (fusion, evaluation,
    avoidance, reason-giving),
    19–20
fears and aversions, 172
feedback loops, 82
fibromyalgia, 94
fight or flight. see sympathet-
    ic arousal
flexibility, psychological,
    21–22, 78, 88–89, 255–56
flow, 70
Fox, Michael J., 174, 240–41
Francis, Martha, 188

Frankl, Viktor, 202
FreezeFramer, 152
Fricchione, Gregory, 187
friendships, 165, 296. see also
    relationships
fusion. see cognitive fusion
Futterman, Ann, 262

GAD (generalized anxiety
    disorder), 323–24
gastric activity, 338
Gawler, Ian, 97–98, 264–65,
    311
generalized anxiety disorder
    (GAD), 323–24
genetics, 324–26
Gerson, Max, 98
Get Out of Your Mind and Into
    Your Life (Hayes), 49–50
getting well, attachment to,
    57
Gevirtz, Richard, 348
Glaser, Ronald, 228
goals, 121, 201–2
gobbledygook, 106
Gordon, James S., 212
gratitude
    and cancer, 153
    and caregiving, 311–12
    effects of practicing, 149
    and happiness, 149–51
    practicing, 154–56
Greer, Steven, 183, 184, 185
Greeson, Jeffrey, 67–68
Groopman, Jerome, 278
Gross, James, 48
Grossman, Paul, 79

Hallisy, Julia, 285
Hanson, Bertil, 226

happiness, 86, 149–51, 206, 347

Hawking, Stephen, 198

Hayes, Steven C., 49, 70, 113, 177

headache, 258

heart disease, 224–27, 334

heart health, and MBSR, 96

heart rate variability (HRV), 152–53, 251, 323, 344–47

help, asking for, 191–92, 305–6

helplessness, 5–6, 143

Hirshberg, Caryle, 263

histone markers, 325

Hölzel, Britta, 87, 343

hope, 327

hopelessness, 5–6, 143

Horsten, Myriam, 345

hostility, 186–188, 194

House, James, 208, 221

How Doctors Think (Groopman), 278

HPA axis, 318–319

HRV (heart rate variability), 152–53, 251, 323, 344–47

Hughes, J. W., 345

humor, 237–42

hyperventilation, 344, 348

hypothalamic pituitary axis, 318–19

"I am," 33

identification with illness, 56–57, 60

idiopathic diagnoses, 284

illness, chronic
    attachment to getting well and, 57
    body mechanics and, 164–65
    control and, 5, 61–62
    demographic data, 3
    depression and anxiety and, 58
    effects of, 58
    identification with illness and, 56–57, 60
    living a normal life with, 61
    new symptoms and, 57
    and putting life on hold, 54–56
    support and, 59–60
    and unnecessary suffering, 56–58

imagination, 310–11

immune system, 91–93, 181, 227–28. *see also* autoimmune diseases
    and anxiety, 97
    and stress, 93, 326–27
    and sympathetic arousal, 320

impatience, 90–91

impulsiveness, 18

inaction, 18

inflexibility, 21–22. *see also* flexibility

Ingersoll-Dayton, Berit, 223

insight, 71

insight meditation, 104–5

insurance, and screenings, 275

intention, conscious, 140

intention setting, 128, 132–33. *see also* Valued-Action Practice

internal feedback loops, 82

intimacy, 46

intranets, 287

isolation, 59, 191, 220, 227

Jamner, Larry, 184
Japanese
    and heart disease, 225–26
    Okinawans, 211
Jensen, Mogens, 185
journaling, 83, 154–55,
    188–89, 193
    and goals, 201
    and gratitude, 151
    and self-expression, 193
    and trauma, 48
Journey to Wild Divine, 252
joy, 328
judging/evaluating, 20–21,
    105
    in mindfulness, 71–72

Kabat-Zinn, Jon, 65–66, 74,
    93, 95, 101
Kamiya, Joe, 237
Karmu studies, 232–33
Kaszniak, Alfred, 244
Katz, Roger, 198
Keltner, Dacher, 238, 241
Kemeny, Margaret, 202, 319
Kennedy, John F., 3
Kennedy, Susan, 227
Kiecolt-Glaser, Janice, 12,
    222, 227, 326
King, Laura, 201
Kop, Johan, 187
Krishnamurti, Jiddu, 108
Kristeller, Jean, 67

labeling, 20–21, 105
    in mindfulness, 69, 70
labile personalities, 262–63,
    266
lab techs, 285
Langer, Ellen, 30, 88, 89, 90

language, 33–34, 45
laughing clubs, 239–40
laughter, 238. see also humor
Lehrer, Paul, 348
LeShan, Lawrence, 112, 169,
    182, 198, 200, 203, 235
lethargy, 259
Levenson, Robert, 48
life values. see values
Lightner, Candy, 202, 204
limitations
    belief in, 89
    hiding, 173
Linehan, Marsha, 68–69
Lipton, Bruce, 69
living by choice. see also
    choice
    examples, 130–31
    guidelines for, 132–33
    overview, 128–30
    practices, 132–36
living wills, 292–93
long-term potentiation, 315
love, 231
lovingkindness, 67, 162
loving self-care. see also self-
    care mastery
    attention needed for, 158
    benefits of, 157–58
    body mechanics and,
        164–65
    and caregiving, 303, 308
    choice of, 158–59
    and depression, 58
    and exercise, 163
    gratitude and, 151–52
    in hospital, 159–60
    mindfulness and, 157–59
    needs vs. wants, 161–62
    relationships and, 165
    suggestions for practice of,
        166–67

walking mindfully and, 164–65

Luks, Allan, 208

Luoma, Jason, 17, 171

Lutz, Antoine, 87

Lyubomirsky, Sonja, 149–51, 201, 206, 211

MADD. *see* Mothers Against Drunk Driving

Manne, Sharon, 198

Marlatt, Alan, 67

Marmot, Michael, 225

mastery, 5–6, 74, 121. *see also* self-care mastery
  goal of, 312
  and health, 91
  and "I am choosing" practice, 133

Maunsell, Elizabeth, 229

MBCT. *see* Mindfulness-Based Cognitive Therapy

MBSR. *see* Mindfulness-Based Stress Reduction

McClelland, David, 231, 232–33

McCracken, Lance, 175

McCullough, Michael, 151

McGaugh, James, 78

McKay, James, 231

meaning and purpose
  caregiving and, 308–9
  cultivation of, 203–4
  and depression, 213
  goal-setting and, 201–2
  health and, 198–202
  in illness, 197–98
  in loss of loved ones, 202
  and survival rates, 200

Meares, Ainsley, 97–99

medical appointments, 213–14, 300

medical records, 274, 290–91, 300

medical self-efficacy, 271. *see also* self-care mastery

medication, 154, 173, 259, 260–61, 286. *see also* antidepressants; placebos
  drug packaging, 332
  drug studies, 336–37
  effectiveness of, 340–41
  effects of, 327
  effects on cell function, 316
  marketing of, 341
  and personality changes, 297
  and physician expectations, 339–41
  and recovery, 49

meditation, 84–87, 88, 89–90. *see also* mindfulness practice
  and conscious breathing practices, 347
  and pain, 115–16
  use of term, 72
  vipassana, 81, 88, 104–5, 106, 255
  vs. mindfulness, 90

meditation, Buddhist, 62

meditation, insight, 104–5

meditation, transcendental, 88, 89–90, 92

melatonin, 80

memories, 42, 149

Mendius, Richard, 345

meprobamate, 340

methylation, 325

metta, 85

Millan, Cesar, 164

mindfulness. *see also* mindfulness practice
  aging, 88–91
  alternatives to, 245–47

benefits of, 72–73, 77–78, 84

brain function and, 83–88

cancer and, 95–99

chronic pain and fatigue and, 93–95

cognitive fusion and, 26

defined, 65–71

dissociation/distraction and, 46–47

effects on cognitive decline, 88–91

emotional distress and, 14, 22–23

energy levels and, 80–81

experiential avoidance and, 40

explanatory style and, 73–74, 75

and flexibility, 255–56

formal, 113–14

goal of, 73, 101–2

immune system and, 91–93

importance of, 7–8

inaction/impulsiveness and, 18

informal, 114–15

loving self-care and, 157–59

Mindfulness-Based Cognitive Therapy, 71, 172

Mindfulness-Based Stress Reduction, 79–80, 83–84, 92, 96–97, 103

moods and, 21

new symptoms and, 57

and physiological functioning, 34

as practice, 65–66

prodromes, 81–83

related terms, 71–72

as training exercise, 69–70

vs. meditation, 90

as way of life, 65–66, 73, 98

Mindfulness-Based Cognitive Therapy (MBCT), 71, 172

Mindfulness-Based Stress Reduction (MBSR), 79–80

and brain activity, 83–84

and cancer, 96–97

and immune system, 92

and introduction to mindfulness, 103

mindfulness practice. see also meditation; mindfulness; Valued-Action Practice

caregiving and, 304

formal vs. informal, 106–8

getting started, 103–4

informal, 106–11

mortality and, 111–13

neutral observation and, 102–3

pain and, 115–16

self-acceptance and, 171–72

suggestions, 113–15

symptoms and, 108–11

vipassana and, 81, 88, 104–5

mindlessness, 26

mind-watching, 102–3

mitral valve prolapse, 252

mobile devices, 274

mood disorders, treatment of, 84

moods, 21–22

Moore, Thomas, 233

morbidity and mortality. see also survival rates

and relationships, 220–21

morning sickness, 338–39

morphine, 333–34

Morris, Tina, 184

mortality, 111–13

Mothers Against Drunk Driving (MADD), 202

multiple identity disorder, 262–63, 266

needs
identifying through discomfort, 172–73
vs. wants, 161–62
neuropeptides, 316–17
neuroplasticity, 87–88
neurotransmitters, 316–18
neutrality, 73
neutral observation, 102–3
nice, being, 193
Nicoyans, 211
Nielsen, Lizbeth, 244
nitric oxide, 187
no, saying, 166, 182
non-acceptance, 176–77, 186. see also acceptance
norepinephrine, 83
noticing, 68
noting, in mindfulness, 69

observer, neutral, 73
observing, 68, 70
obsessing, 260
Okinawans, 211
Oliner, Pearl, 209
Oliner, Samuel, 209
Ong, Anthony, 151
openheartedness, 208, 212
openness, 67
opportunity
and caregiving, 299
diagnosis as, 265
illness as, 198
optimism, 209, 213, 309–11
O'Regan, Brendan, 263
Ornish, Dean, 224–25
Ornstein, Robert, 222
Orsillo, Susan, 15, 23
Orth-Gomer, Kristina, 226

outcomes, attachment to, 30

pain. see also discomfort; suffering
acceptance of, 94, 115, 174–75
and ACT, 95
avoiding, 173
dissociation and, 247–48
meditation and, 115–16
mindfulness practice and, 93–95
placebos and, 333–34
pain, chronic, 93–95
panic attacks, 44
Parkinson's disease, 334–35, 339
participating, 70
patient, compliant, 182, 338
patient, empowered, 281–85
patient, use of term, 60
patient advocates, 160, 273–74, 288
patient-controlled analgesia (PCA), 328
The Patient from Hell (Schneider), 282
patient portals, 287
patient support associations, 290
PCA (patient-controlled analgesia), 328
Pelletier, Kenneth, 220
Pennebaker, James, 48, 188, 199–200
peptides, and breathing, 347
personality changes, 297
personality traits, and mindfulness, 74–75
personal life values. see values

pessimism, 310
Peterson, Christopher, 231
Pettingale, Keith, 183
Phongsuphap, Sukanya, 347
photoplethysmography, 152
physician expectancies,
    339–41
physicians
    interviewing, 272
    partnering with, 287–88
    trust in, 338
placebos, 331–39
    beta blockers and, 334
    cholesterol and, 337–38
    depression and, 339
    dopamine and, 334–35
    drug packaging and, 332
    gastric activity and, 338
    meta-analysis results, 337
    morning sickness and,
        338–39
    pain and, 333–34
    Parkinson's disease and,
        339
    and physician expectan-
        cies, 339–41
    side effects and, 329,
        335–36
    studies on, 336–37
    warts and, 335
polygraph tests, 48–49
positive thinking, 264, 309
posttraumatic stress disorder
    (PTSD), 43
posture, 164, 165, 167, 261
power of attorney for health-
    care, 293
POWs, 229
practice, 141–45
practice, altering, 255–68
practices, destructive, 139–40
present experience, 71, 73,
    313

preventricular contractions,
    252
procedures, volume of, 272
prodromes, 81–83, 115
protocols, 282–283
Prozac, 336
psychoimmunology, 181. see
    also immune system
psychoneuroimmunology
    (PNI), 91, 326–28. see also
    immune system
psychotherapy, 80. see also
    Acceptance and Commit-
    ment Therapy
psychotherapy groups, 236.
    see also support/support
    groups
    and loving self-care, 165
    and self-expression, 192,
        194
PTSD (posttraumatic stress
    disorder), 43
purpose. see meaning and
    purpose

Quillian-Wolever, Ruth, 250

rage, 186–88, 194
reactions, 74
reason-giving, 20
recoveries, unexplained,
    263–67
reevaluation, 296
Reeve, Christopher, 174
relationships. see also sup-
    port/support groups
    cancer and, 228–29
    and caregiving, 296, 297,
        299
    elderly people and, 221–24
    health and, 219–20
    heart disease and, 224–27

immune system and, 227–28
Karmu study, 232–33
love and, 231
loving self-care and, 165
morbidity and mortality and, 220–21
POWs and, 229
Roseto study, 229–31
self-acceptance and, 176
self-expression and, 189–90
sense of belonging and, 230–31, 233–34
support and, 234
relaxation, 102, 153
remissions, 97, 263–65
repression, *vs.* suppression, 185–86
research and documentation, 289–93, 300
resonant frequency breathing, 346
respiration, 174, 248–53, 312, 343–49
respiratory sinus arrhythmia (RSA), 250–53, 345–47
retreats, 103–4
Ricard, Matthieu, 22
rigidity, psychological, 41
Rodin, Judith, 88, 89, 90
Roemer, Lizabeth, 15, 23
Rook, Karen, 234
Rosenbaum, Elana, 172
Rosenberg, Ira, 251
Roseto studies, 229–31
RSA (respiratory sinus arrhythmia), 250–53, 345–47
Ruggieri, Paul, 272
rules, unwritten, 19
rumination, 28–29, 72–73, 116

sadness, 172, 258–59
samatha vipassana, 104, 106. *see also* vipassana
saying no, 166, 182
schizophrenia, 262–63
Schneider, Stephen, 282
Schulz, Ute, 209, 225
Schwartz, Gary, 82, 181, 184, 185
screening tests, 276
SDNN (standard deviation of beat-to-beat intervals), 344. *see also* heart rate variability
second opinions, 267, 276–79, 280–82, 283, 299–300
Segal, Zindel, 28, 172
self-acceptance
anxiety and, 175–76
benefits of, 171
breathing and, 174
experiential avoidance and, 170–71
fears and aversions and, 172
lack of, 169–70
medication and, 173
pain and, 174–75
practice of, 177–79
support and, 176
transparency, 173–174
self-care, loving. *see* loving self-care
self-care mastery
biomarkers and, 275–76
defined, 271
and depression, 271
early treatment and, 273
economics and, 276
emergency departments, 273–74
idiopathic diagnoses, 284
interviewing physicians, 272

lab techs and, 285
partnering with doctor,
   287–88
patient advocates and, 288
preparing for medical ap-
   pointments, 286–87
protocols, 282–83
questions to ask, 279–80
research and documenta-
   tion, 289–93
risk and, 285–86
second opinions and,
   276–79, 280–82, 283
self-diagnosis, 274–75
and self-esteem, 271
vigilance and, 284–85
self-compassion, 167
self-concept, 17–18, 27, 45
self-consciousness, 107–8
self-diagnosis, 274–75
self-efficacy, medical, 271. *see
   also* self-care mastery
self-empowerment, 235
self-esteem
   and breathing, 164
   and health, 184
   and self-care mastery, 271
self-expression
   anger *vs.* hostility, 186–88
   asking for help, 191–92
   authenticity and, 181–82
   and cancer, 190
   developing skill of, 192–95
   health and, 181, 182–83,
      190–91
   and immune system, 184
   practice of, 192–95
   relationships and, 190
   saying no, 182
   stoicism and, 183–86
   and survival rates, 182
   writing and, 188–89
self-image, 295
self-knowing, 71

self-pity, 257
self-rejection, 109, 177
self-talk, 109–11. *see also* explanatory style
self-treatment, 81
Seligman, Martin, 209
sense of belonging, 220,
   230–31, 233–34
sensory input, lack of attachment to, 73
serotonin, 317
service. *see also* altruism;
   volunteer work
   and longevity, 211
   practicing, 214–16
   thoughts on, 216–17
shame, 58, 169–70, 173, 184
Shapiro, Shauna, 66–67
Sheldon, Kennon, 201
side effects, 335–36
sign, defined, 274
Simonton, Carl, 112, 198, 201,
   238
sleepiness, 345
smiling, 242, 261–62
Sobel, David, 222
societal values, 18–19
Solomon, George, 181, 182,
   198
Speca, Michael, 79
Specter, Herbert, 30
Spiegel, David, 112
Spontaneous Remission
   (O'Regan & Hirshberg),
   263
standard deviation of beat-
   to-beat intervals (SDNN),
   344. *see also* heart rate variability
stoicism, 183–86

Stoney, C. M., 345

Stop-Breathe-Feel, 250, 312

stress, emotional. *see also* distress, emotional; stress, physiological
and immune system, 326–27

stress, physical, 93

stress, physiological. *see also* distress, emotional
allostatic loads, 320–24
biochemistry of stressful thoughts, 318–20
epigenetics and, 324–26
experiential avoidance and, 47–49
immunosuppression and, 326–27
overview, 11–14
self-acceptance and, 170

StressEraser, 252

Stuban, Sandra Lesher, 312

Suarez, Edward, 187

suffering. *see also* discomfort; distress, emotional; pain; stress, physiological
and acceptance, 175
attachment to getting well and, 57
attributions and, 29–30
causes of, 15–16
cognitive fusion and, 16–17, 27
concepts and, 17–18
core beliefs and, 20–21, 28
depression and anxiety and, 58
experiential avoidance and, 17
FEAR and, 19–20
identification with illness and, 56–57, 60
inaction/impulsiveness and, 18
inflexibility, 21–22

moods and, 21
new symptoms and, 57
rumination and, 28–29
values and, 18–19

suffering, unavoidable, 54

suffering, unnecessary, 54, 56–58

suggestion, power of, 330. *see also* placebos

Suls, Jerry, 187

support/support groups, 208, 209. *see also* relationships
building, 236
cancer and, 228–29
for caregivers, 299, 300, 306–8
chronic illness and, 59–60
elderly people and, 221–24
empathy and, 234
heart disease and, 224–27
immunity and, 227–28
love and, 231
and loving self-care, 165
morbidity and mortality and, 220–21
patient support associations, 290
POWs and, 229
Roseto studies, 229–31
self-acceptance and, 176
and self-empowerment, 235
skill building in, 235
suggestions for, 234–35
and volunteer work, 235

suppression, 47–49, 184–86. *see also* experiential avoidance

survival rates, 89–90
and facing mortality, 112
and meaning, 200
and self-expression, 182

Swami Beyondananda, 69

Syme, Leonard, 220

sympathetic arousal, 47, 48,
    82–83, 319–20
    effects of, 321–22
    and health, 49, 109
    and immune system, 320
sympathy, 310
symptoms
    and behavior, 275
    cognitive fusion and, 57
    defined, 274
    in differential diagnosis,
    274
    and early treatment, 273
    in formal mindfulness
    practice, 114
    in informal mindfulness
    practice, 115
    and loving self-care, 161
    and medication, 260–61
    and mindfulness, 95
    mindfulness practice and,
    108–11
    new treatments and,
    256–57
    treatment of, 327

tai chi, 43
Tan, Stanley, 238
Tecumseh study, 208, 221
Temoshok, Lydia, 185
terminal illness, 60–61
Thera, Nyanaponika, 69
theta brain wave state, 81–82
thoughts
    connection to sensation,
    108
    content of, 35
    relationship to, 35 (see also
    cognitive fusion)
thoughts, categorical and
    judgmental, 33
thoughts, self-critical, 139–40
tics and twitches, 42

TM. see transcendental medi-
    tation
toxins, 326
trance. see altered states of
    consciousness
transcendental meditation
    (TM), 88, 89–90, 92
transparency, 173–74
trauma, 42–43, 46
treatments, alternatives, 299
Tsuji, Hisako, 345
Twohig, Michael, 39, 177

Uchino, Bert, 221
Uhlmann, Carmen, 188
Unden, Anna-Lena, 226
Understanding Patient Safety
    (Wachter), 272
urgent care, 273

Vaillant, George, 209
Valued-Action Practice
    living by choice, 128–36
    loving self-care, 157–58
    practicing awareness,
    141–45
    and self-expression, 193
    taking action, 124–25
values vs. goals, 121
values. see also Valued-Action
    Practice
    ACT's focus on, 57
    and asking for help, 305
    behaving in accordance
    with, 70
    caregiving and, 309
    and choice, 127–30, 135
    and chronic illness, 58
    defined, 70
    and diagnosis, 53
    and experiential avoid-
    ance, 39, 41

focusing on, 121
goals *vs.*, 121
identifying, 122–24, 172–73
life-threatening illness
and, 198
suffering and, 18–19
taking action, 124–25

Van Wielingen, Laura, 80

Vaschillo, Bronya, 170

Vaschillo, Evgeny, 170, 252

victimhood, 59–60, 140, 163

vigilance, 284–85

vipassana, 81, 88, 104–5, 106,
255

volunteer work, 206–7
and depression, 213
and social support, 235

Wachter, Robert, 272

wait-list controlled method,
96

walking, 164–65

Wan, Choi, 187

wants, *vs.* needs, 161–62

warts, 335

websites, 289–90, 300

Wegner, Daniel, 45

wellbeing, 5–8

Wenzlaff, Richard, 45

Wirga, Mariusz, 238

wisdom, 71

Wolf, Stewart, 229–30, 338–39

writing, 48, 49–50. *see also*
journaling

yoga, 43

About the Author

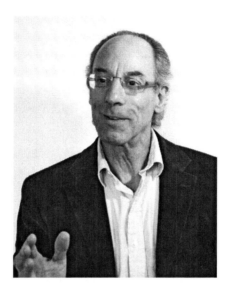

In 1990 Larry Berkelhammer embarked on a project to discover the most evidence-based mind training practices shown to improve health and wellbeing. The project turned into an amazing journey filled with surprising revelations, such as the discovery that by approaching life as an opportunity to master ourselves, we cultivate resilience and accrue all its benefits. The journey has included rigorous and extensive personal training, qualitative action research projects, and professional training with several world leaders in the fields of psycho-neuroimmunology, psychophysiology, and psychooncology. Dr. Berkelhammer's psychotherapy clients, all of whom were living with serious chronic medical conditions, benefited from the varied practices he learned through these endeavors. After retiring from practice in 2010, he spent the next three years writing *In Your Own Hands* in order to inform many more people of these life-altering practices.

A dedicated practitioner of the mindfulness-based practices described in the book, today Larry continues to focus on empowering people with chronic medical conditions to live with increased health and wellbeing. He currently teaches a class called Mastery of Aging, is an advisor to Marin Center for Independent Living, plays an active role in the work of the Empowered Patient Coalition, and teaches through articles, videos, interviews, presentations, and sharing information on his website, http://www.larryberkelhammer.com, and dozens of other blogs. He lives with his wife, Irma Botvin, in San Rafael, California.

CPSIA information can be obtained at www.ICGtesting.com
Printed in the USA
BVOW04s2030300514

354969BV00006B/125/P